TAI CHI CHUAN
A COMPARATIVE STUDY

BY VINCENT CHU

DISCLAIMER

Please note that the author and publisher of this book are NOT RESPONSIBLE in any manner whatsoever for any injury that may result from practicing the techniques and/or following the instruction given within. Since the physical activities described herein may be too strenuous in nature for some readers to engage in safely, it is essential that a physician be consulted prior to training.

First published in 2010 by the Tai Chi Company.

Copyright © 2010 by Vincent Chu

All rights reserved. No part of this publication may be reproduced or utilized in any form or by any means, electronic or mechanical, including photocopying, recording, or by any information storage and retrieval system, without prior written permission from the Tai Chi Company.

ISBN: 0-9841909-0-2

Distributed by:
Tai Chi Company
33 Harrison Avenue, 2nd Floor
Boston, MA 02111

First Edition
Printed in the United States of America

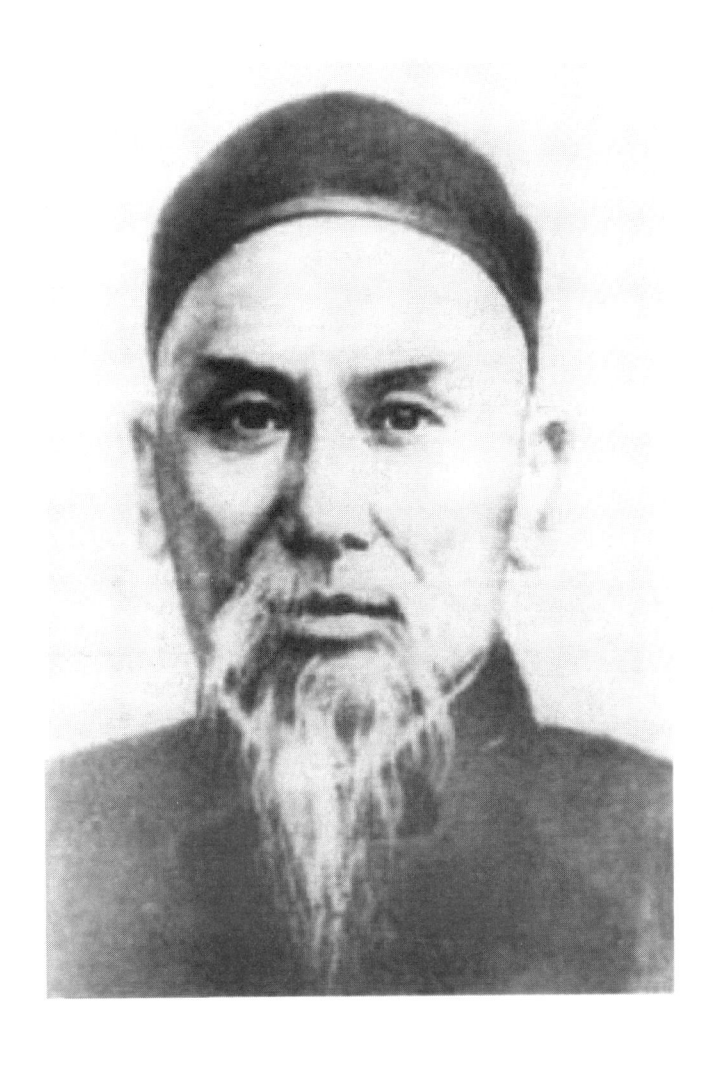

Great Great Great Great Grandmaster Yang Lu Chan (Yeung Lu Sim)

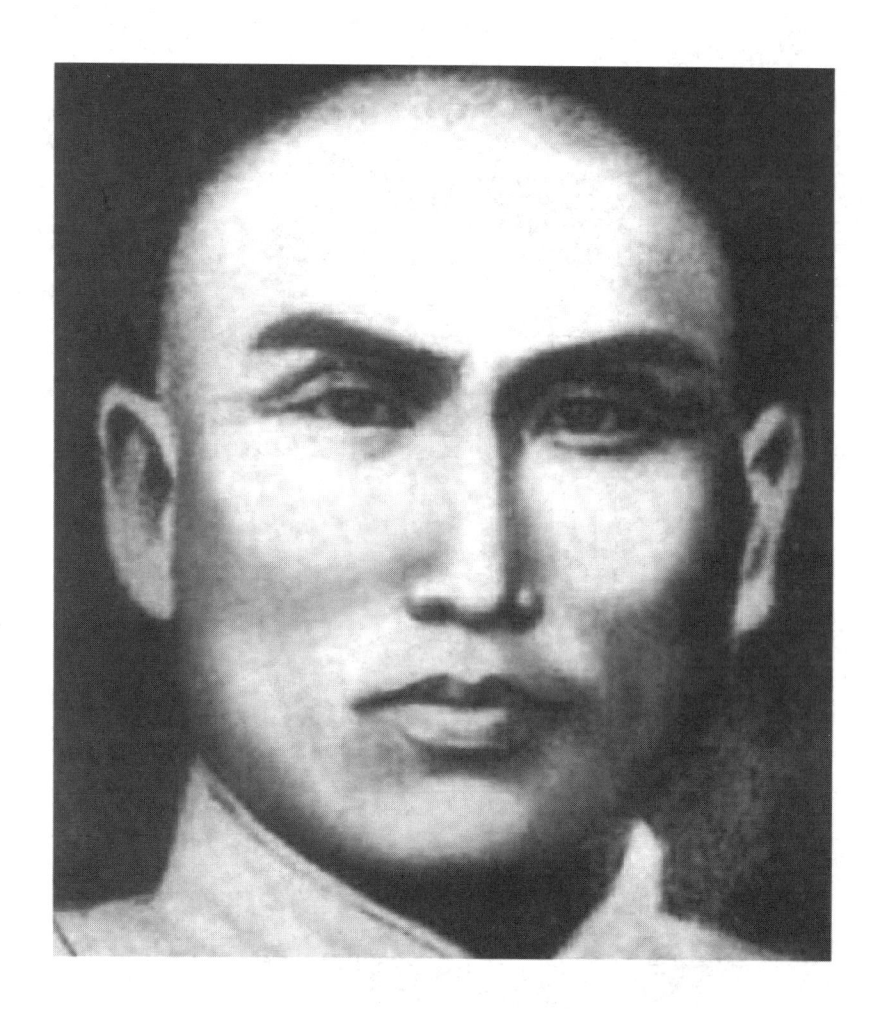

Great Great Great Grandmaster Yang (Yeung) Ban Hou

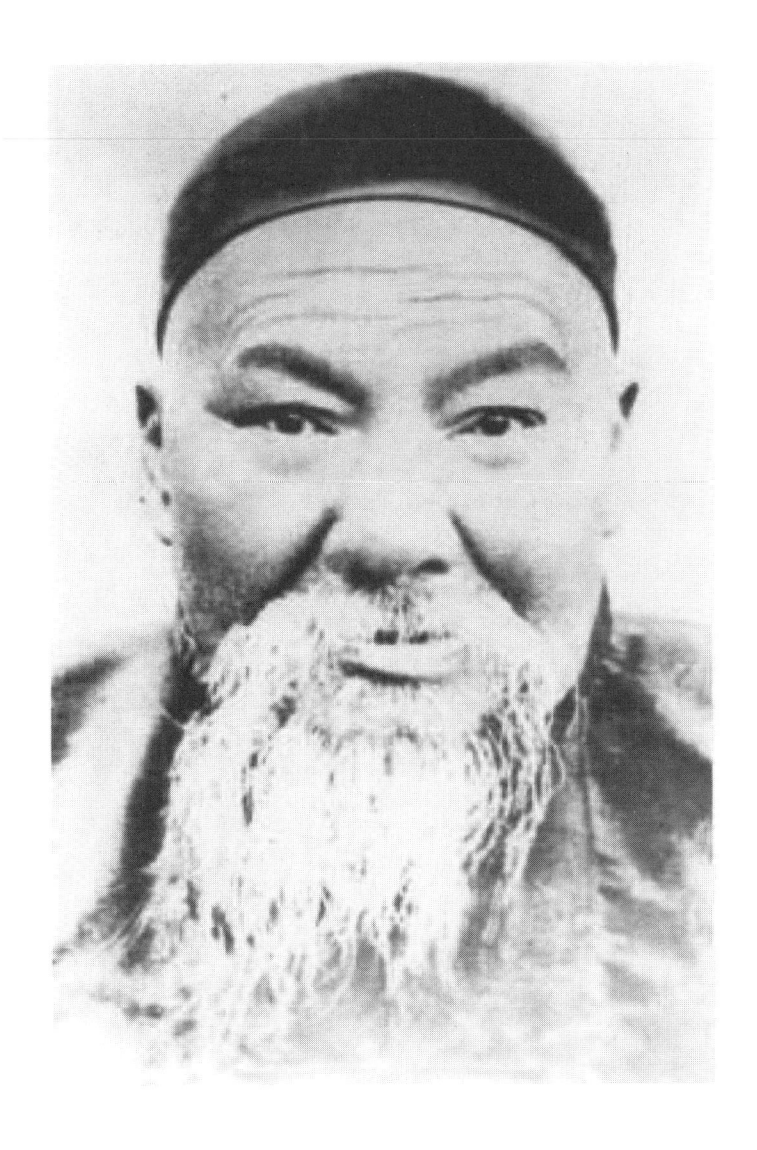

Great Great Great Grandmaster Yang Jian Hou (Yeung Kin Hou)

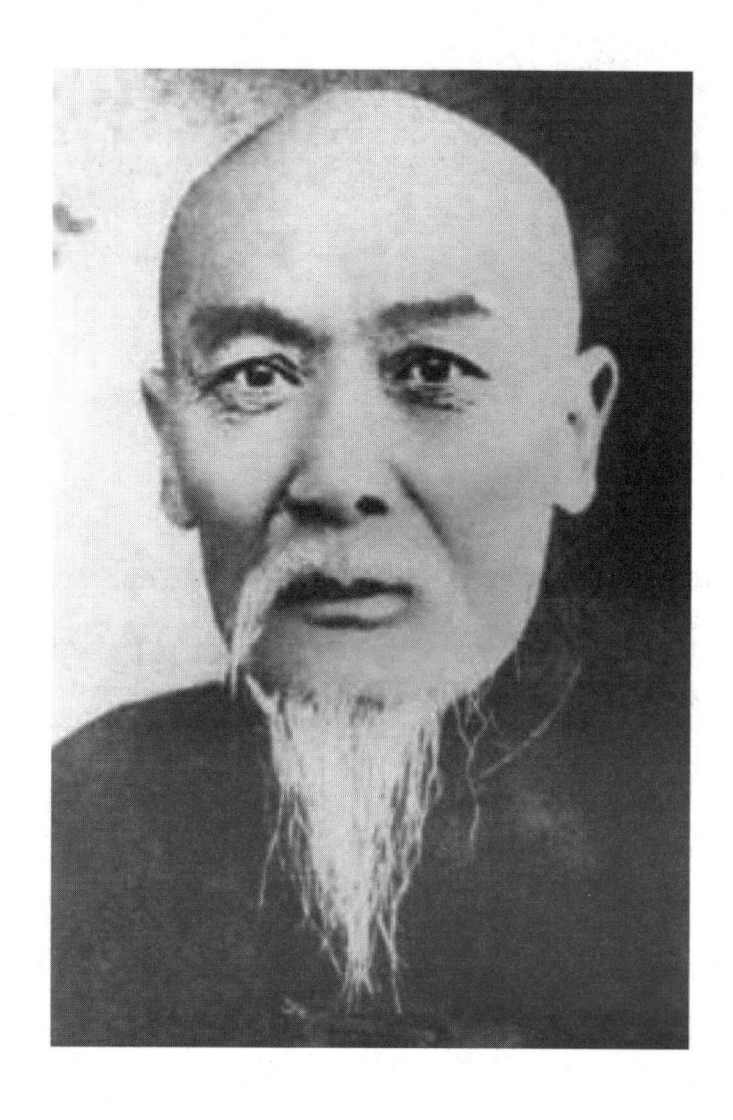

Great Great Grandmaster Yang Shao Hou (Yeung Siu Hou)

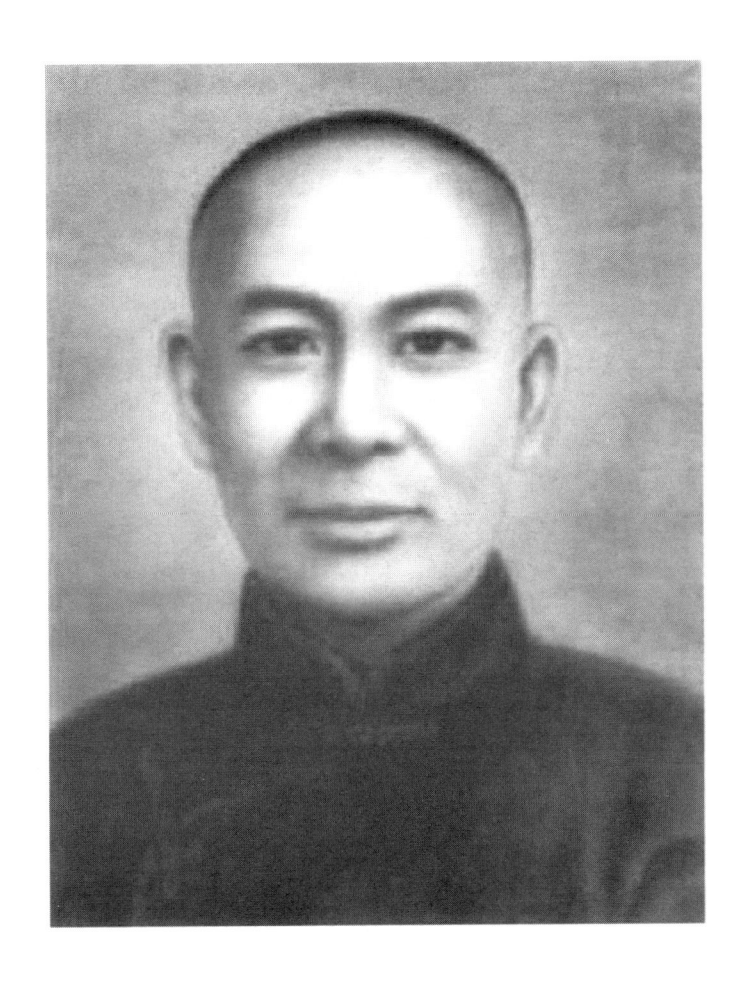

Great Great Grandmaster Yang (Yeung) Siu Yuan

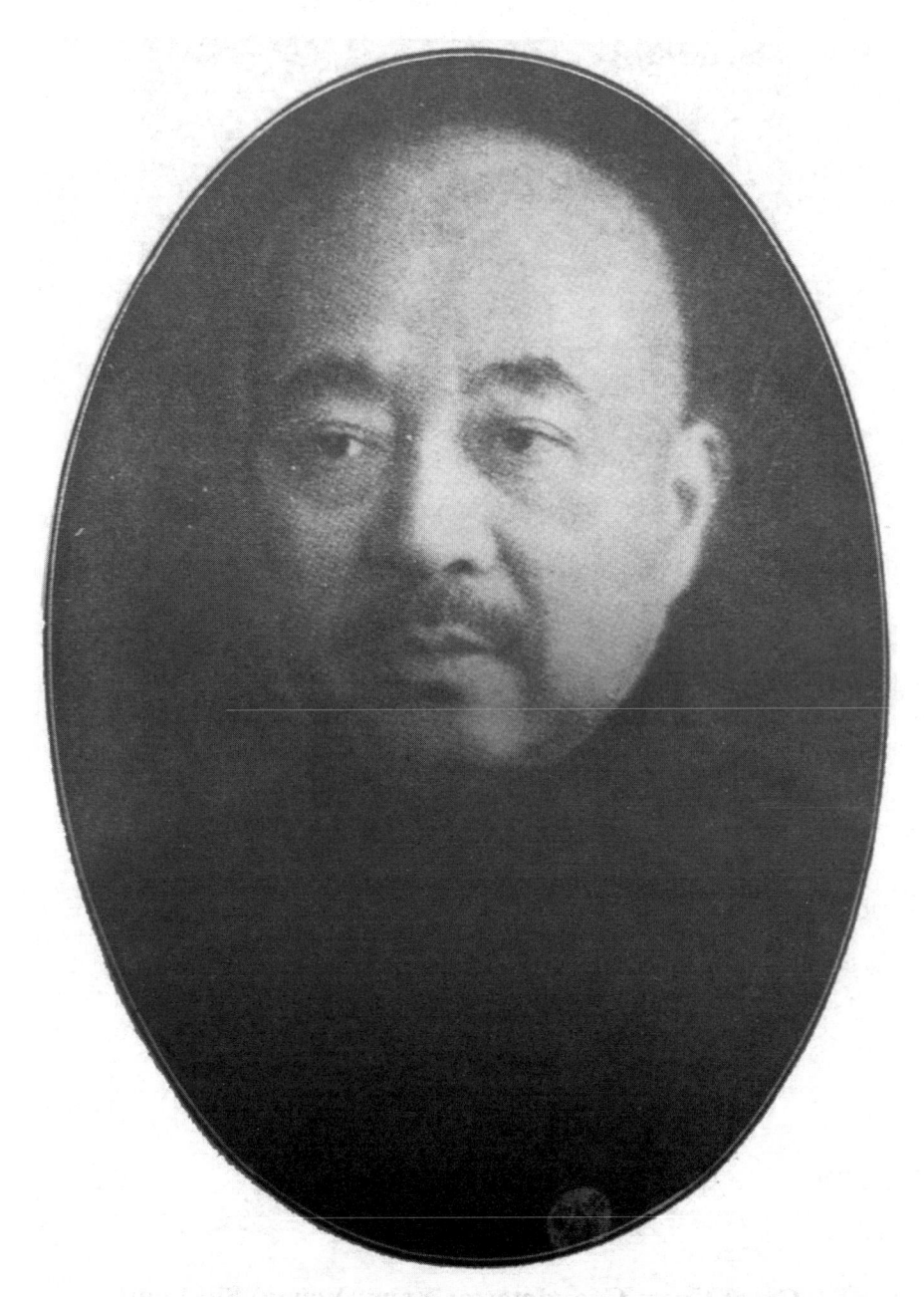

Great Great Grandmaster Xu Yu Sheng

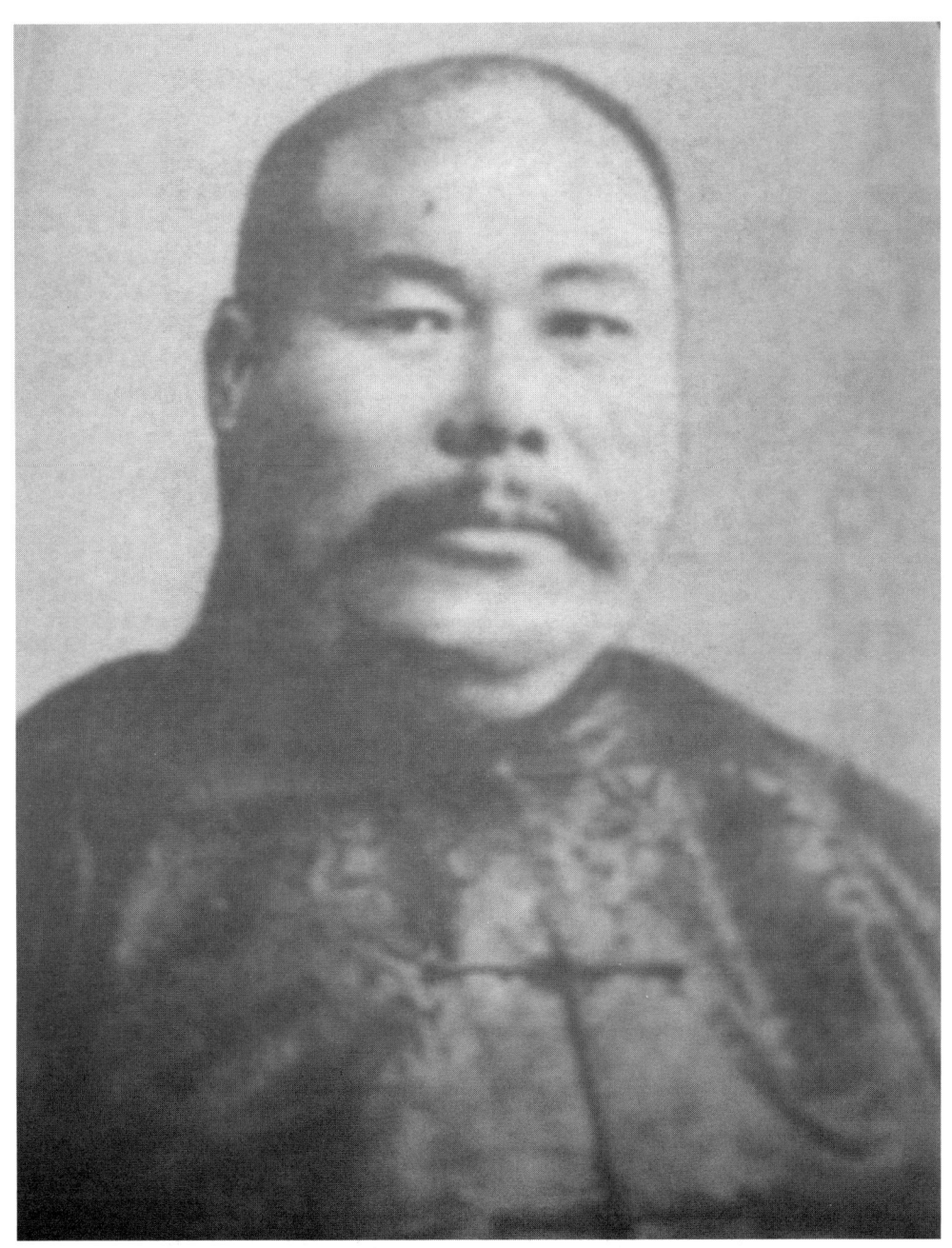

Great Great Grandmaster Yang Cheng Fu (Yeung Ching Po)

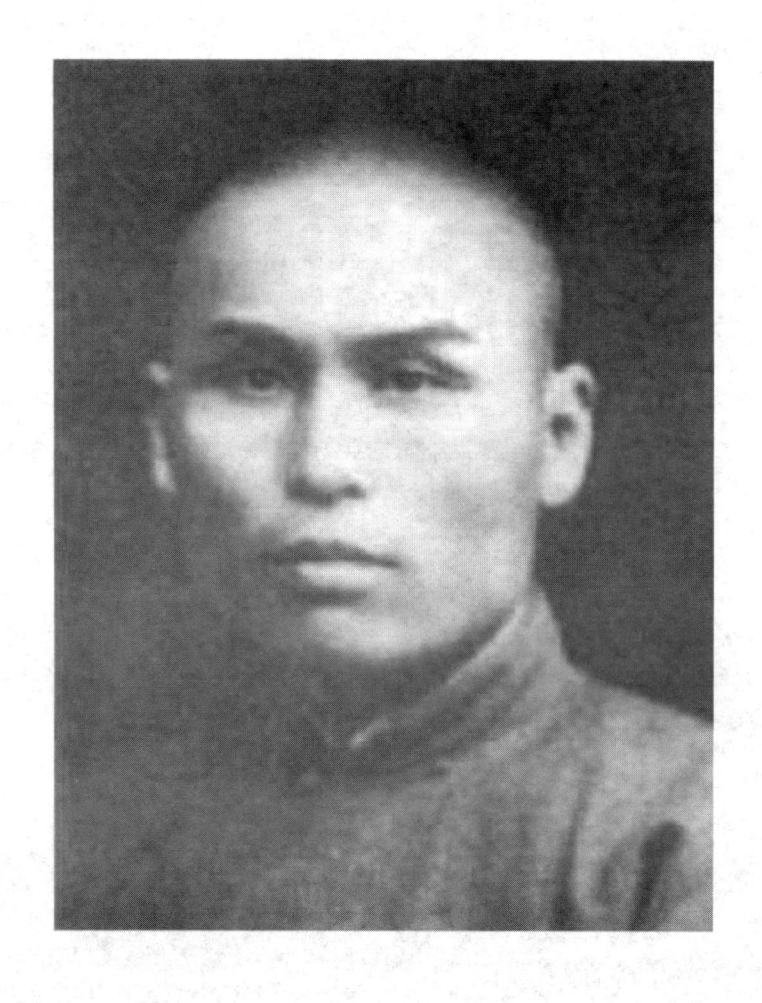

Great Great Grandmaster Yang (Yeung) Siu Pang

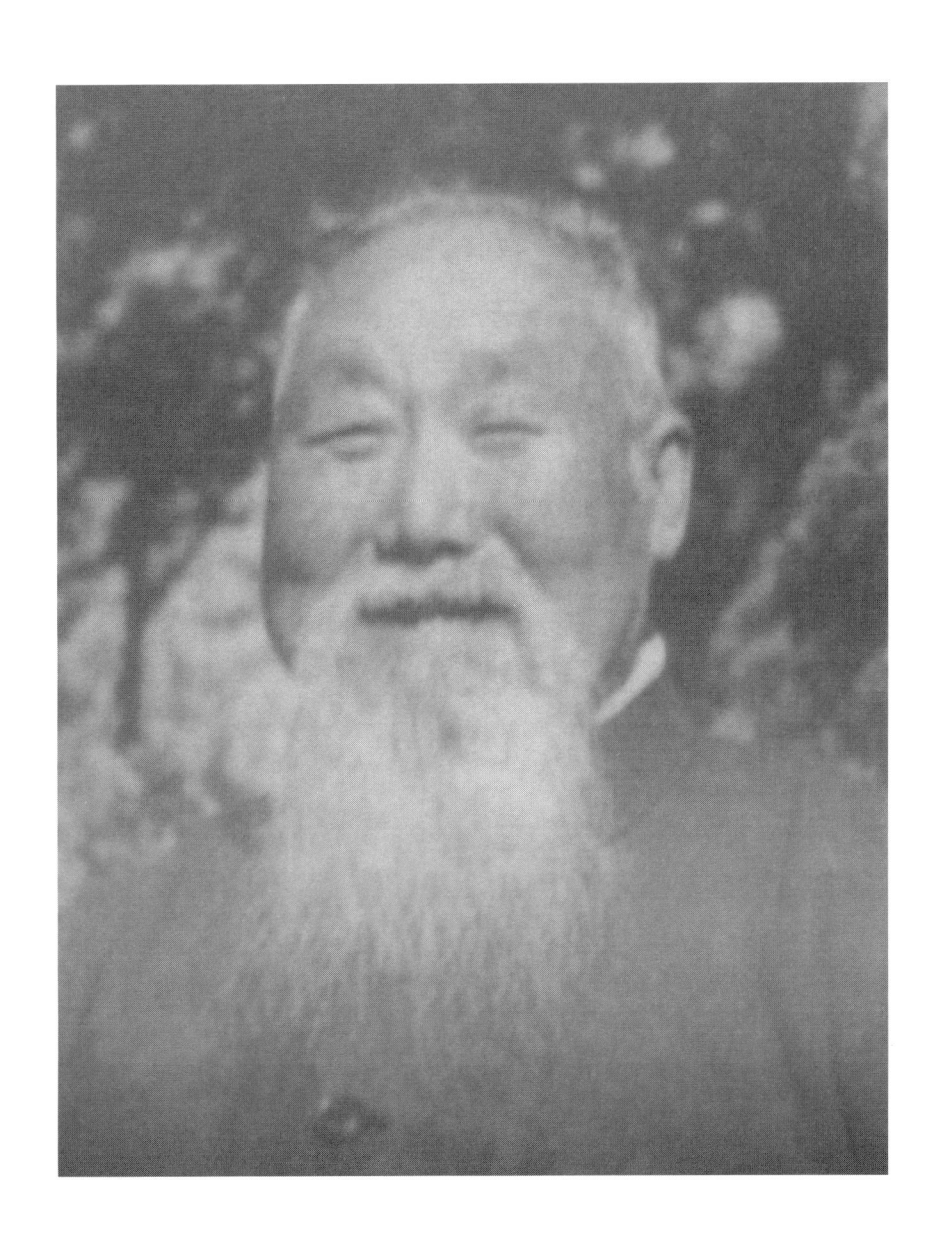

Great Grandmaster Cui Yi Shi (Tsau Li Shu)

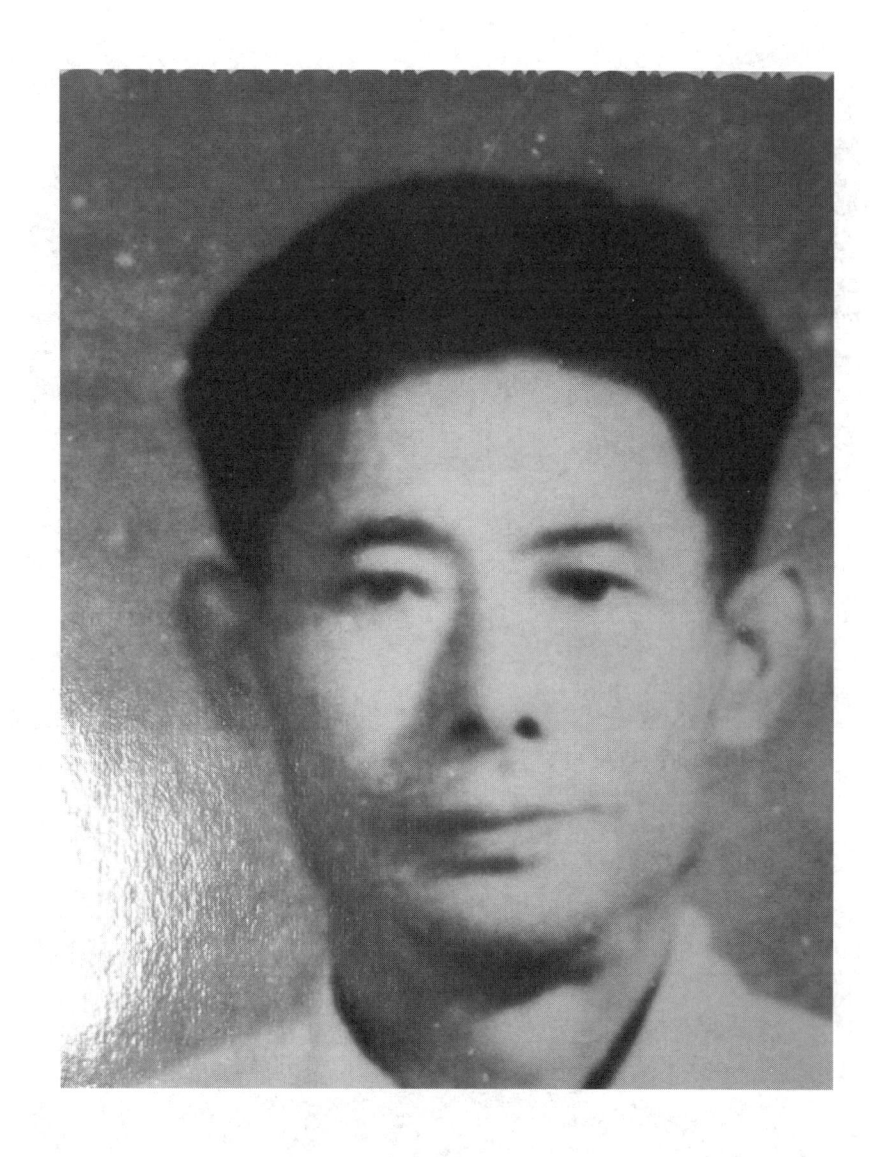

Great Grandmaster Zhang Fu Chen

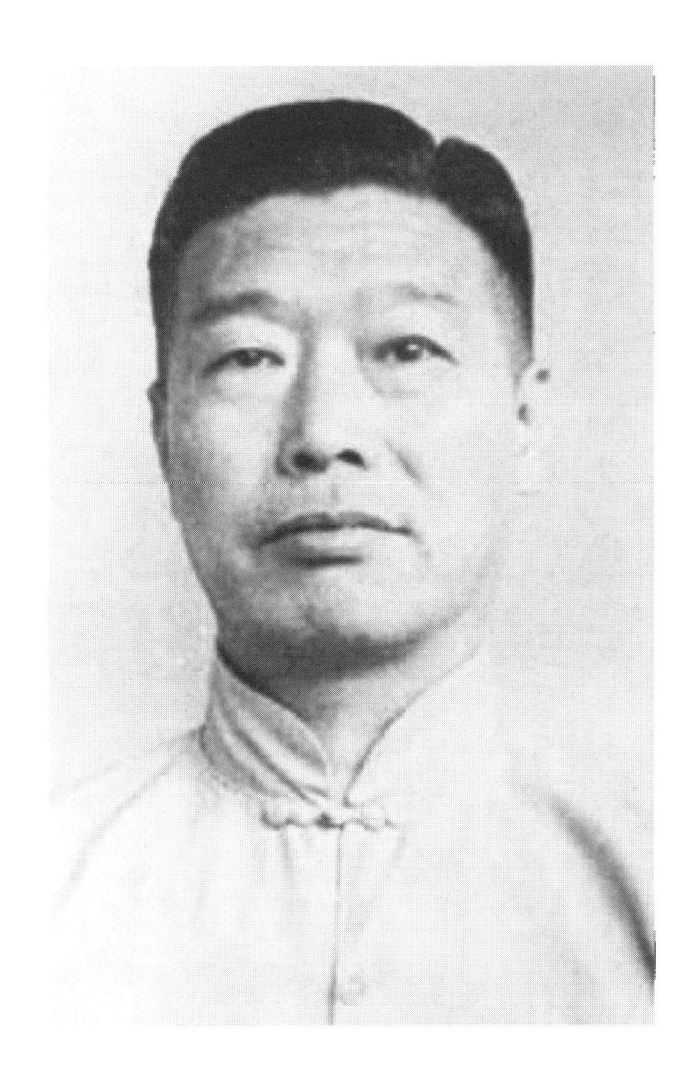

Great Grandmaster Yang (Yeung) Sau Chung

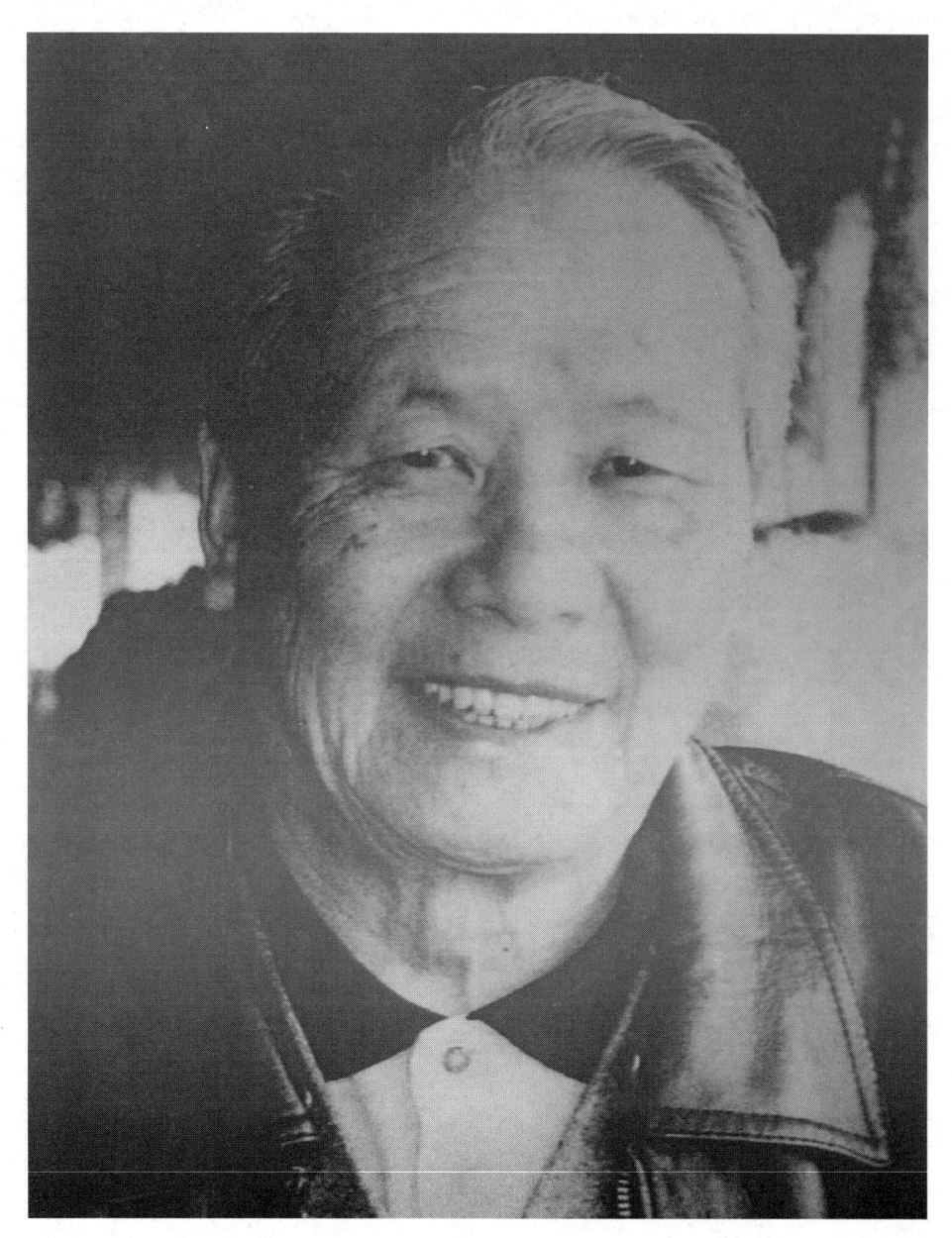

Grandmaster Fang Ning

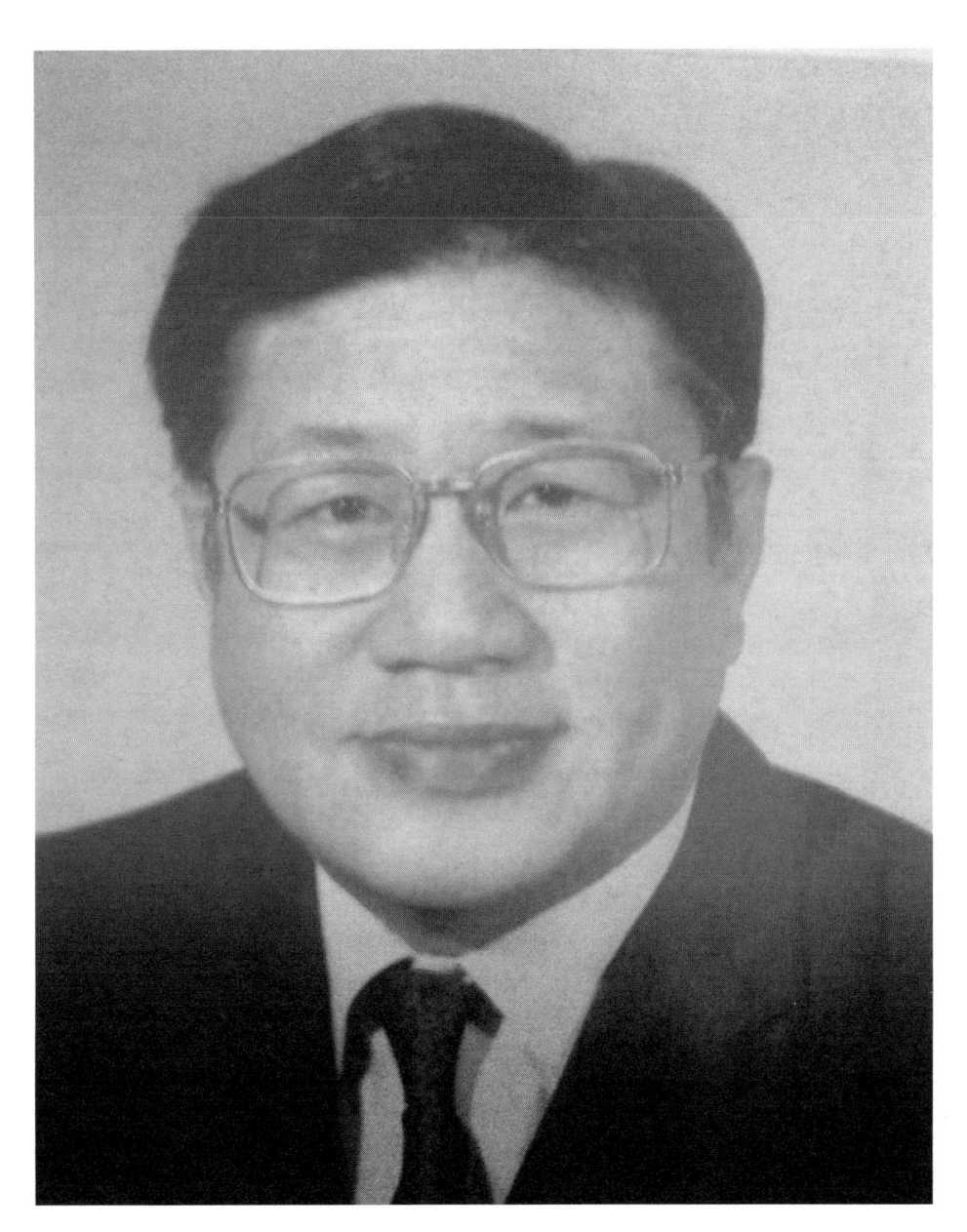

Grandmaster Ip Tai Tak

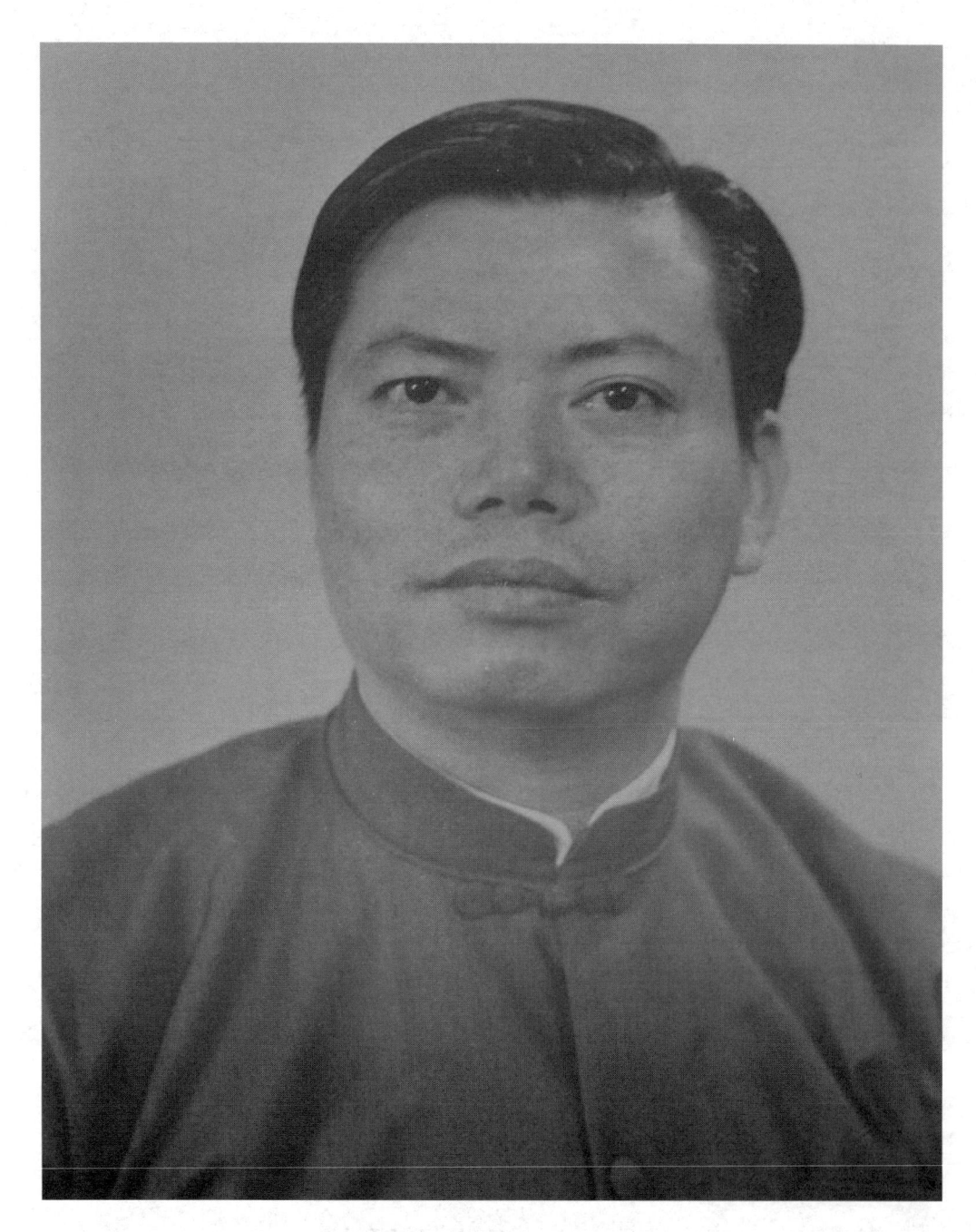

Grandmaster Chu Gin Soon

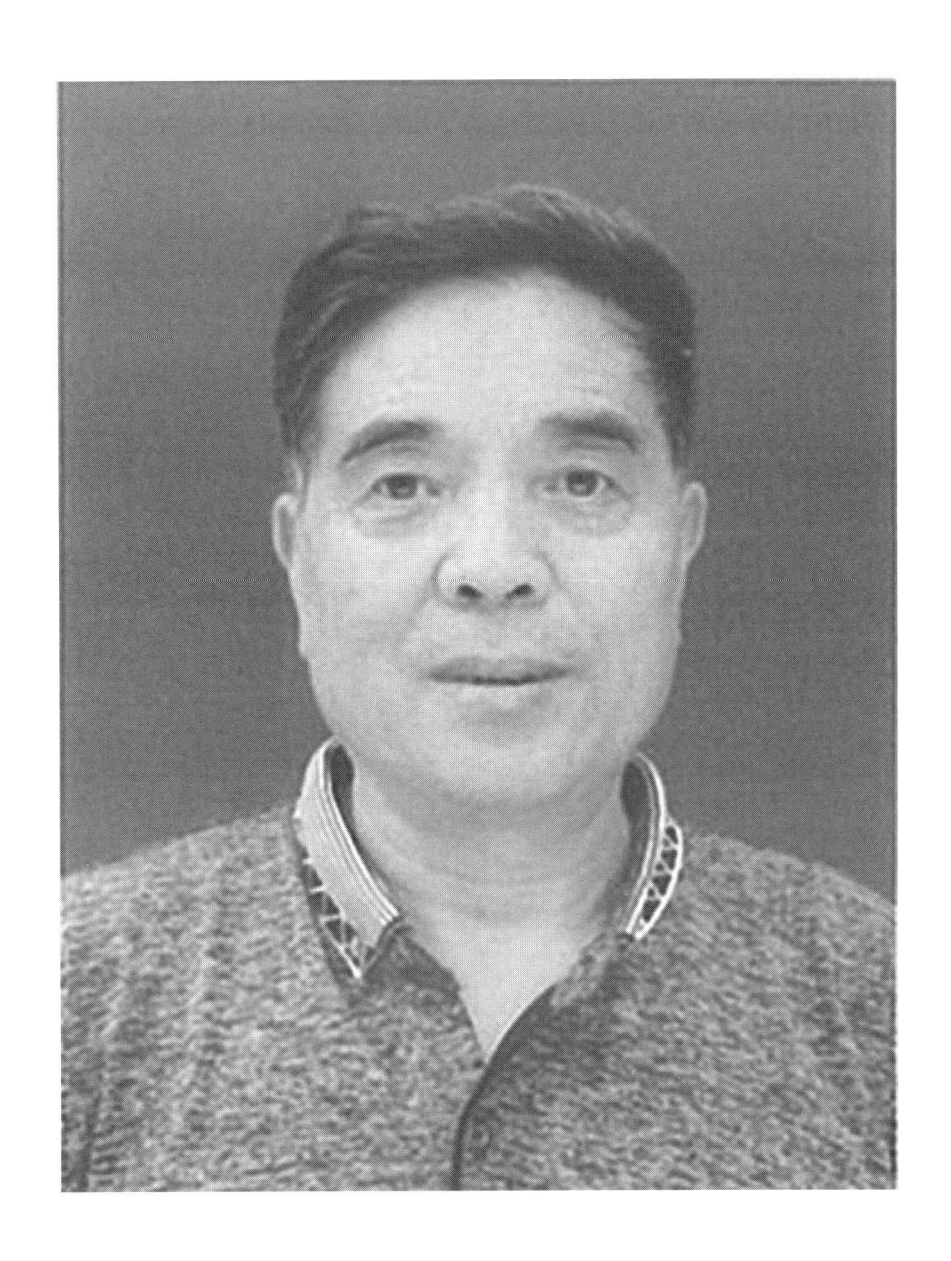

Grandmaster Liu Xi Wen

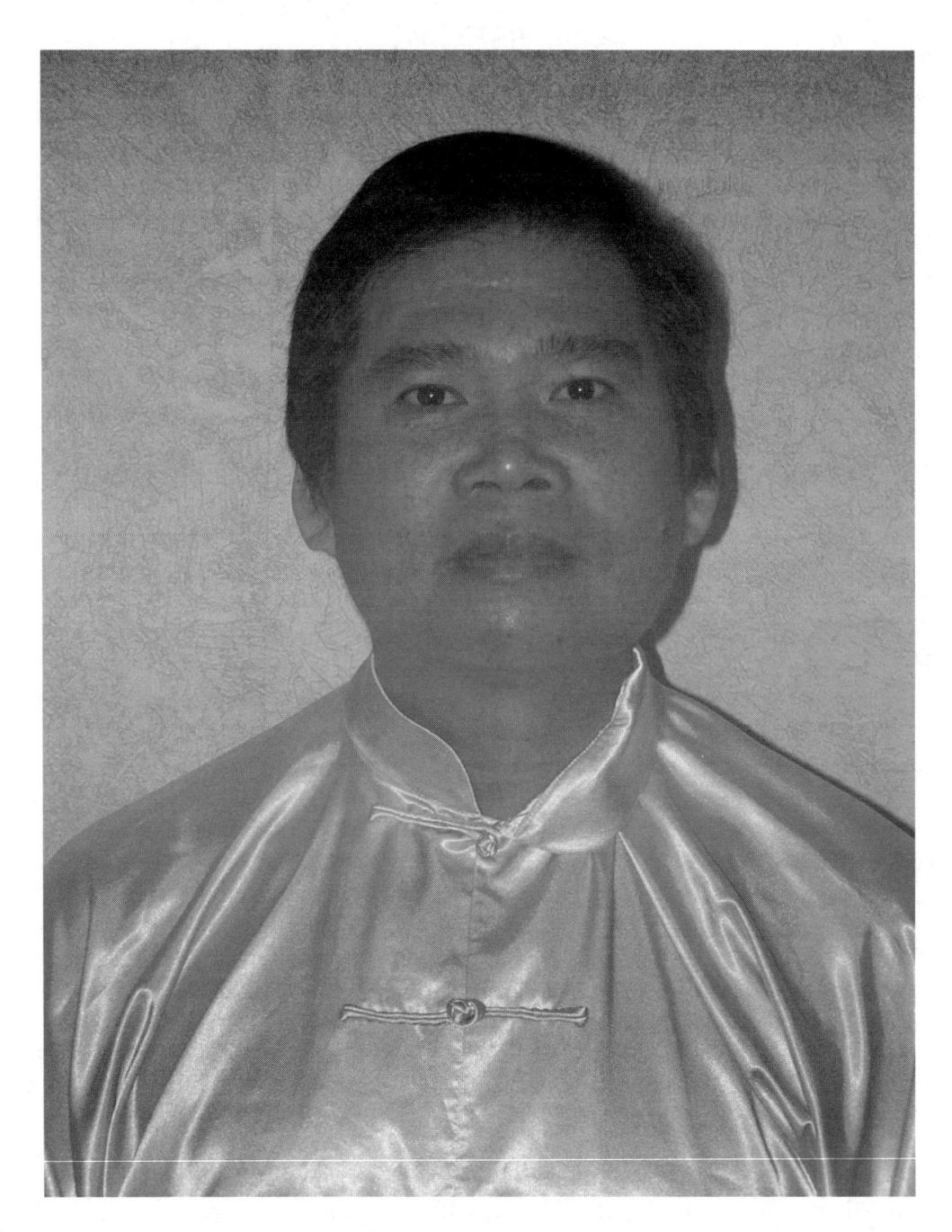

Author Vincent Chu

Acknowledgements

Wang Tsung Yueh has written that there are many incorrect methods of practicing Tai Chi Chuan. In order to learn the correct method, one has to find a knowledgeable teacher and receive an oral transmission. I would like to thank my Tai Chi Chuan teachers, Ip Tai Tak, Gin Soon Chu, Liu Xi Wen, Ou Wen Wei, and Fang Ning, for having been so generous in the passing of their knowledge to me. Their teachings have lead to a better understanding of what the Classical Yang Family Tai Chi Chuan System is, and without their contribution this book would not have been possible.

Special thanks also go to my students Bob Krygowski, Tony Zhu, and David Gabbe, who were the data managers and photographers for this book. I would also like to thank Mike Arsenault, Robert A. Anderson, and Barbara Mintz for their valuable contributions to this book.

I would further like to give my heart-felt gratitude to Colin McMonagle and Rene Navarro, who edited this work despite their busy schedules.

Contents

Portraits of the Masters

Acknowledgements

1	Introduction	1
2	Chinese Martial Art Forms	7
3	The Tai Chi Chuan Solo Form: Design and Development	22
4	Functions of the Tai Chi Chuan Solo Form	27
5	The 43 Movement Large Frame Solo Form	32
6	The 42 Movement Medium Frame Solo Form	166
7	The 48 Movement Small Frame Solo Form	269
8	The Three Emphases	371
9	Envoi	377

About the Author

The Gin Soon Tai Chi Chuan Federation

Chapter 1
Introduction

Today there are many styles of Tai Chi Chuan, and no two practitioners practice the solo form in the same way. This is true even among the Yang Family members. Many students wonder why this is and want to know the correct way to practice the Tai Chi Chuan Solo Form.

In the Tai Chi Chuan system, the solo form is a series of physical bare hand movements that maneuver the body for martial techniques and fine tune the body for martial fundamentals. Depending on the practitioner's intention, a movement can be executed in many different ways to achieve these results. Thus it is said that Tai Chi Chuan is a multi-functional art.

It is also said in the *Tai Chi Chuan Classics* that the solo form is for the body and push hand exercises are for application. The body is the center of the four limbs' movements. It is the key to unifying all physical movement. Some of the fundamental results of practicing Tai Chi Chuan include better coordination, chi circulation, powerful striking, improved flexibility, balance, vitality, physical endurance and mobility.

There are many methods to train the body to achieve these results. In Tai Chi Chuan, *jia* refers to family, style, and frame. We often encounter this word in association with *lao jia* and *xian jia* in Tai Chi Chuan books. The word *lao* refers to old or traditional, and *xian* refers to new and contemporary. When people say that Yang Lu Chan practiced the *lao jia*, it means that he practiced the traditional 108 movement solo form created by Zheng San Feng. Zheng San Feng's 108 movement solo form emphasized martial art usage more so than the styles commonly seen today.

A. Three Levels of Martial Art Skills

Generally, martial art skill is divided into three levels: the beginner level, the intermediate level, and the advanced level.

The beginner level refers to the stage when one learns to grasp the basics or fundamentals. The student trains to develop some skills involving the eyes, hands, feet, and body, and to acquire some benefits in bodily health. This is the foundation or the stage of developing the body.

The intermediate level is reached when the student has had several years of practice. The student has built a strong foundation. The eyes, hands, feet (stepping) and internal substances are able to act together in movement. This is the enlightenment stage, or the stage of developing the intent.

The advanced level is reached when one has had several decades of practice. The practitioner has spent a great deal of time in search of the application and power of each movement. All the movements are done with ease. The hands are able to move with lightening speed. Stepping is quick like the wind and the eyes shine like a shooting star. When the intent wants to move, the whole body moves together. This is the stage of developing the spirit.

a. Beginner Level

This is the stage of physical practice. It is the stage to practice the basics of martial art training. The main characteristic of this stage is that one practices the basics such as hand, leg, and waist movements, and the beginner's hand and weapon forms. The purpose is to build a solid foundation for more advanced training later. A student must remember three things here to be successful: seriousness, persistence, and perseverance. This stage is also known as body development. This is because the student mostly works on the basic movements of the hands, feet, waist and body, and also on standing, all to condition the body for more difficult movement later on.

b. Intermediate Level

After one has mastered the fundamentals, one will go on to the next step of intent development. The difference between body development and intent development is as follows:

- Body development involves many maneuvers to fine-tune the body, combined with following all the rules and regulations described in the *Tai Chi Chuan Classics*.
- Intent development involves practical application combined with following all the rules and regulations described in the *Tai Chi Chuan Classics*, but at the same time, one finds ways to stretch out the perimeter of these rules and regulations to improve one's skill.

Therefore, it is said that body development is working on the technical component, and intent development is working on the *chi,* or internal power component, in martial art training. A complete style or system of

Chinese martial art must include *gong*, training for both the body and intent components to foster the student's skills. There is a saying that it is not enough just to have *chi*: a skillful practitioner must have *gong* as well. When one has both *chi* and *gong*, the strike will be so powerful that the opponent will be terrified.

Martial artists who understand the relationship of *gong* and *chi* have said, "The fist relies on the chi, the chi relies on the gong, and the gong relies on the chi." From this, one can see that in order to succeed as a martial artist, one must find the solution to developing both the *gong* and *chi* components.

c. Advanced Level

In order to advance to a higher level, one must begin the energy training, or *chi kung*. From energy training, one will develop a skill so profound that no words can correctly describe it. My father, Gin Soon Chu, said that all the movements are fueled by *chi*, or energy. The speed of a movement involves the energy level, not the physical level; the result is fast and devastating. The *Tai Chi Chuan Classics* refer to this stage in the following statements: "No feathers can be added and no fly can land." "Nobody knows me, I alone know others." What is the difference between spiritual development and intent development? Spiritual development is the continuation of intent development and is the step of *chi* accumulation. The essence of spiritual development is that the brain will unconsciously practice the solo form all the time, so that all responses will become a natural reflex whenever one faces danger. This is also known as an inborn ability. A practitioner develops the nervous system to the peak of sensitivity so that an automatic response occurs without any conscious thought.

B. Three Frames of the Classical Yang Style of Tai Chi Chuan

The term *nei jia*, or internal art, was first used by Wang Tung Yee in 1669. He said:

> The Shaolin External Martial Art System is famous for the fist; it is used mainly for controlling others. There is an alternative *nei jia* system; it is based on the static to overcome the dynamic. The opponent falls down as soon as there is contact. It is different from the Shaolin external martial art system. Therefore, it is called *nei jia*, or internal art.

Internal art is as difficult to describe as is its founder, Zheng San Feng, a twelfth century Taoist priest who lived at Wudang Mountain in China. The story goes that he studied *The Bone Marrow Classic* and *The Tendons Changing Classic* of the Shaolin external martial art system in his youth. When he grew up, he combined that with the teachings of Taoism and came up with a series of exercises later known as Tai Chi Chuan 13 Techniques or 108 movements. It is the result of eight hand techniques: ward off, roll back, press, push, pull down, split, elbow and shoulder strike. The 13 Techniques are also known as 8 Gates and 5 Step Techniques, the latter including 5 directions: left, right, advance, retreat, and center. These are also known as 5 Elements. They correspond to metal, wood, water, fire, and earth. There are people who call this correspondence Eight Gates and Five Steps Equal 13 Techniques.

To facilitate students training in Tai Chi Chuan as a martial art, the Yang Family members developed the 108 Lao Jia Tai Chi Chuan Solo Form into four major solo forms, or frames, each with its own distinctive characteristics to prepare and arm the practitioner for combat. Yang Cheng Fu developed the famous and most popular Large Frame Solo Form from the traditional 108 movement form. The objective of this frame is to stretch the body's tendons and ligaments and to develop the flexibility of all the joints so that the body is able to meet the highest demands of the martial arts. Large refers to the large degree of circular motion in each movement. The Large Frame Form emphasizes the fine tuning and conditioning of the body's joints. Therefore, it is also known as the "enter the door form," or a form for the beginner.

Yang Chian Hou developed the Middle Frame Solo Form, or transitional form, from the traditional 108 movement form. The objective of this frame is to prepare the student for the more difficult Small Frame Solo Form. The Middle Frame Form emphasizes martial fundamentals. He enlarged the movements of the Small Frame Form so that students could grasp the mechanics of the movements, as well as offensive and defensive variations. Middle refers to the stage of transition. The movements comprise large and small frame degrees of circular motion. It is known as a training form.

Yeung Sau Chung developed the Medium Frame Solo Form from the traditional 108 movement form. The objective of this frame is practicing the obvious application and mobilization of power. Medium refers to the degree of circular motion involving the body's joints, not as large as in the Large Frame Form and not as small as in the Small Frame Form. It is the distance that enables one to quickly execute an offensive or a defensive maneuver.

Therefore, the Medium Frame Solo Form is also known as an application form.

Yang Pan Hou and Yang Lu Chan emphasized the Small Frame Solo Form in their teachings from the traditional 108 movement form. The objective of this form is stretching the muscle groups for *chi* circulation and close quarter martial usage. Small refers to the small degree of circular motion in each movement. The circle is so small that most of the movement is based on the rotation of the waist and coiling of the body. The emphasis is on *chi* circulation and application. Therefore, it is known as an advanced style and is generally practiced among senior and more experienced practitioners.

C. Multiple Disciplines of the Tai Chi Chuan Solo Form

The Tai Chi Chuan Solo Form can be practiced by people of all ages with many different physical conditions. It depends on the objectives of a practitioner. Generally, practicing the solo form is divided into four categories based on the practitioner's objectives. This is similar to the four seasons of the year when all living things grow in a complete life cycle: birth, growth, maturity and death. Since Tai Chi Chuan is a multi-functional art, one must practice the solo form accordingly to achieve all functions. A practitioner who inherited transmission generally goes through four stages of Tai Chi Chuan training to maximize its benefits. This is why many Tai Chi Chuan practitioners are still able to execute a powerful strike in their senior years.

We know that spring is a time for planting seed and the beginning of life. In Tai Chi Chuan training, this is the time to develop strong fundamentals. The objective of the solo form at this time will be based on how to improve these martial fundamentals. Summer is the time for growth. In Tai Chi Chuan training, this is the time for development, for the acquisition of skills. Autumn is the time for harvest. In Tai Chi Chuan training, this is the time for skill maturation and benefit. Winter is the time for storage. In Tai Chi Chuan training, this is the time for the reservation of *chi* to maintain good health. From this, we can see that Tai Chi Chuan training and development are different at different times of a practitioner's life. One should practice the Tai Chi Chuan solo form accordingly. A successful training method begins with the physical body to build strong fundamentals and advances into the spiritual training of the *chi* and intent at a later date. This is similar to education: one begins with the primary school knowledge, then progresses to secondary school knowledge and collegiate knowledge in due time.

There are many disciplines for practicing the solo form, but the sequence, principles, concepts, and philosophy remain the same. The significant difference is in the objectives and the execution of each movement. In this book, I will introduce three condensed versions of classical Yang Style Tai Chi Chuan solo forms with similar sequences but distinctive characteristics. In order to better learn these three Tai Chi Chuan forms, a student must focus on and master one movement at a time, and adhere to this method throughout the training session. One should digest one solo form before going on to the next solo form. From a martial art point of view, a skillful martial art practitioner should engage in many different types of training disciplines and situations to prepare the body to expect the unexpected in a combat environment. I introduce three forms in this book to warn and alert students that there is no one true way to do things and advise them to keep an open mind for possibilities. Grandmaster Yeung Sau Chung told me in 1984:

> The practice has to be alive! You have to practice the solo form with lightness, heaviness, softness, hardness, fastness, slowness, big circle, medium circle and small circle. If the solo form practice is concentrating on hardness, the *chi* will come up from the *dantien* to the four limbs. If the practice is concentrating on softness, the chi will return to the *dantien*. Hardness without softness is not enough strength. It is easy to break. Softness without hardness is not enough power and intensity. In a movement with only a fast component and no slow component, one is not considered to have control of the movement. A movement with slow motion but without a fast component indicates that the practitioner's skill is not very high. Hardness does not mean stiff, and softness does not mean weak. Strike fast without hesitation. The striking is slow but does not miss the target. This is the correct execution.

From a health maintenance exercise perspective, one training discipline selected according to one's health condition will do the job, for we know that any physical activity will improve body endurance. However, we know that by nature people generally are not satisfied with what they have. We have to progressively engage in new goals and training disciplines to build stronger and healthier bodies, and at the same time, maintain interest in Tai Chi Chuan training, fulfilling human nature by engaging in alternative Tai Chi Chuan forms.

Chapter 2
Chinese Martial Art Forms

A. Introduction

Martial art forms are the entry level of Chinese martial art curriculum. They teach students the fundamentals of martial art. This is equivalent to calligraphy. First, one follows someone's calligraphy sampler to learn all the brush strokes and later writes calligraphy without the sampler to develop his or her calligraphy style. Martial art training is the same. One begins with forms. All Chinese martial art systems and styles have very distinctive forms. Generally, a form can be done alone, with a partner, or with one or more weapons. Each movement is created and executed based on the martial art's offensive and defensive meanings.

The development of a martial art form is the result of many generations of praxis and training. A good form has many effective martial art techniques and tactics, applications and variations. Therefore, a good form is generally kept secret and not revealed to the public. Some forms emphasize strong and powerful techniques, while others emphasize soft and yielding techniques.

B. What is a Martial Art Form?

A form comprises posture, which is commonly called frame. A posture comprises technique. A technique is composed of the hand and feet movements. Put another way, a form is the warehouse of the hand and feet movements, the techniques, the body positions, and the steps. It is also the warehouse of the combination of many variations of hand and feet movements, techniques, body positions, and steps. Therefore, it does not matter if the form has a long or short movement; it must involve all body parts.

Generally, form has technical elements and mechanical elements. Mechanical elements are divided into composition technique, segment technique, and complete sequence technique. The relationship among them is that they are independent, connected, and related to each other, respectively.

   a. **The Technical Element**
   The technical element refers to the different components of fundamental techniques in martial art. This element involves techniques of the body, such as eye movements, hands, stances, steps, overall body position, and weapons. A powerful strike must have a

technical element that combines the following components: input from the intent, spirit, breathing, power, and rhythm.

    i. Hand
    This refers to the hands completing all techniques and positions of the bare hand and weapon forms.

    ii. Step
    This refers to the feet completing all the techniques and positions in motion.

    iii. Leg
    This refers to the legs completing all the lower body techniques and positions.

    iv. Body Position
    This refers to the position of the torso, including the different positions of the torso in motion.

    v. Eye
    This refers to the movement of the eyes in coordination with the movements of the body and hands.

    vi. Intent
    This refers to the controller or coordinator of all the conscious activities.

    vii. Spirit
    This refers to the internal expression of the movement, generally projected outward by the eyes.

    viii. Breathing
    This refers to the breathing, and breathing method, applied in coordination with the movement. Generally, there are two breathing methods used by martial art practitioners. In the deep breathing method the abdomen goes outward when one inhales and goes inward when one exhales. The second method is called shallow breathing. Here the abdomen goes outward when one exhales and goes inward when one inhales.

ix. Power
This refers to the power expressed in various physical movements.

x. Rhythm
This refers to the control, understanding, and execution of the following concepts in the solo form: static and dynamic, empty and full, hard and soft, fast and slow.

b. The Mechanical Element
The mechanical element refers to different types of movements in a solo form. It is properly assembled by various technical elements. The mechanical element includes composition techniques, segment techniques, and complete sequence techniques.

i. Composition Techniques
This refers to the technique following certain body mechanics. It is a bare hand or weapon movement following a certain objective or mission, to combine the techniques together. After one has learned these combination techniques, practicing composition techniques will facilitate learning some of the more difficult movements later. An example of a composition technique would be "Brush Knee." "Brush Knee" involves the hands, feet, and body working together.

ii. Segment Techniques
This refers to a series of composition techniques put together. An example would be combining "Brush Knee" with "Play the Guitar."

iii. Complete Sequence Techniques
This refers to a series of segment techniques put together. A complete sequence is executed with the beginning movement, transitional movement, and ending movement. Practicing the complete sequence can improve the proficiency of each martial art technique as well as the condition of the practitioner. Complete sequence techniques are considered a complete routine and could involve one or more moves depending on the objective of the routine.

C. The Basic Rules

Martial art has a long history in China. Throughout Chinese history, there have been many experienced and knowledgeable people overseeing the development and propagation of this wonderful art.

Chinese martial art has highly emphasized the concept, "Internal substances are harmonized with external substances." This is but the experience of demonstrating the relationship and connection between martial arts skill and power. From the solo form's essential elements, we can see these relationships clearly. Chinese martial art is based on internal substances and external substances.

External substances refer to the movements and positions of the eyes, hands, body and feet. Internal substances refer to the spirit, *chi* and power.

The body's every movement is controlled by the nervous system, influenced and restricted by the internal organs. A movement is perfectly executed only when it is able to coordinate with the internal substances. At the same time, the internal substances will be improved and enhanced by the action of the external substances.

Internal and external substances are connected and complementary. External harmonies are dictated by the internal harmony. Internal harmonies depend on external harmony. From a technical perspective, one should begin with the training to transform the external substances so the internal substances can be in harmony. The martial art is the practice of this combination; therefore, when the internal substances harmonize with the external substances the intensity of the martial art strike is stronger. One often hears that a teacher only shows a student the movement, but it is up to the student to discover how to apply the information correctly. The Chinese martial art's internal three harmonies and external three harmonies are based on the ancient Chinese philosophy called "Man and Universe Harmony."

D. The Fundamentals

When one is performing a bare hand or weapon form, one must have correct body position and variation. The hands and eyes should coordinate, the spirit concentrate, and the energy flow smoothly. The breathing should be proper, the rhythm clear.

All of these different attributes are united. They should occur together, connected and complementary.

a. **Posture**
   This refers to a completed physical movement. It is a static position in space.

b. **Technique**
   This refers to the movement of specific body parts. A technique dictates the following:

   i. The proper positioning of different body parts
   ii. The proper and accurate movement of the different body parts when one is in motion
   iii. The proper and accurate discharge of power when one is in motion

c. **Body Position**
   The body can display many positions. Generally, this refers to the different positions and variations of the torso when one is engaged in offensive and defensive maneuvers.

   The body position is not isolated. It connects to all the body parts that are engaged in offensive and defensive maneuvering. Since the torso is the major connector between the upper and lower body, when one is in motion, the torso must move according to the feet. When the feet step forward, the body must follow. When the body moves, the feet must step to provide support. This type of execution is correctly expressed in coordination, balance, and the interaction of hard and soft. When completing each body position, one should pay closer attention to the waist and feet. When the hands and feet move, the body should move accordingly to provide support. In order to place the body position properly, one has to research, analyze and understand the offensive and defensive meaning in each movement. This is especially true among the transitional movements.

d. **Eye Movements**
   This refers to the eyes moving in coordination with the hand and body movements. The eyes are the window of the spirit. Therefore, people often say that eyes and hands must go together to express the internal substances' meaning, so that when the eyes are there, the hands should be there as well. In solo form practice, if one does not correctly apply the eye movements, the body movement has no spirit, and the form is lifeless. If the eye movements are incorporated in each technique, one

is able to express the true meaning behind each technique. The eyes serve two functions in the solo form: to focus and to follow. To focus is for the eyes to concentrate on a specific subject or direction. It is often applied at the completion of a movement. To follow is for the eyes to follow a specific part of the body or weapon until a movement is completed. It is often applied at the beginning of the movement all the way to the end. The principle is generally to have the eyes and the hands coordinate together.

Coordination of the eyes and hands is one of the critical criteria to determine the correctness of a movement. If the hand and eye movement is not correct, it affects the spirit's revelation and the quality of the movement itself. When a movement is missing either component, it is not a perfect movement.

e. **Spirit**
This refers to the condition of the concentration in martial art's offensive and defensive meanings when one is executing a movement during the bare hand form or weapon form. It also refers to the understanding and involvement of the martial art's offensive and defensive meanings, rhythm, power, breathing and gracefulness.

f. **Power**
This refers to a specific type of power in martial art. It is generated under the control of intent, mind and *chi*. It is commonly referred to as *jin* among the practitioners of Tai Chi Chuan. It has soft and hard components.

The delivery of this power should not be stiff or too hard. The power is not measured by large or small. Its measure is based on following through the technique in execution. When discharging power, one should pay attention to coordination and integration so that the internal and external substances work together.

g. **Breathing**
When one is practicing the solo form, the breathing should have a specific standard, control and rhythm. Therefore, in practice, the breathing should function according to the nature of a movement. In general, inhale when executing a rising and opening movement, and exhale when executing a falling or closing movement. Based on the

nature of a movement, additional breathing techniques are divided into lifting, suspending, concentrating, and sinking.

i. Lift Breathing
This refers to the diaphragm contracting, expanding the chest cavity and shoulders stretching outward. When one is executing this lift breathing technique, the *chi* comes upward. The center of gravity will come up as well. This technique is often used when one is in a lower position going to a higher position.

ii. Suspending Breathing
When inhalation is almost complete, one forcefully repeats another quicker and shorter inhalation. This action allows the air to remain in the chest cavity longer to support completing the movement. This technique is often applied at the end of a high or low position.

iii. Concentration Breathing
After completing the inhalation, one delays the exhalation to better coordinate with the movement and deliver more power. In general, this happens when one is executing a strike movement. In striking, one speeds up the exhalation so that inhalation and movement go together. This technique can increase the amount of power discharged.

iv. Sink Breathing
This is a deep breathing technique. When the abdomen sinks, the chest relaxes. This will lower the center of gravity, facilitating balance. It is often used when one is in a lower position.

One can see that a proper breathing technique provides many benefits in a movement's completion. It makes the movement look better and improves body condition, position, and the internal organs. These techniques require a knowledgeable teacher's oral instruction to prevent any damage to the body.

h. **Rhythm**
The rhythm in martial art refers to the pace of executing the movement. It is often demonstrated in speed, transformation, and orientation. It involves the following concepts: dynamic and static, empty and full, hard and soft, fast and slow.

How to properly treat these connections and relationships directly affects the rhythm and the quality of the form. If one is unable to correctly treat the form's rhythm, the form is not good and it does not have much to offer. In demonstration, if a form does not have any light movement, it cannot reveal any heavy movement. If the form does not have any soft movement, it cannot reveal any hard movement. If there is no slow movement, it cannot reveal any fast movement. Therefore, one must execute each movement with distinction. When one is able to express the meanings of these concepts of soft and hard, dynamic and static, fast and slow, and empty and full correctly, the rhythm is very obvious; the form is very good, attractive to the eye and offering many functions. A further explanation of these concepts follows.

i. Static and Dynamic
In the form, static and dynamic are important elements. The movement in the form should be based on the number of movements divided into static and dynamic. This division will reflect the dynamic and static movements of the form.

In the dynamic condition, all the movements should be connected and continuous. One movement properly follows another movement without any stop. One should be able to clearly distinguish these static and dynamic concepts in execution and in discharge power. A spectator should be able to see this distinction clearly.

In the static condition, externally, the body is remaining still but the muscles are in a certain dynamic condition. Based on the nature of movement, one should apply a correct breathing technique to energize the body. The eye concentrates to demonstrate the mental condition and the martial art's offensive and defensive meanings.

ii. Empty and Full
This is another very important concept in Chinese martial art. Empty is lightness, variation and yielding. Full is hardness, intensity and alertness. Empty and full are always within the same movement.

The concept of empty and full in martial art is always guided by internal substances and external substances. The relationship between the internal and external substances is initiated by internal substances and manifested by external movement. Only when one has comprehended the concepts, and distinguished empty and full internally, can one execute the movement properly with power.

   iii. Hard and Soft, Fast and Slow
The concepts of hard and soft, fast and slow appear on the physical level as speed. These concepts are inseparable. It is common that when the movement is soft, it is slow, and when the movement is fast, it is hard. When one is in motion, based on the degree of transitional empty and full concepts inside the body, the nervous system mobilizes the muscles to relax or contract so that one is able to execute a movement either hard or soft, fast or slow.

E. The Benefits of Form Practice

Chinese martial art forms, whether bare hand forms, weapon forms, or two-person forms, have two major characteristics. They function as a performance art and as training for martial art fundamentals. They were created based on the martial art's offensive and defensive tactics that have the rhythm of static and dynamic movements, empty and full body weights, hard and soft power, and fast and slow speeds. To compose a form that has competitive martial art, health maintenance exercise, and performance art characteristics is no easy task. A good form contains the contributions of practitioners from many generations. Forms generally provide the following five benefits:

a. **Improved Body Condition**
When one practices the martial art forms, it can improve and strengthen one's body condition, not solely the physical body but the mental body as well. Physically, it benefits the body's joints, bones, muscle groups, ligaments, and tendons. It also improves the functioning of all internal organs and blood and *chi* circulation. Moreover, it elevates one's spirit.

b. **Improved Offensive and Defensive Skills**
The major characteristic in martial art forms is its combat function. When one practices the forms, the health condition improves, as do all the martial techniques such as striking, punching, kicking, etc.

c. **The Training of One's Temperament**
Martial art form training is a slow and sometimes boring process. It requires a lot of dedication, perseverance, discipline, and consistency. With years of training, one will develop good character traits such as a

strong will, a hard work ethic, patience, discipline, devotion, a good martial ethic, trustworthy confidence, humbleness, and so on.

d. Entertainment
Besides their value as a combat art, martial art forms have performance value as well. One can appreciate the graceful movement along with power and speed when one is demonstrating or viewing the forms.

e. Encourage Exchange of Skill, Establishment of Friendships
Martial art forms involve much information and theory. One can learn, share, and exchange practical experiences with other practitioners.

F. Teaching the Form
It is often said that martial art teaching is more difficult than scholarly teaching. In martial art teaching, a teacher has to both lecture on and demonstrate the movement. One can imagine that to be a good martial art teacher is not an easy job.

Traditionally, martial art teaching is taught by modeling. A teacher lets the students stand behind and follow what the teacher does. Therefore, it is necessary for a student to have a good teacher offering clear explanation and demonstration.

a. Two Methods of Learning
There are several methods of learning. One can learn strictly from lecture, within a group, or be self-taught. However, since martial art is a type of physical activity, the best method of learning is by behavior modification. Over the years, martial art teachers have recognized that there are but two methods best suited to teach this subject. Therefore, a teacher usually transmits the information by demonstrating one or several movements at a time along with explanation, all depending on the difficulty of the movement and the learning ability of the student.

i. One Movement at a Time
In this method, we treat each movement as one unit. One has to learn one movement, understanding completely all the techniques, applications, and variations as well as the transformation inside the body before progressing to the next movement. Although this method of working step by step requires time to complete the sequence, when one does complete it, one must understand all the

information and the body be comfortable with it. This method is perfect for someone without any previous martial art knowledge.

ii. Emphasis on Movement
In this method, one learns the complete sequence in a very short time. Later, one practices a segment of the sequence at a time, to understand the transformation inside the body and each movement's application and variation. This method is better for people who have previous martial art knowledge.

b. **Practice**
After one has learned the complete sequence (the movements, techniques, and postures), to better digest the application and improve skill, one has to practice the solo form daily. When one is in practice, one should pay closer attention to the coordination and interaction of the different parts of the body. This practice can reveal the application of the movements and provide insight for improving one's skill. After one has practiced the solo form a thousand times, the logic and reason will reveal itself.

c. **Disassembly**
Although one has learned each movement, technique, and posture, this is still not enough for use in martial combat. One has to disassemble each movement and practice each individual technique separately. One not only has to practice a technique, such as a shoulder strike, elbow strike, hip strike, knee strike, kick, or step, but also take a movement apart so one will understand the visible and the hidden technique.

d. **Variation**
There are many styles that divided the same solo form into many training objectives. Each solo form training fulfills a specific objective. Generally, a solo form has a large posture called the Large Frame Form, which is often demonstrated to the public. It has a performance art characteristic. The solo form also has a medium posture called the Medium Frame Form, which is often used as a combat art. Each movement is executed properly as defensive and offensive martial maneuvers. A solo form with a small posture is called the Small Frame Form, and it is often practiced as a *chi* circulation to improve health.

Forms have direct connection to the defensive and offensive martial tactics. If a student is engaging in martial art training and following the described procedure, skill and comprehension will improve.

G. Criteria for a Well-Executed Form

A well-executed martial art form must have the following five elements: the movements have to be accurate and stable, the offensive and defensive tactic of each movement has to be performed clearly and completely, the execution of each movement should deliver sufficient power, the rhythm should be clearly performed, and each movement should be energized with high spirit and concentration.

    a. Accurate and Stable Movements

Any physical performance done correctly is graceful and pleasurable to watch. To be done flawlessly, a performance must be invested with much practice. This is why people say that practice makes perfect.

First, all the movements should be accurate. A form is composed of many technical and mechanical elements, and each of these is composed of movements. A movement is a building block for the form. When we say the form should be performed with accuracy, we are referring to the accuracy of each movement from static to dynamic and from fast to slow motion. Body position has to be proper. Hand and feet movements have to follow the rules. For example, in the static posture, the head must be upright, the neck straight, and the shoulders sunk; the upper body is relaxed and the lower body is stable. When one looks at this posture, it has offensive and defensive value. In the form, there are many movements, and each movement has a specific feature and requirement. The quality of the movement is centered on the hands, feet, stepping, etc. To perform these basic movements properly, follow the criteria to determine the quality of the form.

Second, all the movements should be stable. Often, a movement ends by a speedy motion. Therefore, when one is executing a movement, it should be speedy when it is in a dynamic condition, and it should be stable when it is at the static condition. Many people say that the dynamic condition is the soul of martial art, and static posture is but the shell. One can see that performing a movement properly requires stability with speed.

b. **Offensive and Defensive Techniques Should be Performed Clearly and Completely**
Technique refers to the offensive and defensive tactics of each movement. A performance of a movement without any decided martial technique renders the movement a merely calisthenic exercise.

First, the technique has to be clearly defined. One has to be able to demonstrate the meaning of each movement such as push with the palm, punch with the fist, and strike with the elbow. All these techniques require specific movement and coordination from the body and feet so that the power can be delivered to the target.

Second, the technique has to be completely executed. This means from the beginning to the ending motion of execution, one has to clearly execute the technique with good coordination. A well-executed technique generally requires coordination from many body parts.

c. **Delivery of Sufficient Power**
Physical power and martial art power are two completely different concepts. Physical power refers to the power that fuels all physical activity. This requires some tension from the involved muscle groups. Observable tension gives spectators a sense of a performer's power. Martial art power often refers to *jin*, and it is often demonstrated in a discharge or martial strike.

First, the *jin* delivery requires well-coordinated parts of the body. Chinese martial art has many systems and styles, and each system and style has its own methods of training for discharge power. However, they all share the theories of "Three Sections" and "Six Harmony." In the "Three Sections Theory," the hands and feet are the root section, the elbows and knees are the mid-section, and the shoulders and hips are the head section. These six body parts are inter-related in motion. Therefore, this is also known as the "Six Harmony Theory."

Second, the *jin* has to have substance. Discharge power is based on coordination and intensity and requires these to demonstrate its substance. The substance is expressed in its power delivery. For example, when a punch has substance, it should be a powerful punch because it is well-coordinated with the feet, hip, waist, shoulder, and hand.

d. **Clear Rhythm**
The rhythm in martial art forms manifests as dynamic vs. static, light vs. heavy, fast vs. slow, and upward vs. downward motion.

i. Dynamic vs. Static
Dynamic vs. static is a special quality in martial art. When one is performing the movement, one has to move very fast. When one has completed the movement, one has to completely stop like a mountain. This reveals the basic rhythm of martial art.

ii. Light vs. Heavy
Light vs. heavy must be well-defined in performing the form. It is like two kinds of music. One is marching band music, and the other is chamber music. People describe these two types of rhythm as heavy like a crushing hammer and light like falling leaves.

iii. Up vs. Down
Up vs. down refers to the performance of the movement in space. This is like musical dynamics; sometimes the volume goes up very loud and sometimes the volume goes down very quiet. Martial art movements are generally performed at three heights. They are high, medium and low. This is also referred to as high plane, medium plane and low plane. From the mechanical perspective, the movements of all three planes should be clearly demonstrated. However, coming from the technical perspective, the high movement has a sense of supporting the sky. The lower plane movement is nimble like a swimming fish, and the medium plane movement is stable like a rock.

iv. Fast vs. Slow
In martial art activity, all action should be done quickly. This is obvious. However, this is not like a machine that has only one speed. It should be like a piece of music that has many rhythms. Therefore, when one is performing a form, based on the specific techniques, some movements should be done quicker than others. Technical meaning dictates speed.

e. **Energized with High Spirit and Concentration**
There is a common expression among Chinese martial art practitioners: "Externally, one is training the ligaments, bones and

skin. Internally, one is training the *chi*." *Chi* refers to energy. When one is demonstrating a movement, one should pay close attention to complete it with all the necessary requirements of a perfect performance. Concentration refers to paying close attention to each movement and its transformation. This can be facilitated through the expression of the eyes. Eye expression is generally happening in two ways. The eyes are following the hand movement, or the hand movement is following the eyes' guidance. When the movement completes, the eyes are focusing on a specific target. This gives the impression that although the movement has completed, the *chi* and intent continue.

Chapter 3
The Tai Chi Chuan Solo Form: Design and Development

A. Introduction
Tai Chi Chuan is an internal Chinese martial art. Practicing Tai Chi Chuan emphasizes body and power development. This is different from Chinese external martial arts, which emphasize technique and the control of others. From this distinction, Tai Chi Chuan has but one bare hand solo form with many variations to train both the body and martial art skill. This is why when one asks an experienced Tai Chi Chuan practitioner about issues relating to Tai Chi Chuan as a martial art, the answer commonly refers to its solo form.

It is true that Tai Chi Chuan has only one bare hand solo form. However, based on a practitioner's personality, objective, and intention, the same solo form can be practiced differently. This is comparable to a medical prescription. A prescription is altered according to a patient's condition. An experienced doctor understands what to prescribe. The same is true with an experienced Tai Chi Chuan practitioner. Next time you see someone practicing the Tai Chi Chuan Solo Form differently from you, you'll know why.

B. The Traditional Solo Form
Some complain that the Tai Chi Chuan Solo Form is too long and too difficult to remember or that it is not the right routine for today's busy and stressful society. Consequently, practitioners have come up with shorter and easier versions of the form. These new versions, while easier to learn and more accessible to the public, have lost many of the original intentions.

The movements of the solo form created by Zheng San Feng are a combination of old and new, simple and complex, and easy and difficult. One can see this in a movement that involves stretching and relaxing, up and down, fast and slow, repetition and variation, following the principle of Yin and Yang. Movements do not just simply repeat themselves. Rather, along with the repeated movements are many new and different movements in between so that they act as an alert and provide a sense of spiral repetition. This spiral implies moving ahead. For example, take the movement of "Brush Knee and Twist Step." It first appears in the first section of the solo form. It is done five times: once after "White Crane Spreads its Wing," three times after the first "Play the Lute," and once more after the second "Play the Lute." In the second section, "Brush Knee and Twist Step" is done four more times: twice after "Turn Around and Kick," and twice more after the two instances of

"White Crane Spreads its Wing." From this sequence of repetitions, we see that the movement of "Brush Knee and Twist Step" is not only reviewed, but also connected into the contexts of other movements. This process of repeated movements followed by new movements throughout the solo form alerts practitioners that attention and concentration must be observed at all times.

Ward off, roll back, press, and push are the four directions. Split, pull down, elbow strike, and shoulder strike are the four corners of the hand techniques. The solo form highlights the most essential movements first by beginning with the four directions, as in "Grasp the Bird's Tail." This sequence is then repeated several times, in the second and third sections. It is common knowledge among practitioners that if there is no "Grasp the Bird's Tail" in the solo form, it is not Tai Chi Chuan.

Although there are hundreds of movements, there are actually only 37 sets of completely different movements. The solo form repeats some of these 37 movements several times. The number of repetitions is based on the importance of the movements. For example, "Grasp the Bird's Tail" appears seven times, "Step Forward and Punch" and "Repulse Monkey" both appear six times, "Brush Knee and Twist Step" appears nine times, and "Single Whip" ten times. These movements have a lot of functional value. They are choreographed repeatedly into the solo form so that the practitioner can understand them thoroughly.

Tai Chi Chuan is also known as "Chung Chuan," or "Long Form," to symbolize the ocean waves. It is a process of infinite phenomena. One can see the solo form as being like an ocean wave in three ways: (1) Each single movement flows into the next movement, like one tide flows into another. (2) A group of movements comes together to form a segment that has new and repeated, simple and complex, and easy and difficult movements. This is like several tides connecting together so that one comes after another. (3) The solo form is divided into three sections. The second section is longer and more complex than the first section, and the third section is much more complex than the second section. This is like one wave growing larger and higher than the last one. In the first section, there is simplicity, but important movements are highlighted. In the second section, the movements use more of the body, from palm strikes to kicks, and so on. The third section contains more movements than either previous section, and also incorporates many complicated body maneuvers in the movements. The first section is like a low tide, the second section is a higher tide, and the third section is the highest.

The three sections composing the solo form are also comparable to a good novel. There is an introduction, a climax, and a conclusion. Each section has its important movements: "Brush Knee and Twist Step" and "Grasp the Bird's Tail" in the first section, all the kicking techniques of the second section, and the more difficult movements of the third section. The movements of "Step Forward to Form the Seven Star," "Retreat to Ride the Tiger," "Turn Around Lotus Kick," and "Pull Bow to Shoot the Tiger" are a difficult series. In a novel, a good conclusion is very important. It generally summarizes what the author wanted to present. The form concludes with the familiar movements of "Step Forward and Punch," "Seal Tightly," and "Cross Hands." This same sequence of movements ends each section and completes the whole circle with "Closing Tai Chi Chuan."

Tai Chi Chuan is the physical interpretation of the philosophy of Tai Chi. We see that the composition and structure of the Tai Chi Chuan Solo Form aim to achieve the following objectives:

1. The solo form points out the philosophy of Tai Chi Chuan by demonstrating the movements according to the following:
    a. The beginning and ending movements are the same. The solo form is a complete circle.
    b. It is not always the same movement that follows a repetition, and all the movements do not go in one direction. In one set, the movements go backward and forward three times. This provides a sense of spiral motion and advancement.
    c. All the wave motions described above symbolize continuity.
    d. There are repeated and new, fast and slow, and easy and difficult movements. This is the interpretation of Yin and Yang.

2. The solo form points out the essence of the art of Tai Chi Chuan by demonstrating the movements according to the following:
    a. Begin with the movement "Grasp the Bird's Tail" to highlight the importance of ward off, roll back, press, and push.
    b. Repeat the important movements several times in one practice so that a practitioner will become intimately acquainted with them and comprehend their usage.
    c. The movements following the repetitions are not always the same so that a practitioner will pay closer attention to practice.
    d. The routine is not done strictly in one direction, as is common among external styles; rather, it goes back and forth three times. This provides a sense of "folding" for leverage and flexibility.

Thus, we can see why it is so difficult to learn the solo form. It is designed to answer the question: What is the solo form? It exists for the practitioner to explore, to experience, and to adapt. Throughout history, many practitioners have attempted to improve it, but the essential framework has remained the same.

C. The Condensed Solo Forms

Now we see that the traditional Tai Chi Chuan Solo Form involves a rich body of meaningful knowledge. We see why it is so difficult to learn and remember. It is through this knowledge and its meaning that one sees Tai Chi Chuan's value. However, acquiring this value may seem disadvantageous in today's fast-paced society. Although the solo form offers much knowledge and meaning, for many it is too long to practice, too complex to remember, and too difficult to learn.

In the last several hundred years, Tai Chi Chuan was practiced strictly among a small group of people. This is partly because of the disadvantages mentioned above. Consequently, properly modifying the traditional solo form is the trend of Tai Chi Chuan's development. In the past hundred years, there were many experienced practitioners who distinctively modified contemporary Tai Chi Chuan solo forms. The developmental history of Tai Chi Chuan confirms that it is necessary to modify the traditional solo form, but how to modify it properly is a very difficult task. It takes much time and many experiences. It cannot be done by one person or in a short time.

I have been teaching Tai Chi Chuan at Brookline Adult and Community Education Program since 1984 and have assisted my father at the Gin Soon Tai Chi Chuan Club since 1975. I understand first hand the learning difficulties for a new student of Tai Chi Chuan. Over the years, I developed an abbreviated 22 technique Medium Frame Solo Form for the beginning students in the program and included it in my first book "Beginner's Tai Chi Chuan" published in 2000. For the intermediate students, I developed The 43 Techniques Large Frame Solo Form, The 42 Techniques Medium Frame Solo Form, The 43 Techniques Middle Frame Solo Form, and The 48 Techniques Small Frame Solo Form. These four forms share similar movements and sequencing. However, each movement is executed according to its respective form's frame perimeter. I omitted some of the repeated movements from the related traditional solo forms so that these condensed solo forms can be done in less time and learned quickly. And yet, they are long enough for the body to properly exercise with each practice. I introduce the Large, Medium, and Small Frame Forms in chapters 5, 6, and 7 of this book.

D. The Beginners' Solo Forms

With the recent surge of interest in Tai Chi Chuan, the student's pool of available forms and styles has increased; differences reflect cultural backgrounds, objectives, and physical health conditions. I feel it is necessary to have proper introductory courses for these students. Therefore, I have developed an additional five abbreviated solo forms for students with no previous experience in Tai Chi Chuan. All these beginners' solo forms feature a reduced total number of movements. With fewer movements, it is easier for the students to learn and practice; the qualities of Tai Chi Chuan remain the same.

The abbreviated solo forms are the Eight Techniques Medium Frame Solo Form, the Twelve Techniques Large Frame Solo Form, the Fourteen Techniques Middle Frame Solo Form, the Fifteen Techniques Small Frame Solo Form, and the Twelve Techniques Returning Tai Chi Chuan.

Chapter 4
Functions of the Tai Chi Chuan Solo Form

A. Introduction
Over the years, many students have asked me variations of the following question: How can the slow movements of Tai Chi Chuan be considered a martial art? The question is understandable since a martial art is supposed to move fast and with power and Tai Chi Chuan seems to do the opposite.

B. The Multiple Functions of Tai Chi Chuan
The slow Tai Chi Chuan Solo Form has many functions. It has been used quite successfully as a healing regimen for sick people who were chronically ill. It has been found to be a meditative and quieting influence, an extremely relaxing routine in the face of modern stress. It has also been cited as a means of communicating with the environment, nature, and one's self. Although it is true that this discipline has other goals like centering, relaxation, health, and longevity, Tai Chi Chuan is first and foremost a martial art. Precisely because it is slow, the Tai Chi Chuan Solo Form allows the practitioner's body to be more relaxed, loose, and nimble. To the Tai Chi Chuan masters, that is the ideal body to cultivate, one that is at ease, fluid, and alive. A body that is hard, tight, and inflexible is associated with death. When the Tai Chi Chuan practitioner fights, he is alert, supple, and sensitive. At the same time, his body responds to any situation however unpredictable. And it is definitely easier for the teacher and the student to fine-tune the body and correct the posture if the movement is slow rather than fast. There is also better awareness of the body dynamics when the movement is slow.

The slow Tai Chi Chuan Solo Form also teaches a new vocabulary. It is a beginning. The body starts to learn a different way, a relaxed way, of fighting. Inherent in the slow movements are certain combative techniques that can be developed through pushing hand exercises. The solo form is an excellent means of teaching and learning the combative techniques.

It is often said that the movements were originally single postures and that somebody put them together as a sequence. Even now, instructors still demonstrate a single and isolated posture for fighting, but the intention is only to demonstrate the correct position. If the instructor also shows the martial application, the student should not believe that that is the only application of the movement or posture. Instructors often demonstrate a fighting technique in class, but that is only to give an idea of one of the many applications of a movement. The demonstration should in no way limit the possibility of other applications in each movement nor inhibit the movement's potential or the student's understanding and development. It is usually said that the applications are infinite. There are refinements and variations. With a shift of the body, the application may change, though the posture is basically the same. One can see this in the following three chapters.

Many people have misinterpreted the slow movement of the solo form as the combative form. Among Tai Chi Chuan practitioners, it is often said that the slow form is for the body while the push hand exercises are for application.

After we master the body by going through different positions to achieve total relaxation, every movement becomes nimble and has offensive and defensive meaning. A practitioner will no longer rely on any individual movement's application. At this point, all responses will be based on the opponent's movements. Any part of the body can be used as a weapon for yielding or discharging power. That is why practitioners often say that when the intention is there, the *chi* will be there too, and the power will not be far behind.

As a new practitioner in this art, one may be confused or overwhelmed with the information of the following chapters. The variations of Tai Chi Chuan Solo Form training are guided by two main objectives: to improve the martial art fundamentals, and to improve the body condition, so that one is healthy and ready to engage in martial art activity.

With these objectives in mind, the high demands that Tai Chi Chuan places on the body parts are understandable. After all, Tai Chi Chuan is a difficult art to understand because it incorporates many subjects, including philosophy, fine art, body mechanics, physics, and health maintenance. It is difficult to practice because of its unique characteristics. There are many people who practice Tai Chi Chuan for health. There are many people who practice Tai Chi Chuan as a martial art as well. In order for the second group of people to acquire martial skill, one should pay closer attention to body parts in training.

C. Tai Chi Chuan as a Martial Art
1. The Hands
In martial art combat, the hands are the first line of defense. The movement of the hands dictates the outcome. Therefore, one should train the hands well. There are many techniques in Tai Chi Chuan that use the hands. The hand is the most flexible and mobile part of the body. The hand functions as follows:

a. The hand is the extremity of the arm. When the arm moves, this extremity must move first.
b. Moving the hand increases concentration and power in the hand.
c. Moving the hand increases balance, coordination and relaxation.
d. When the hand is mobilized with power, it is quick and powerful.
e. When the hand has power, it is accurate.
f. When the power is in the hand, it is able to respond quickly to launch a second strike.
g. The hand is the extremity of the arm. The fingers are the extremity of the hand. When the hand moves, the fingers move first. If one executes the technique in this order, it is easy to catch the target. Otherwise, the technique is no good.

2. The Elbows

In Tai Chi Chuan movement, or other physical activity, the elbow is always in motion outward and stretching the shoulder. It functions as an anchor as well. The root of the elbow is the shoulder. If there is no root at the shoulder, there is no power at the elbow. Relaxing and lowering the shoulder supplies power to the elbow.

In Tai Chi Chuan practices, the five bows in a posture are emphasized. The five bows are located as follows: the bows in the two arms, in the two legs, and the bow of the body. The elbow is the arc of the two bows of the arms. One should always keep it ready. The elbow has the following functions:

a. It supports the hand's movement.
b. It aids in body balance.
c. It supports in stretching the arm.
d. It is able to launch a powerful strike that is very difficult to block. Therefore it is a very good weapon for close quarter combat.

3. The Shoulders

Although it is emphasized that one should relax the body in Tai Chi Chuan training, the standard of relaxation is based on the condition of the body's warding off *jin*. People find it difficult to relax the body because they are unable to relax the shoulders. When one points the elbow to the side, the shoulder comes up. When one points the elbow downward, the shoulder sinks. When one has power in the hand, the shoulder stiffens. When there is no power in the hand, the shoulder is loose. When one is confronted with the techniques of pull down, seizing, hitting, and take down, a natural response is to maintain body balance. This response causes the shoulders to go up and the feet to lift off the ground, losing the root. When the shoulders go up, the opponent easily controls you. The correct response is to sink the shoulders by lowering the elbows so the arms have root, and then one is able to apply a correct response to neutralize the threat. Therefore, the major function for the shoulders is to maintain body balance by lowering them, so that the *chi* can sink down to the *dan tien*. The shoulders are also effective weapons in close quarter combat.

4. Relax the Chest
To relax the chest, one has to keep the chin down and the eyes looking forward. "Relax the chest" and "stretch the back" are two sides of the same coin. If one can relax the chest, one is able to stretch the back and have power. The *chi* sinks to the *dan tien*, the body is balanced, and the bow on the body is ready to launch. If the chest is not relaxed and the back is not stretched and has no power, the chest cavity is filled with air. It is not natural. The upper body becomes heavier than the lower body, so the body has no balance. Therefore, relaxing the chest and stretching the back are important components of body balance and mobility.

5. The Waist
The waist is the most important part of the body. It is the reservoir of *chi* and the center of body movement. If the waist is not flexible, the upper and lower body are not coordinated. When the waist is injured, one will find it is very difficult to move an inch. Therefore, throughout history, exercising the waist has been and will remain a necessary and fundamental exercise in Chinese martial art training.

6. The Hips
The feet are the root of the body. They support all the body's activity. When the hips are relaxed, the *chi* is able to sink down and the legs become stronger. The *Tai Chi Chuan Classic* points out that the power comes from the movement of the feet. When the hip is relaxed, the foot will be connected to the rest of the body and the power able to travel upward to the waist, shoulders, hands, and fingers. Relaxing the hip functions as follows in martial art activity:

a. It can neutralize some or all incoming power.
b. It can lower the center of gravity, thereby stabilizing the body.
c. It can increase the waist rotation; the body becomes nimbler and better coordinated.
d. It is a component in issuing power.

e. It contributes to body position, stepping, and mobilization.
f. It stretches the tendons and ligaments of the legs.

7. The Knees

The function of the feet as root is based on the position of the knee. If the knee is not positioned correctly with the toes, there is no root at the feet, no mobilization or support. When an experienced practitioner looks for correct posture, he is looking for the relaxation of the hip, knee and toe alignment, a round groin, a straight back, and eyes looking forward or following the hands. If a posture does not look comfortable, The *Tai Chi Chuan Classic* recommends looking for answers at the waist and feet. In other words, it recommends looking at the waist rotation, and the knee and toe alignment. When the knee is aligned with the toes, one has empty and full weight distinction on the feet.

8. The Feet

Tai Chi Chuan pays attention to all bodily movement. It does not matter if it is large or small. When the body moves, it involves muscle contraction and extension. Over the years, I have heard students complain that the body aches due to the comprehensive muscular movements of Tai Chi Chuan.

A simple movement of turning the head to the left or right is actually working on the neck muscles. When one is lifting the toes up, pointing the toes, lifting the heel, or turning the foot, one is turning and stretching the tendons, ligaments, and muscles of the feet. When the feet are stronger, stability and mobility are better, and the body is able to move with ease.

After one has understood the significance of the body parts involving movement, one should come to understand the principles behind the many variations of a single posture. After all, martial art activity has numerous possibilities.

A knowledgeable Tai Chi Chuan practitioner does not talk about application all the time. Rather, he talks about internal power, how to develop more of this internal power, and how to incorporate this internal power into a strike. When the body is loose and relaxed from practicing the Tai Chi Chuan solo forms, internal power will be developed from the bodily coordination. This internal power does not come from tension in any part of the body. It is the result of total body coordination developed through the Tai Chi Chuan Solo Form practices. It is very explosive, so explosive that it can send somebody ten or twenty feet away.

Chapter 5
The 43 Movement Large Frame Solo Form

A. Introduction

The Large Frame Solo Form introduced in this chapter is based on Yang Cheng Fu's teaching. Yang Cheng Fu created this form based on the Middle Frame Solo Form, or Transitional Solo Form, of his father Yang Chien Hou. Yang Chien Hou realized that it was very difficult for a student to develop martial art skill from the Small Frame Solo Form, so he modified the form by enlarging the motion of the movements, by making the stances lower, and with a few other adjustments as well.

Today, there are many Tai Chi Chuan solo forms available to and practiced by Yang Style Tai Chi Chuan practitioners, and they all call their forms the 108 Movement Solo Form. This does not mean that the solo forms they practice have 108 movements; rather, they trace their solo form's root back to the original solo form practiced by Yang Lu Chan. In Chinese culture, 108 is one of the infinite mystical numbers.

The major characteristic of the Large Frame Solo Form is its large circular motion. Its function is to open all the body joints by stretching the ligaments and tendons so that a practitioner is able to execute a strike quickly in combat. The philosophy and importance of the circle is transmitted among practitioners: "To learn the art, begin with the circle. To be good in skill, perfect the circle."

Yang Lu Chan's teacher, Chen Chang Hsin, was known as the "King of Tombstone" because of his upright posture in Tai Chi Chuan practices. If the body is in an upright position, it has support from all directions. At the same time, one is able to engage an enemy in combat from all directions. Therefore, when the practitioner's body has upright position, it also means it has mobility.

Yang Cheng Fu lived at a time of transition in Chinese history. The country and its people called for the martial art community to strengthen the people's spirit by modifying the combative art into a health art. Yang Cheng Fu was one of the pioneers who met this challenge. He modified his father's Middle Frame Form to the Large Frame Form to improve one's blood circulation, the first step to better health. Therefore, the health benefit is the third major characteristic of the form.

So, practicing the Large Frame Solo Form serves two functions. It opens the joints by stretching the ligaments and tendons to improve the practitioner's martial skill and power, and the large motion also improves blood circulation to better one's health. It is a perfect solo form to improve one's body condition. Therefore, the Large Frame Solo Form is also known as the beginner's form.

B. The Principles of the Large Frame Form

Traditional Chinese martial art training has internal and external trainings. Internal training trains the intrinsic energy, or *chi*, and external training trains the muscles, tendons, ligaments, and bones. The Tai Chi Chuan Large Frame Solo Form is a method of training the tendons, ligaments, and bones. This is why the Large Frame Form was the first solo form Yang Cheng Fu emphasized and taught to his students. It is a form to build martial art fundamentals.

The fundamental body requirement in martial art discipline is for the body to be so soft and flexible it's as if there is no bone. When the body is soft and flexible, one can quickly and easily change its position, direction, and technique to an advantageous posture. Lao Tzu said, "Extreme softness overcomes extreme hardness." When the body is soft and flexible, as if there is no bone, one can easily manipulate the body and maximize its function.

We know that in order to have a soft and flexible body, the body must engage in a series of stretching exercises to loosen the joints and warm up the muscles. People who have not engaged in martial art training are not prepared and cannot apply their body to the vigorous physical activity of martial art. Therefore, a martial art practitioner must strengthen the body by engaging in some type of exercise to enhance or transform the tendons, ligaments, and bones to prepare the body for this type of activity. Tendons and ligaments are connective tissues between muscles and bones. They are everywhere in the body. The shoulders support; the hands grasp; the feet walk; and the tendons, ligaments and bones make the body nimble.

Although the tendons, ligaments, and bones are important to the body, there are many diseases that weaken them. Therefore, one must exercise them to make them strong and powerful enough for martial art activity. Although the names may not be the same, one can see that all Chinese martial art styles have some kind of exercise to serve this purpose.

People say that the body can be hard as a rock; this is the function of the bone. The body is nimble because of the function of the joints which connect all parts of the body together. The joints are the spaces between two bones. They are the centers of rotations and movements. If the joints are strong, one cannot bend them when they are straight, and one cannot straighten them when they are bent.

In order to make the joints flexible and attain a larger range of motion, one must open these joints by stretching and working the tendons and ligaments, as well as the bones, connective tissues, and cartilage.

This is the reasoning behind the Tai Chi Chuan Large Frame Solo Form. Chinese martial art training combines internal and external attributes. Internal attributes refer to *chi*, or intrinsic energy. External attributes refer to physical movement. The martial skill is divided into many levels. At each level, there are corresponding exercises available among different Chinese martial art systems. When a practitioner is at a certain level, one practices the exercises according to that level. Therefore, practitioners should select the appropriate exercise for their particular level. If one follows this rule, skill will increase tremendously.

The External Approach
A new student is usually unable to unify the intrinsic energy. It is better for him or her to select exercises such as stretching the body, arms, and legs and rotating the waist. Such exercises focus on the condition of and power from the tendons, ligaments, muscles, and bones. The result of this training is the execution of movements quickly and powerfully. Yet although the movement is powerful, it is difficult to control; therefore, it is better for one to make the movement softer and slower in the beginning so it is easier to control and the power is hidden. This is the work for the next step of the internal approach. It is a significant transformation.

The Internal Approach
The intent is to guide the intrinsic energy to circulate among the joints, while externally the body moves in a large circular motion. This combination is what Yang Cheng Fu called internal substances harmonizing with external substances in his "Yang's Ten Important Points."

After one has practiced following this internal approach for a while, internal and external attributes will move together. This is described as, "When the intent is there, the *chi* will be there. When the *chi* is there, the power will be there as well."

Chinese martial arts emphasize that hard power must have a soft component; otherwise, it is easy to break. Soft power must have a hard component; otherwise, it cannot get the job done. A technique that has movement as well as intrinsic energy is the best combination for martial art application. Although it is necessary to have both a physical movement and intrinsic energy, due to the degree of combination, one practitioner's skills and achievements differ from another's. In the external approach, the primary emphasis is on power from the tendons, ligaments, muscles, and bones while the intrinsic energy is secondary. In the internal approach, the primary emphasis is on the intrinsic energy while the power from the tendons, ligaments, muscles, and bones is secondary. One can see that the powers generated from these two approaches are different. Martial art practitioners favor the power generated from the internal approach based on its natural characteristics of control, sharpness, and penetrating ability. When one is engaged in Tai Chi Chuan Large Frame Form training, one is already training in the internal approach; whereas, most martial art practitioners have to begin from the external approach and work their way to the internal approach.

The Fundamentals
All Tai Chi Chuan solo forms follow the same philosophy. They are guided by the same principles and concepts. They differ in the execution of each individual movement. It is this difference that distinguishes the three frames' forms that I introduce in this book from each other. Therefore, in order for one to master this art, to have better health, better skill, and more understanding, one must spend time practicing the fundamentals to build a stronger foundation. In the Tai Chi Chuan Large Frame Solo Form, the most distinguishing characteristic is the open movement and spiral motion involving the whole body.

Tai Chi Chuan fundamentals include movements of the hands and eyes, body position, stance and stepping. It is often said that when one executes a hand technique without moving the feet, one is looking for trouble. In executing a movement, if the head is looking down like a dog and the body is stretching like a cat, one's skill is very poor. Therefore, one must spend time practicing the fundamentals.

1. Basic Hand Techniques and Positions

Tai Chi Chuan involves many hand techniques. It is necessary to get them right so that the movements will be performed and executed correctly in martial application. The hand methods are divided into the fist *(fig 1)*, the palm *(fig 2)*, and the hook *(fig 3)*. The common Tai Chi Chuan techniques are ward off, roll back, press, push, pull down, split, elbow strike, shoulder strike, palm strike, punch, and hook.

figure 1

figure 2

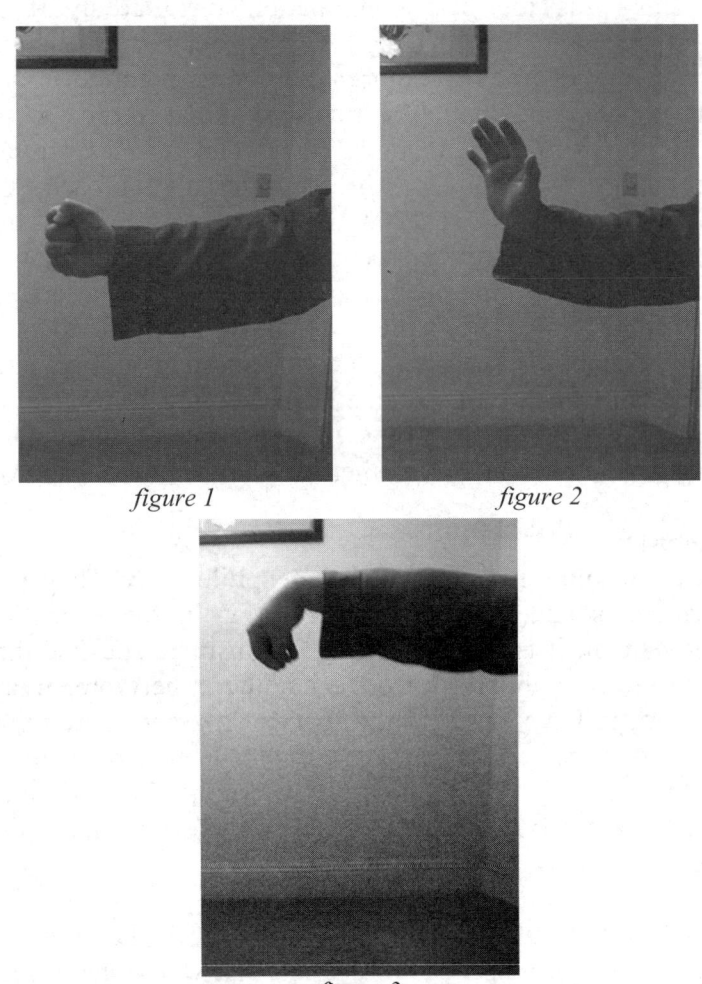

figure 3

When closing the fingers into a fist, the fingers should not be too tight. When forming the palm strike, bend the wrist so that the power will go directly into the palm's center.

a. **The Fists**

The fist is a most important weapon in bare hand combat. There are several techniques involving the fist in Tai Chi Chuan. Here is the list of the common fist techniques:

Hidden Fist: The fist rests by the waist. It is face up.

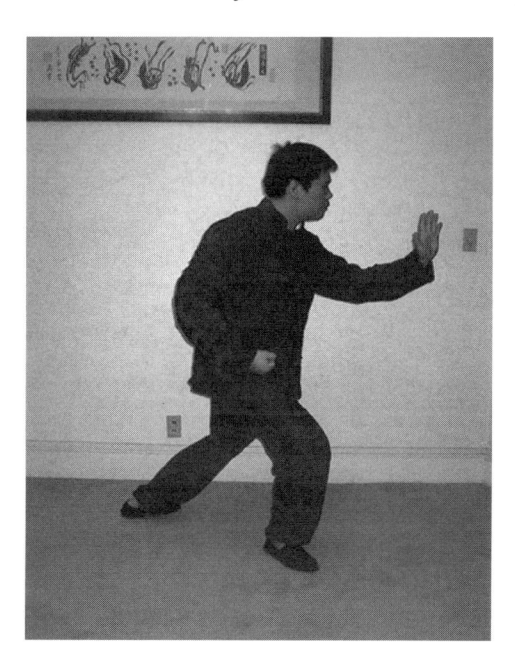

i. Thrusting Fist: The fist rests by the waist then goes forward. Its position is not higher than the shoulder and not lower than the chest. When by the waist, it faces up. When it goes forward, rotate the arm inward.

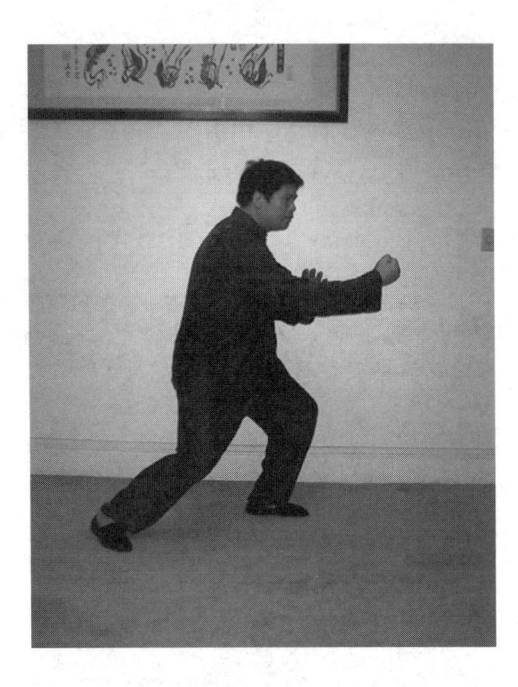

ii. Downward Fist: The fist rests by the waist then goes downward. It faces either to the left or right. It arrives level to the front knee.

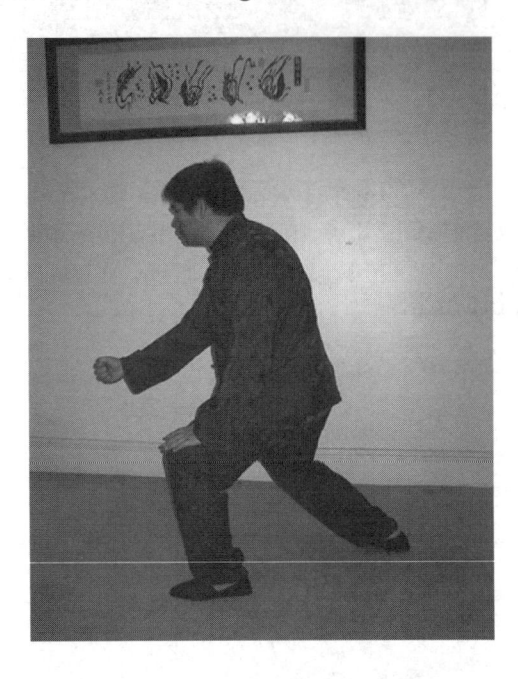

iii. Parry Fist: The fist comes up in an arc. It begins with the fist face down, then transitions to face up as it moves to the front or side.

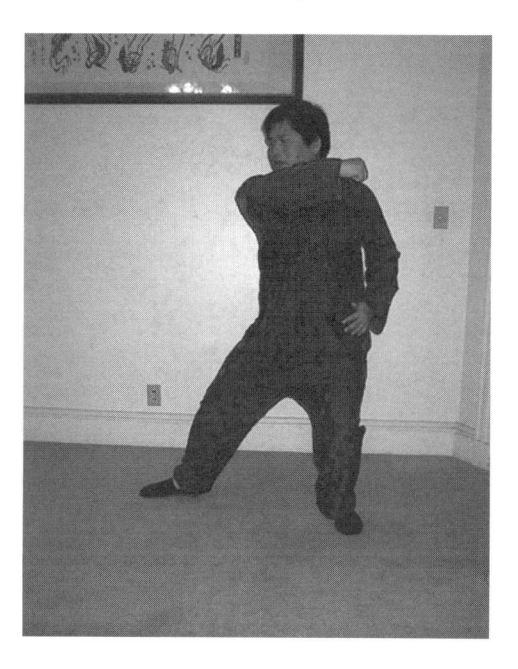

iv. Back Fist: The fist moves upward then downward in an arc. It begins with the fist face down and ends with the fist face up.

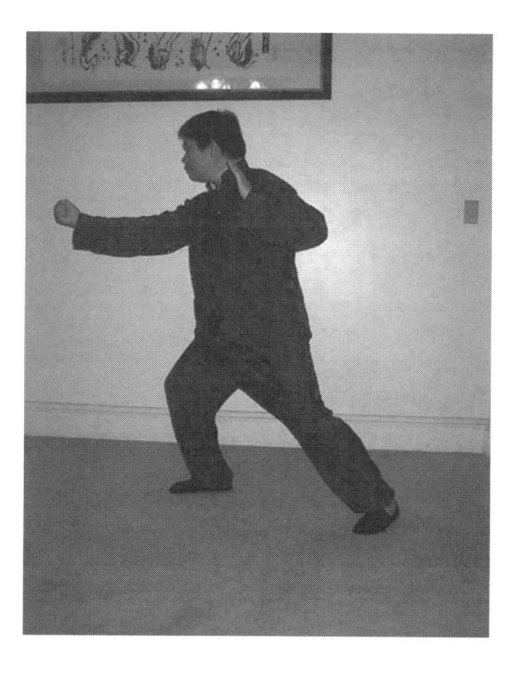

v. Double Fist: The two fists go upward to ear level.

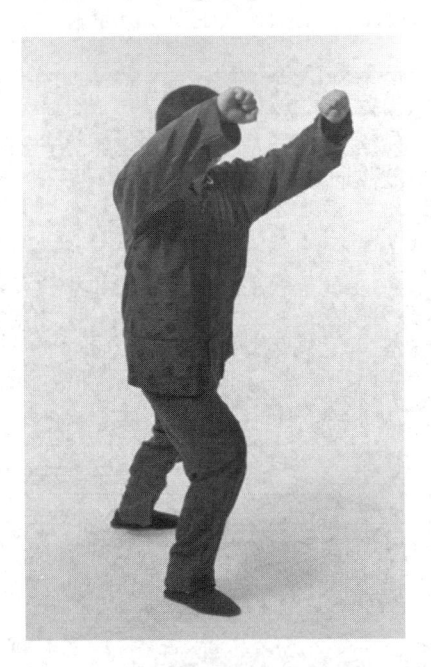

vi. Horizontal Fist: The fists move horizontally to the left or right.

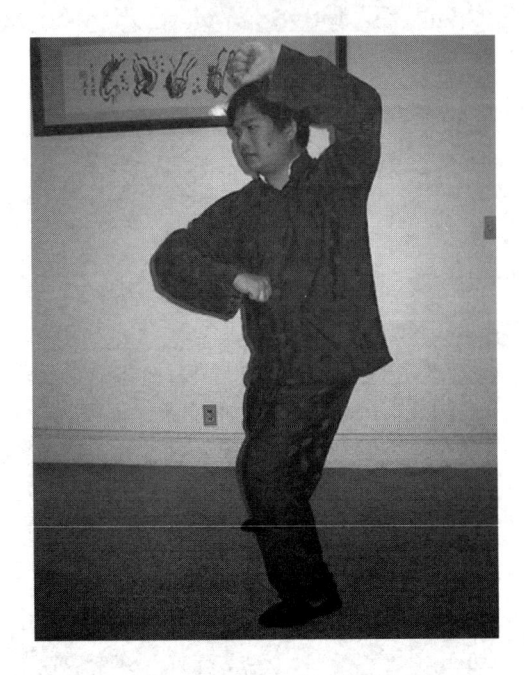

b. **The Palms**

Although the name implies that Tai Chi Chuan uses the fist, most of the hand techniques in Tai Chi Chuan employ the palm. Internal martial arts practitioners recognize that a palm can easily be transformed into more options than a fist. Here is the list of the common techniques involving the palm:

i. Single Palm Push: Bend the elbow and wrist with the fingers pointing up. The palm is pushed forward on level with the shoulder.

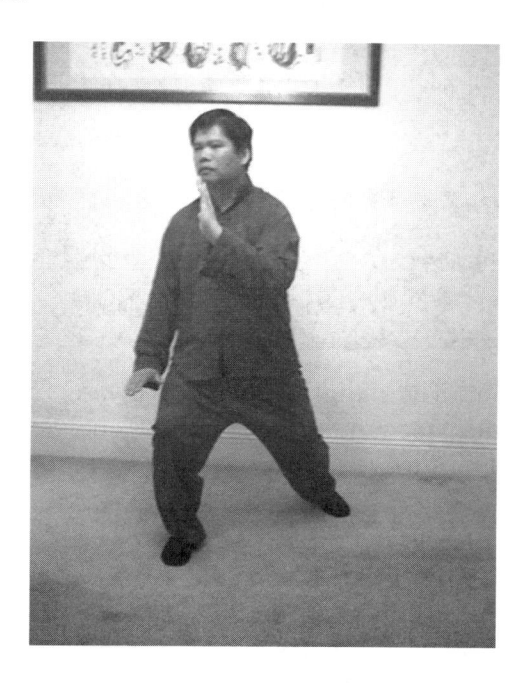

ii. Double Palm Push: The two palms push forward from the shoulders with the fingers pointing up.

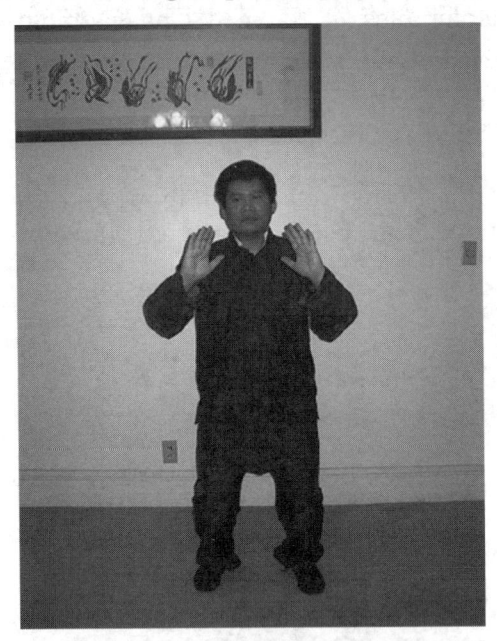

iii. Brush Palm: The palm brushes downward from the center of the body to the side of the body. Here, the lower palm shows the completed motion.

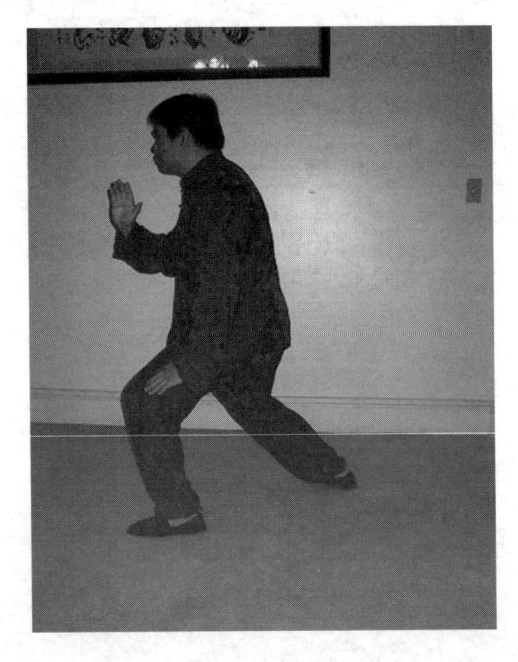

iv. Intercepting Palm: The palm comes from the side of the body to the chest with the palm facing up. The fingers are pointing to the side.

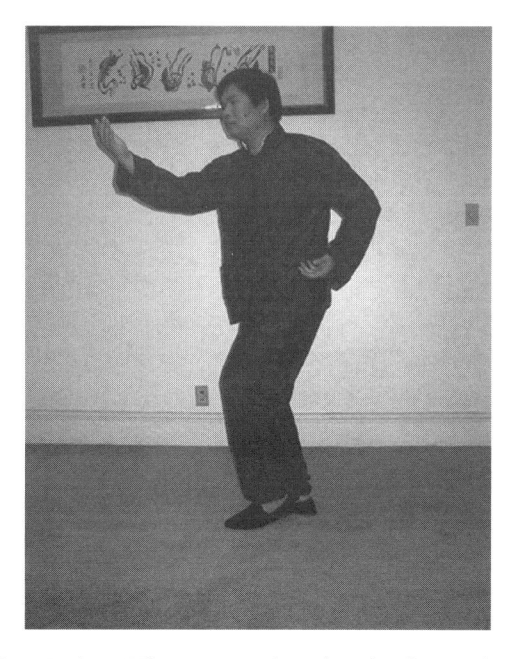

v. Separating Palm: The two palms begin from the center of the body; then separate into two sides with the palms facing away from the body and the lower fingers pointing up.

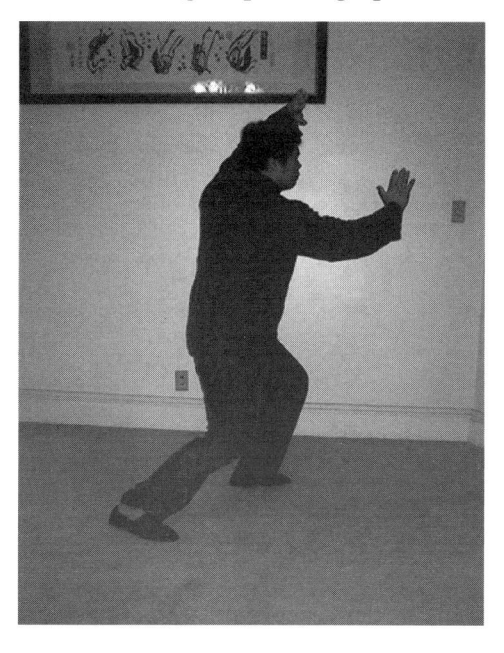

vi. Diagonal Separation Palm: The two palms begin from the center of the body then separate into top and bottom.

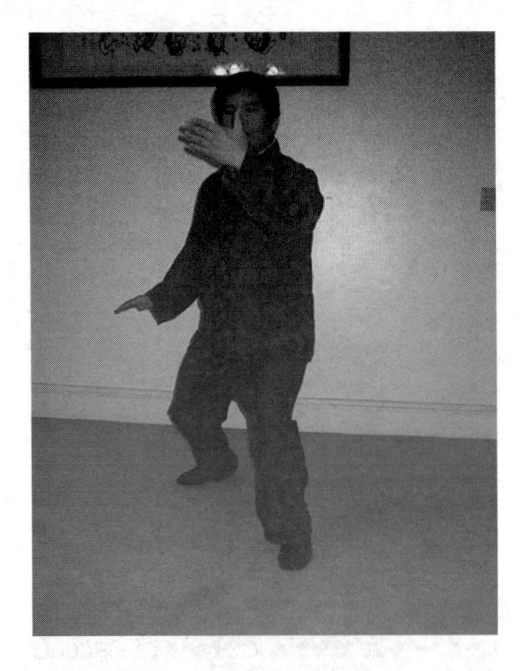

vii. Vertical Cloud Palm: The palms move vertically; the lower exchanging places with the higher and vice versa.

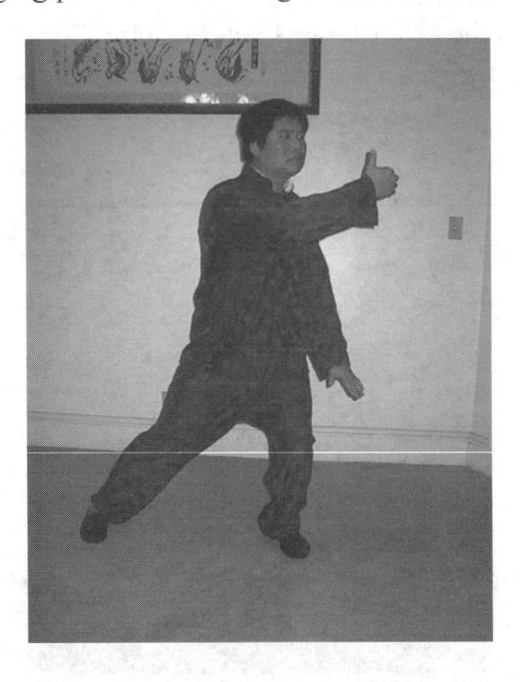

viii. Horizontal Cloud Palm: The palms move horizontally from left to right or right to left.

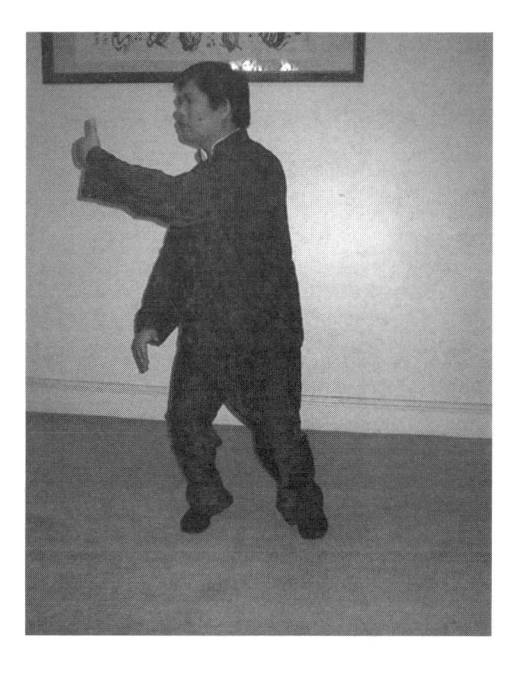

ix. Thrusting Palm: The palm thrusts directly forward with the fingers pointing diagonally upward.

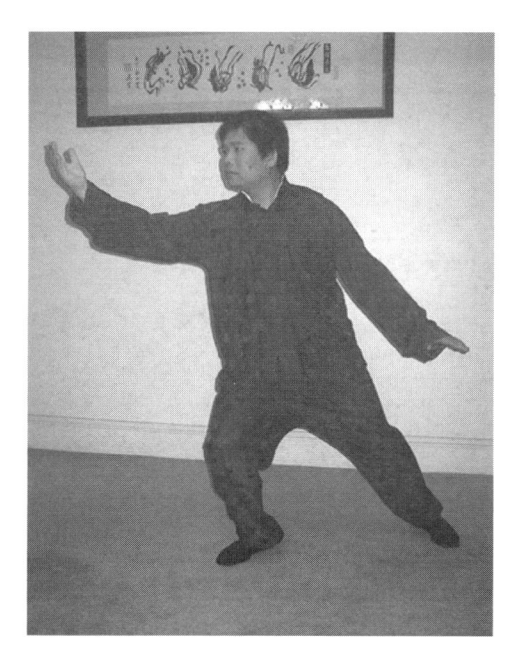

x. Blocking Palm: The palm goes upward above the head, facing out.

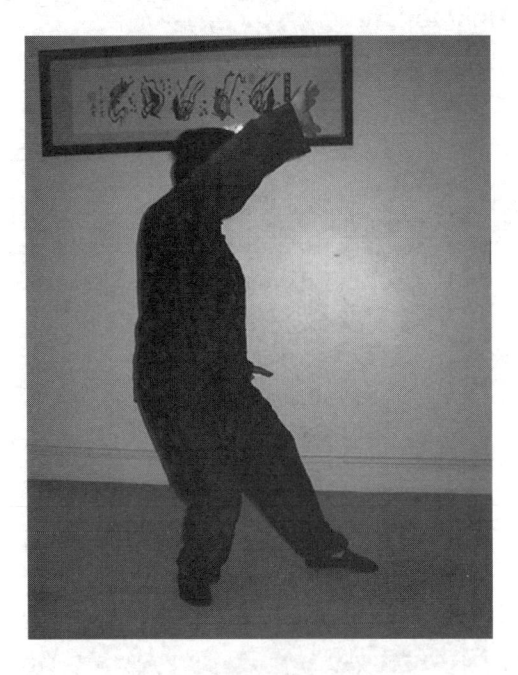

xi. Embracing Palm: The palms face inward with the fingers pointing to the sides. The wrists intersect.

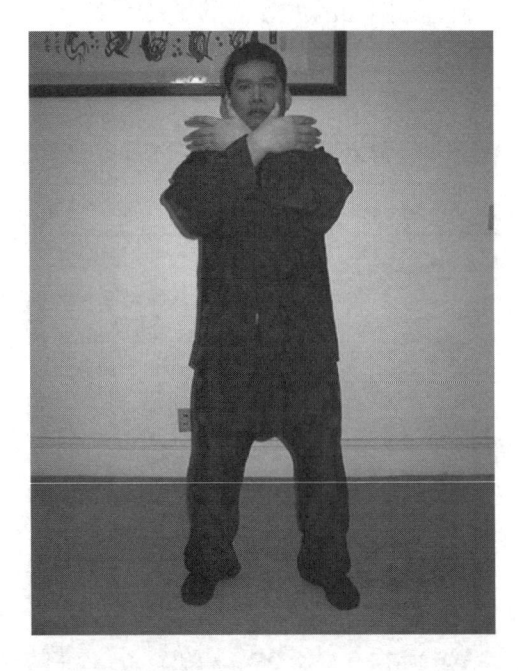

xii. Downward Palm: The palm goes down with the fingers pointing downward.

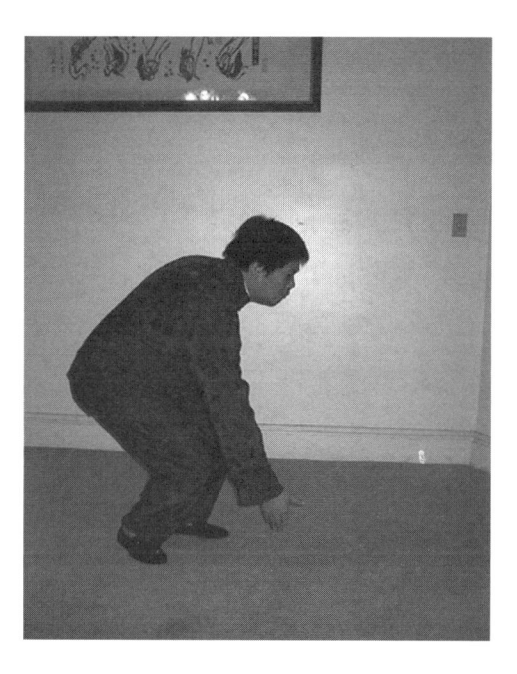

xiii. Lift Palm: The palm goes upward with the fingers pointing up.

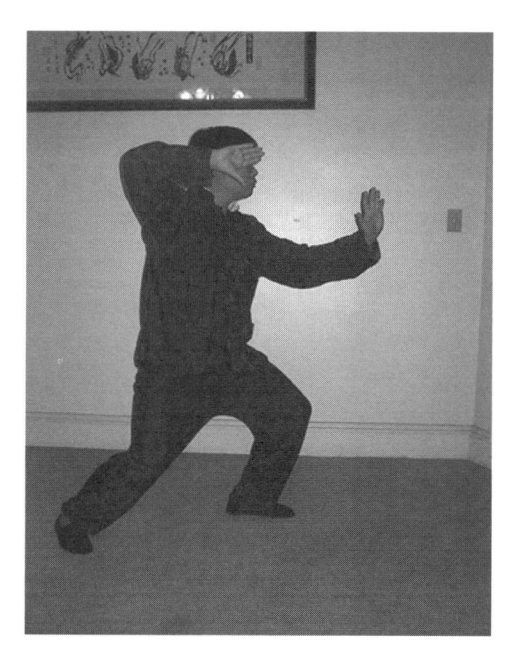

xiv. Yin Yang Palm: One palm faces up, and the other palm faces down.

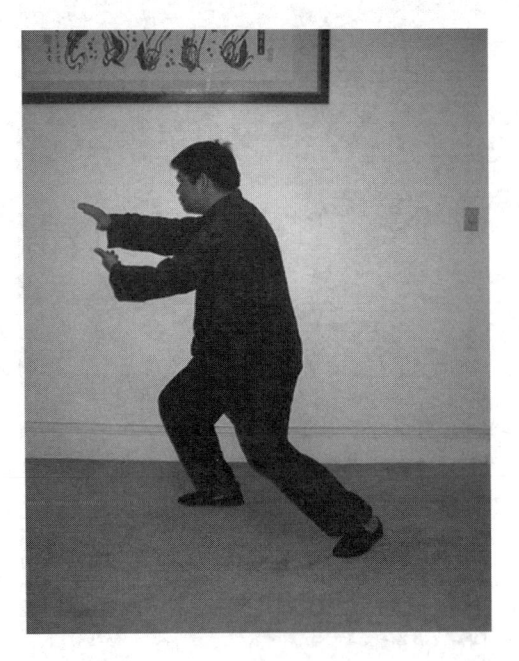

c. **The Arms**

In Tai Chi Chuan, the arm movements are often incorporated to execute the techniques of split, shoulder strike, and elbow strike. Some of the common arm movements follow:

i. Embracing: The palms face inward while the arms encircle.

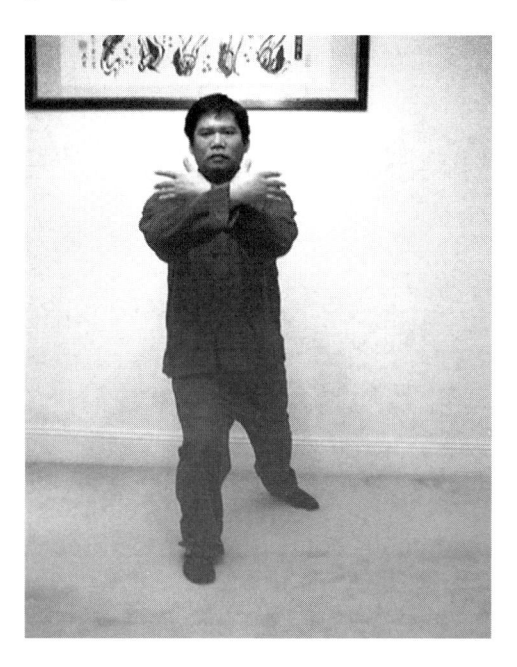

ii. Push: The two arms come together in front of the chest.

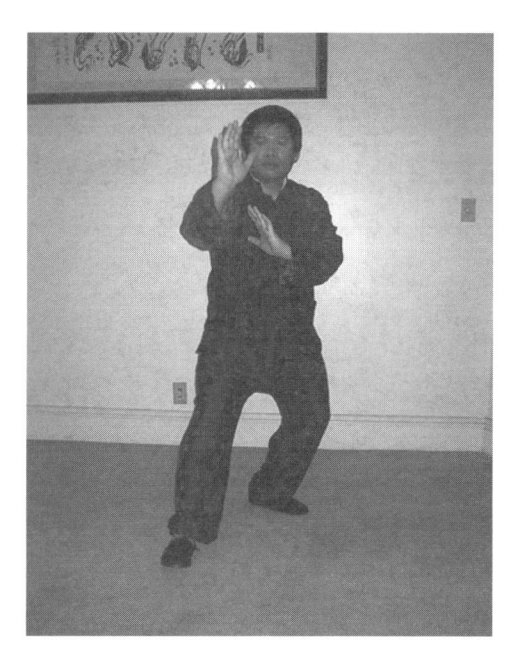

iii. Separation: The two hands separate into front and back.

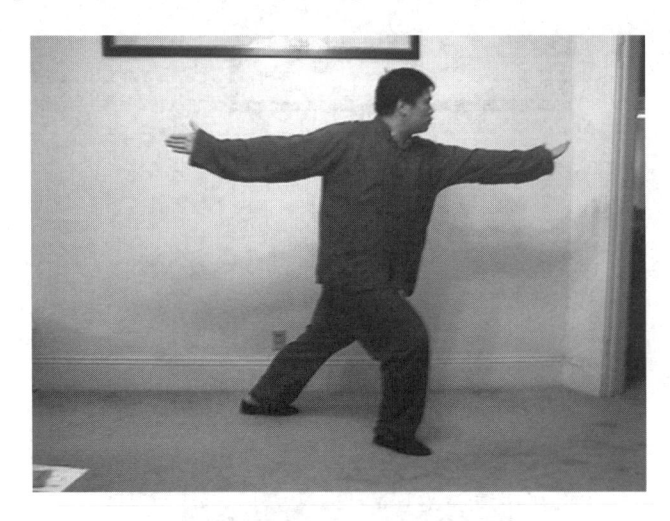

iv. Split: The two hands come together then separate to the sides.

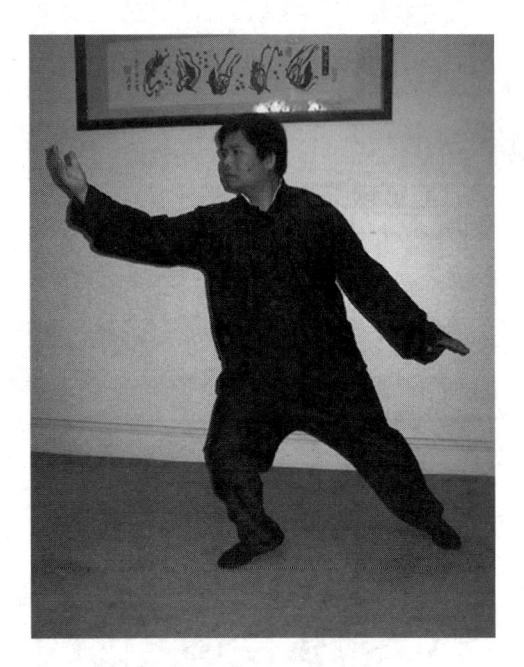

2. **Eye and Body Techniques and Positions**

   a. **Eye Position**

   As in all Chinese martial art systems, the eyes are very important in Tai Chi Chuan. They are related to the expression of *chi*, spirit, and power delivery. In practice, it is necessary to concentrate the spirit and mind. Each movement should coordinate with the intent and be natural so that the hands, feet, and body work in unison.

b. **Body Position**
   i. The head always remains upright with the eyes looking forward and far off so the spirit can reach to the top of the head. This means the head remains upright following the intent. When the top of the head is slightly lifted upward, the jaw tilts inward, and the tongue touches the hard palate. The trunk is upright as if there is support from all directions. The nature of this posture is like supporting a glass of water with the head or like a rope suspending the head from the crown so that the glass does not fall and the water does not spill.
   ii. The neck is relaxed and straight. There is no tension on the neck muscles so that it is easy to rotate the neck to either side without stiffness.
   iii. The shoulders are relaxed and sunk. If the shoulders do not sink, the blood flow is inhibited, and the *chi* will not rise. This will inhibit the whole body from sinking downward to a better rooting.
   iv. The elbows should sink and point downward. Otherwise, as mentioned above, they cause the same problem as the shoulders.
   v. The chest should be relaxed and natural so that the *chi* can sink to the *dan tien*, an area three inches below the navel. Make sure the chest does not thrust outward or sink inward.
   vi. The back should be spread evenly so that the *chi* can penetrate into the bones. It is said that as long as one has the chest relaxed, the back is automatically raised.
   vii. The waist should be relaxed so that it is flexible. All Tai Chi Chuan solo form movements are initially based on the rotation of the waist. Therefore, the more flexible and loose the waist, the better and more efficiently one will be able to execute the solo form movements.
   viii. The hip and buttocks must tuck under so that all the postures are connected. Otherwise, if a posture is not properly connected, issuing power is difficult. Therefore, the hip should be relaxed and sink to get a better balance, and the buttocks should not be protruding to the sides. Overall, the body should be relaxed and natural with the coccyx in a straight and upright position so that all the movements are nimble and start from the waist.

3. Step and Stance

Step and Stance are important aspects of Tai Chi Chuan training. Stance refers to body posture, and step is the movement from one body posture to another. Stance training refers to some of the stationary postures in the Tai Chi Chuan Solo Form, and step training refers to movements with bodyweight transition in the Tai Chi Chuan Solo Form. In Tai Chi Chuan training, when a beginner is unable to master the stance and step trainings, it is difficult to maintain body balance, correctly execute the movement, and progress in training. Therefore, stance and step skills are the basic requirements for body balance and mobility. They are so vital that all martial art systems require beginning students to spend many years on stance and step skill training before being allowed to learn any routine. In the high standard of Tai Chi Chuan practices, principles such as walk like a cat and pulling silk from a cocoon require a lot of movement control and coordination. If the stance and step skills are not strong and correct, one cannot practice the principles properly.

a. Stance Position

In the Tai Chi Chuan Large Frame Form, both knees are bent. It is like one is sitting on an empty chair with the trunk upright. There are several different types of stances. A list of the common stances follows:

i. Forward Bow Stance:
Bend the front leg with the foot flat on the floor. The knee does not pass beyond the toes. The back leg is bent, its knee aligned with the toes. Generally, 60% of the body's weight is on the front leg, and 40% of the body's weight is on the back leg.

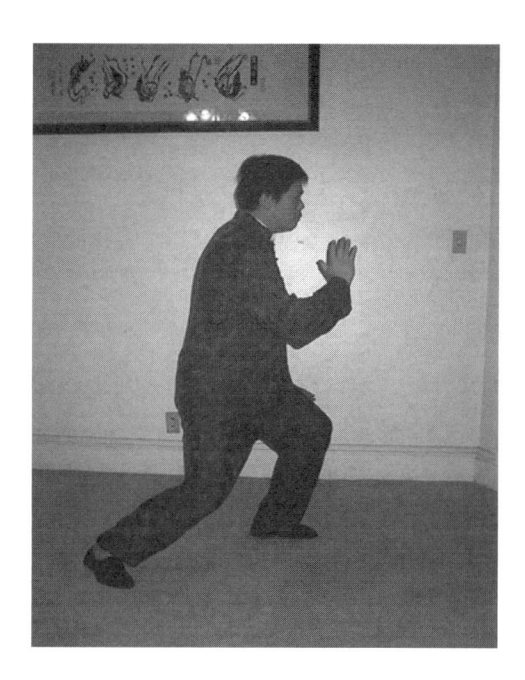

ii. Backward Bow Stance:
   Bend the back leg with the foot flat on the floor and the knee pointing to the same direction as the toes. The front leg is bent with the knee aligning to the toes. Generally, 60% of the body's weight is on the back leg, and 40% of the body's weight is on the front leg.

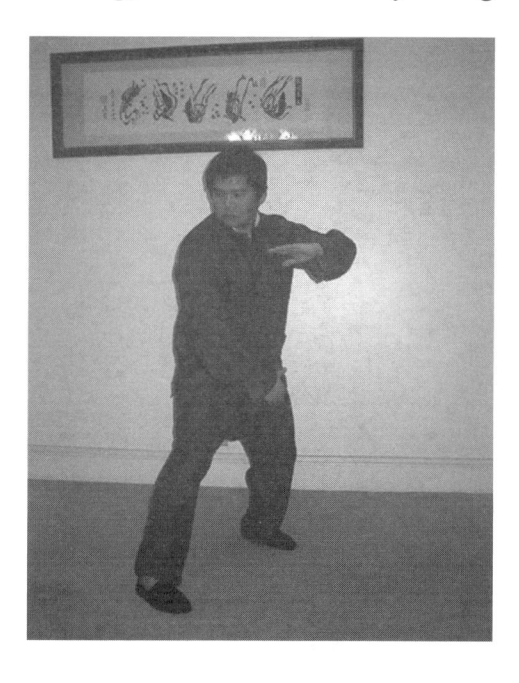

iii. Horse Stance:
Separate the feet as wide as the shoulders. Bend the legs, and line the knees up with the toes.

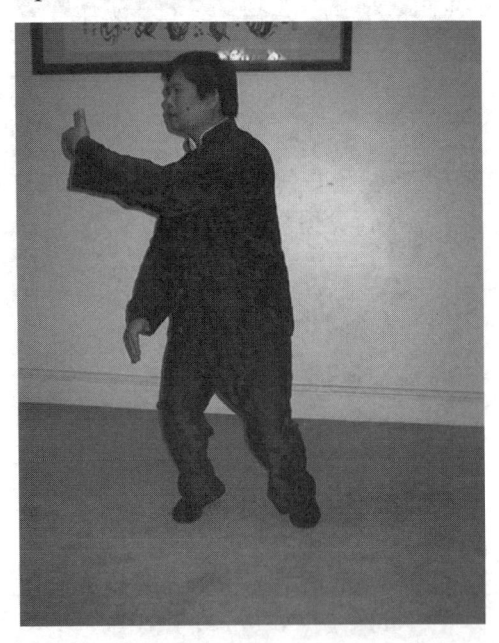

iv. Stand Up on One Leg:
As the name implies, the body weight is supported on one leg with the other leg suspended.

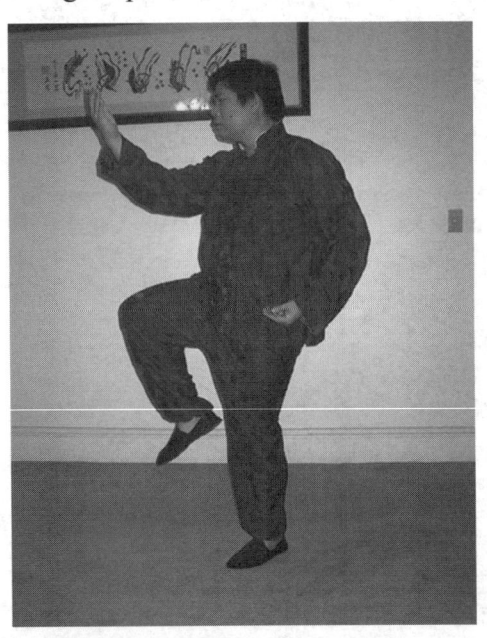

v. Low Stance:
   One leg supports the body weight lower to the ground, and the other leg is extended straight forward.

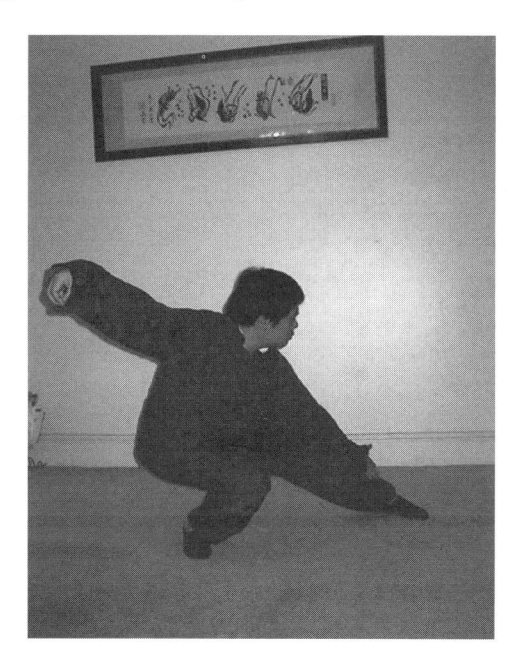

b. Step Techniques

Mobility is very important in all Chinese martial art systems. It is the ability for one to get close to or away from an opponent. It is often said that if one is launching a strike without moving the feet, one is looking for trouble. Therefore, moving the feet is very important. It is the soul of martial art.

i. Forward Step:
   The front leg steps forward.

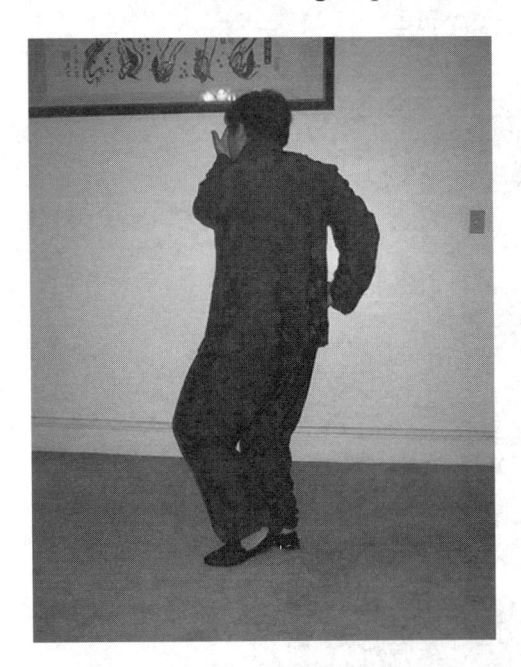

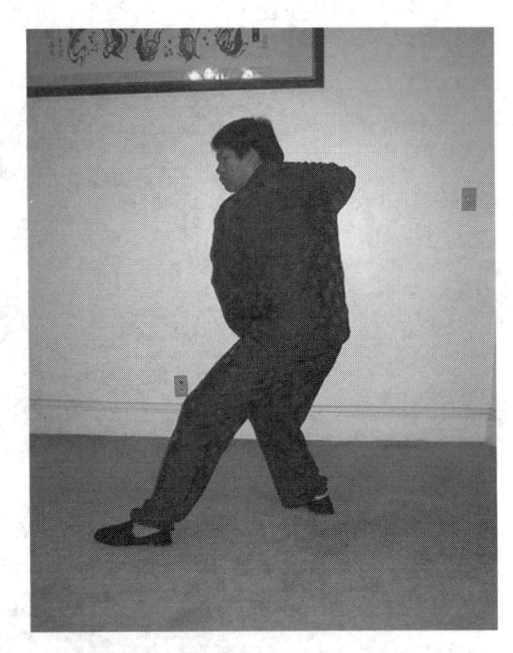

ii. Backward Step:
   The front leg steps backward.

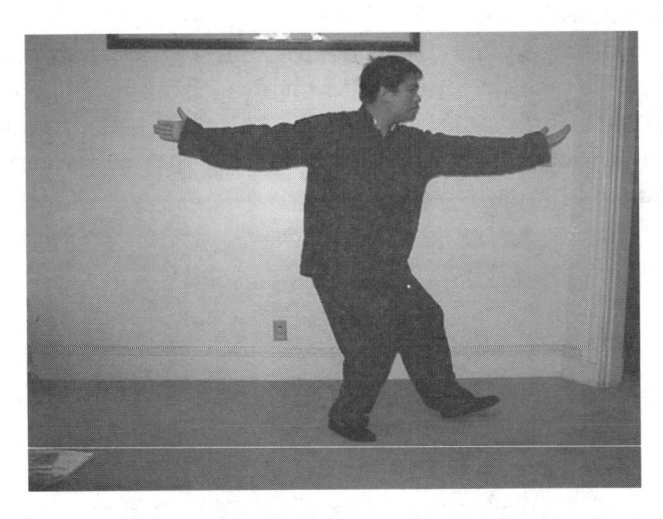

THE 43 MOVEMENT LARGE FRAME SOLO FORM

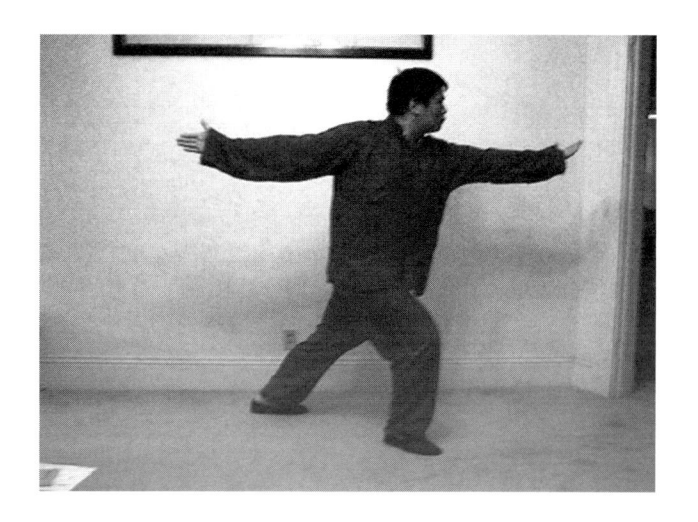

iii. Retreating Step:
   The front or back leg takes a half step back.

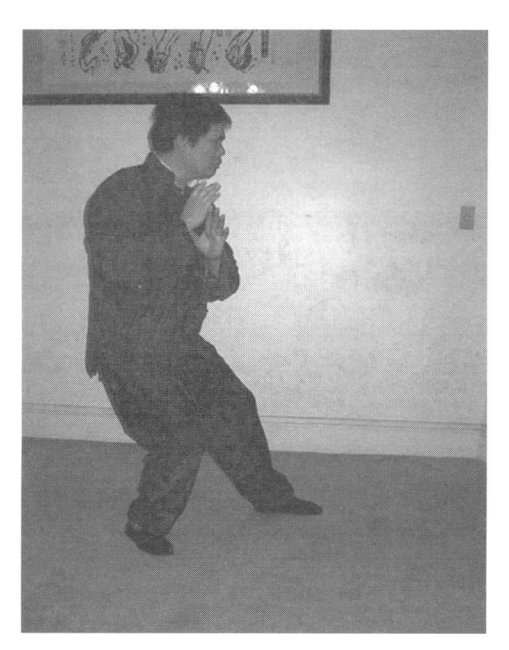

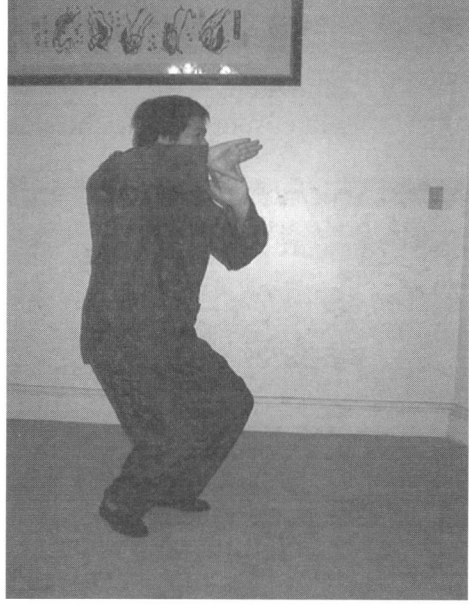

57

iv. Following Step:
   The back leg takes a half step forward.

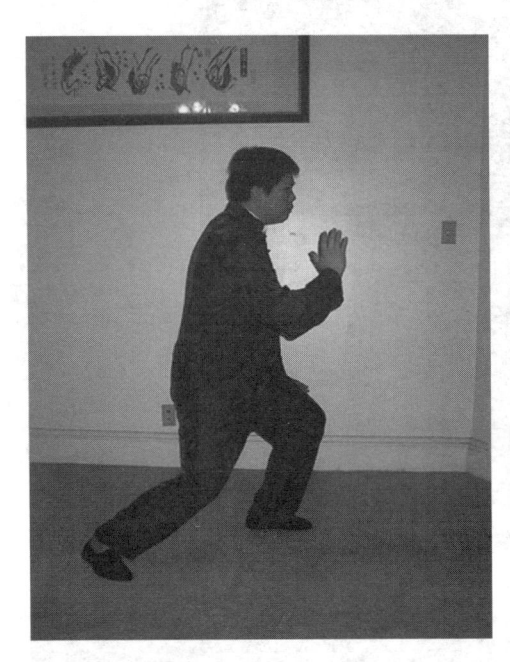

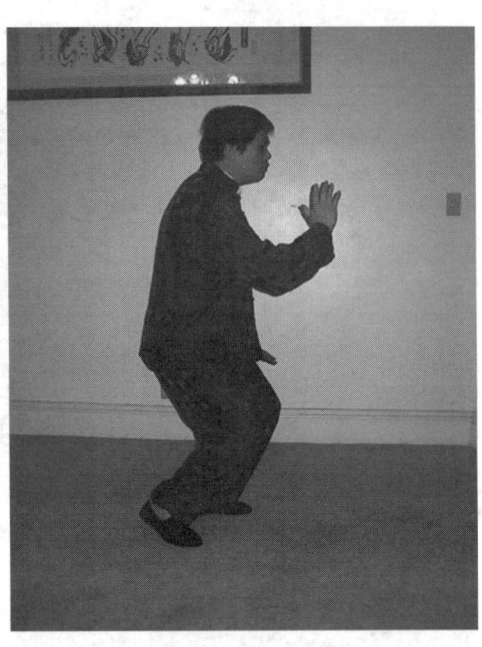

v. Side Step:
   Either foot steps to the side.

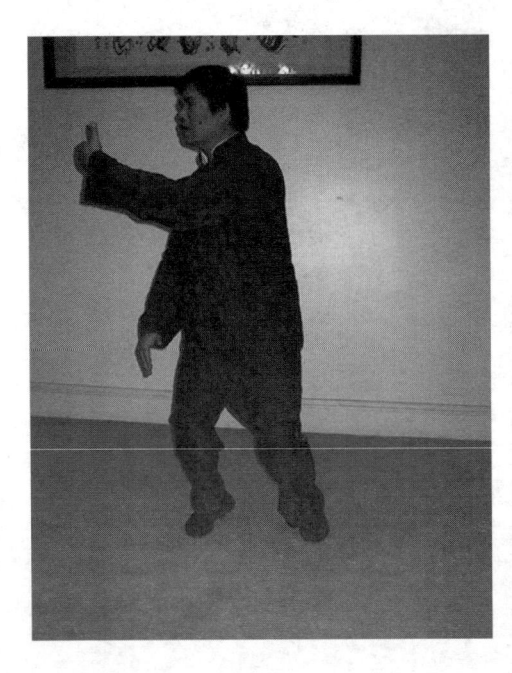

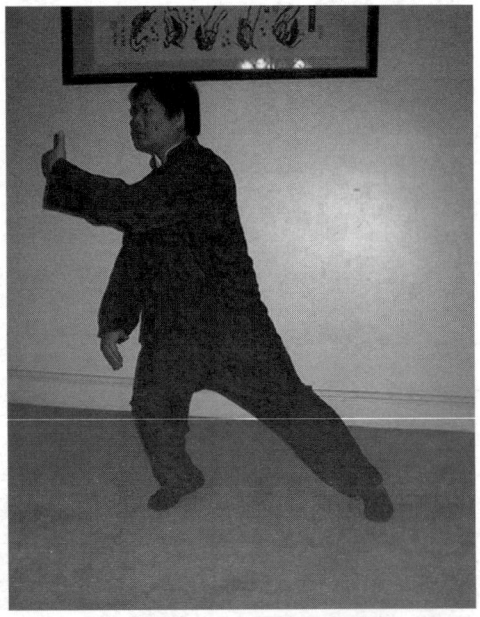

These are the common steps in Tai Chi Chuan. They must be executed slowly and evenly, distinguishing empty and full. When stepping forward, the front foot's heel touches the ground first. When stepping backward, the toes touch the ground first. When shifting the body weight from one foot to another, do it slowly and maintain balance. The distance between the two feet generally corresponds to the width of the shoulders. If the distance is too wide, it affects mobility. If it is too narrow, it will reduce skill and effectiveness. The rotations on the heels and the toes have to be done correctly.

c. Kicking

In Tai Chi Chuan practices, the body is often supported by one leg. Therefore, there are many hidden low kicks in the solo form. The common kicks that one can see in the solo form follow:

i. Separation Kick:
   Kick with the side of the foot. Target the foe's rib cage.

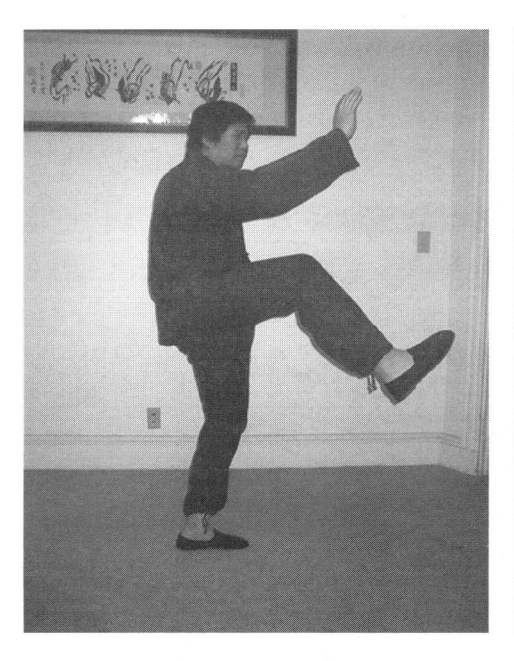

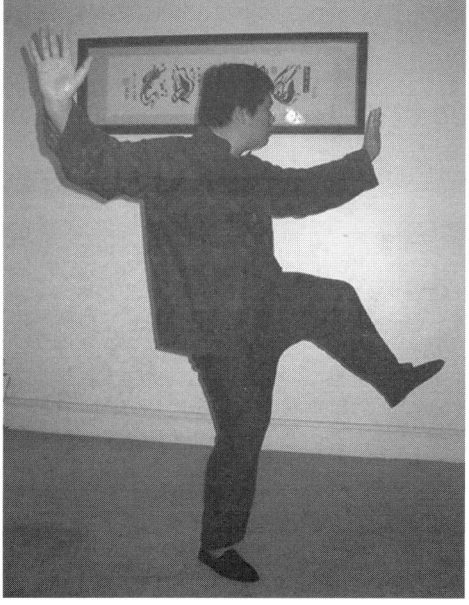

ii. Heel Kick:
   As its name indicates, kick with the heel. One should try to pull the toes inward to expose the heel for kicking.

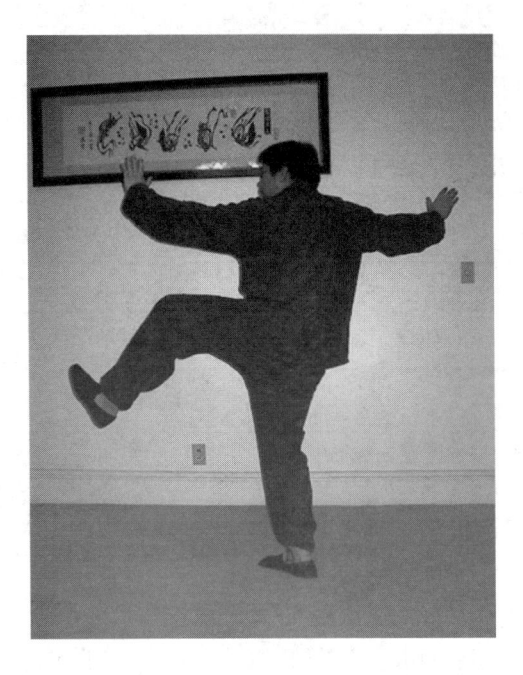

iii. Round Kick:
   This is a kick in a half circle motion by the right leg and foot. The leg and foot sweep upward and across from left to right at chest level or higher. The hands sweep across from right to left, striking the top of the right foot when they meet at the body's centerline.

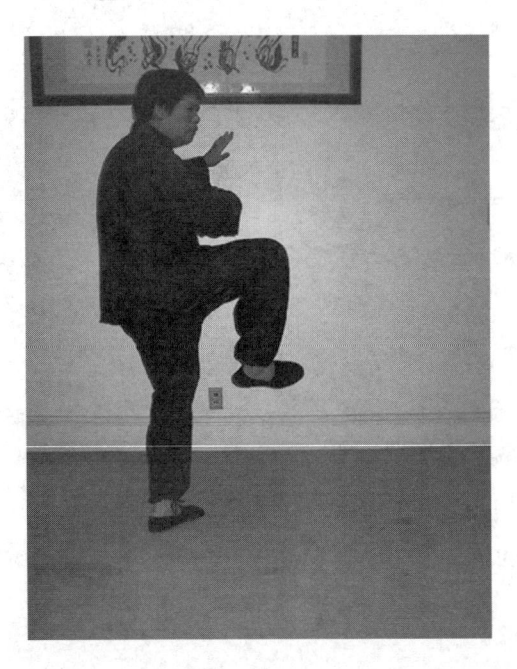

The 43 Movement Tai Chi Chuan Large Frame Solo Form

Initially, I choreographed this condensed Large Frame Solo Form to teach the students in England in 1998. The students there told me that they had practiced the Medium Frame Solo Form for some time and would like to learn something new and different. Since my teaching in England has a seminar format, it is difficult for the students to learn a complete form, yet I wanted to teach them the essence of the Large Frame Solo Form with less time invested on learning the movements. So I taught them the condensed version. The 43 Movement Large Frame Form was derived from the existing 42 Movement Medium Frame Form I developed some time ago. Its presentation follows:

1. Beginning Tai Chi Chuan
2. Grasp the Sparrow's Tail
3. Single Whip
4. Play Guitar
5. Step Forward, Parry, Intercept, and Punch
6. Seal Tightly
7. Cross Hands
8. Embrace Tiger, Return to the Mountain
9. Grasp Sparrow's Tail
10. Diagonal Single Whip
11. Fist under Elbow
12. Step Backward and Drive Away Monkey (three times)
13. Diagonal Flying
14. Lift Hands
15. White Crane Spreads Its Wings
16. Brush Knee, Twist Step, and Push Right Hand Forward
17. Pick up Needle in Sea Bottom
18. Fan Back
19. Turn Around and Chop
20. Right Part the Wild Horse's Mane
21. Left Warding Off
22. Waving Hands Like Clouds (7 times)
23. Single Whip
24. High Pat Horse
25. Side Kicks
26. Fair Lady Works on Shuttles (2 times)
27. Left Warding Off
28. Right Kick
29. Left Hitting Tiger

30. Hit the Ears with Two Fists
31. Left Kick
32. Brush Knee with Twist Step (2 times)
33. Step Forward and Punch Down
34. Step Forward, Grasp Sparrow's Tail
35. Single Whip
36. Lower the Snake Body
37. Step Forward to become Seven Stars
38. Retreat to Ride the Tiger
39. Turn Around with Lotus Kick
40. Shooting Tiger
41. Step Forward, Parry, Intercept, and Punch
42. Seal Tightly
43. Closing Tai Chi Chuan

1. Beginning Tai Chi Chuan

Begin with the feet parallel to the shoulders and the body facing forward *(fig 1)*. Slowly raise the hands up, coming in close to the chest *(figs 2 & 3)*; then turn the palms so that they face forward, and bend the knees *(figs 4 & 5, 5 is the same move from a different angle)*.

figure 1

figure 2

figure 3

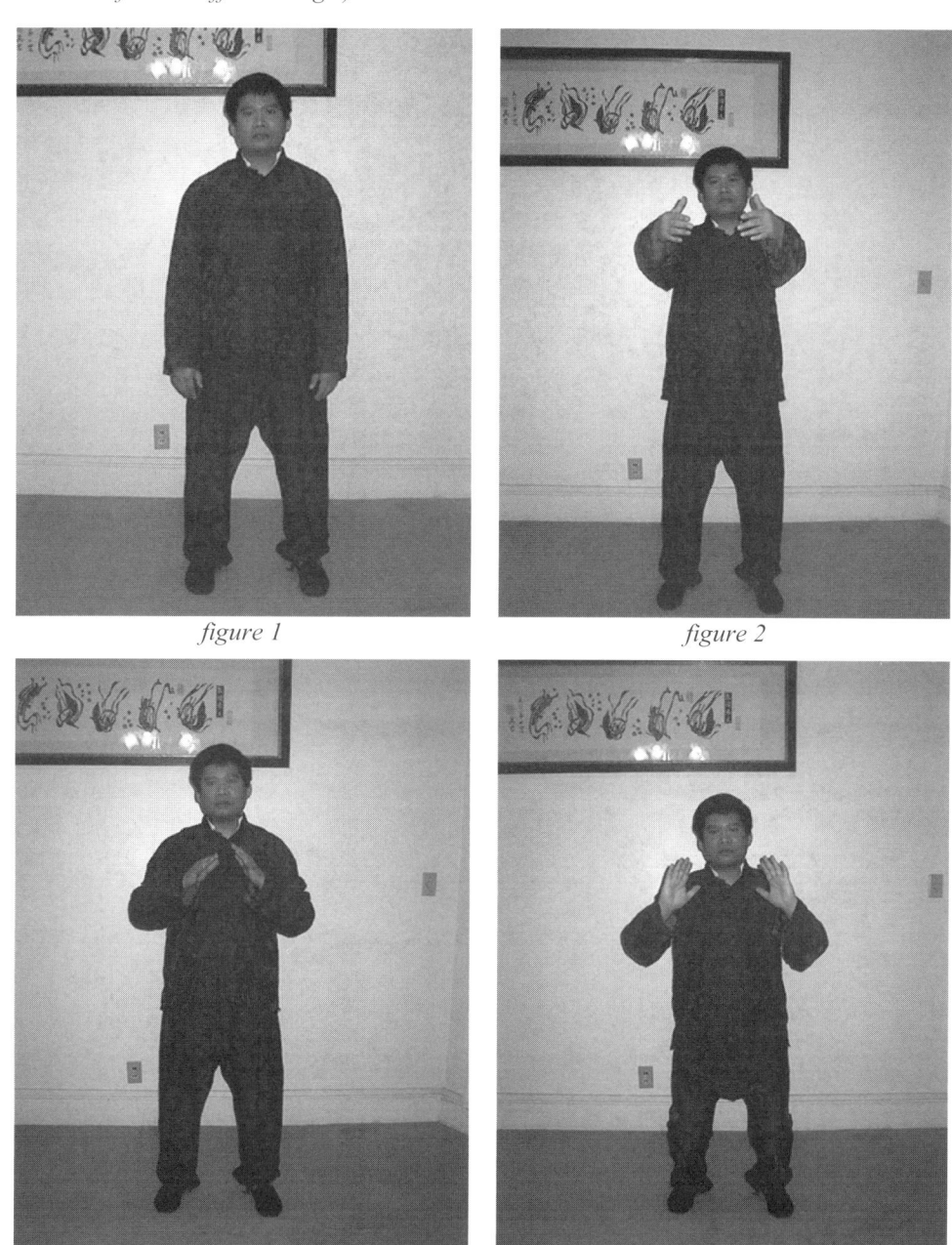

figure 4

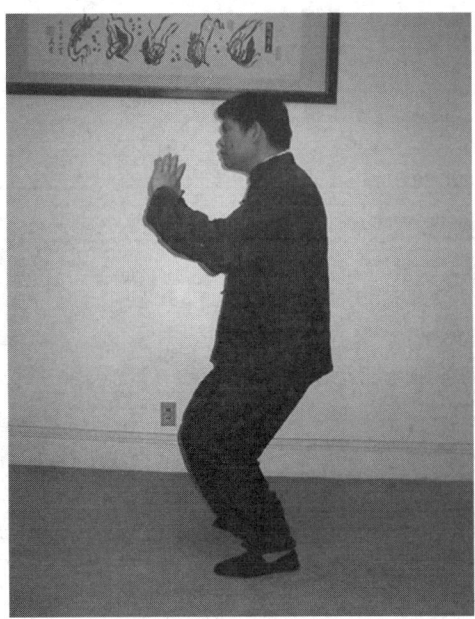

figure 5

Slowly turn the hands to the right side of the body with the left hand arriving below the right, palms facing each other. As the hands move to the right side, the body weight shifts onto the right foot *(fig 6)*. The left hand comes up, and the right hand goes down with the palms facing each other. The movement finishes with the palms facing in *(fig 7)*.

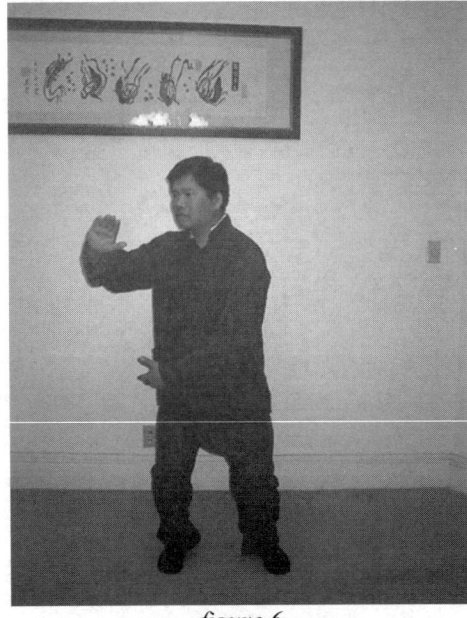

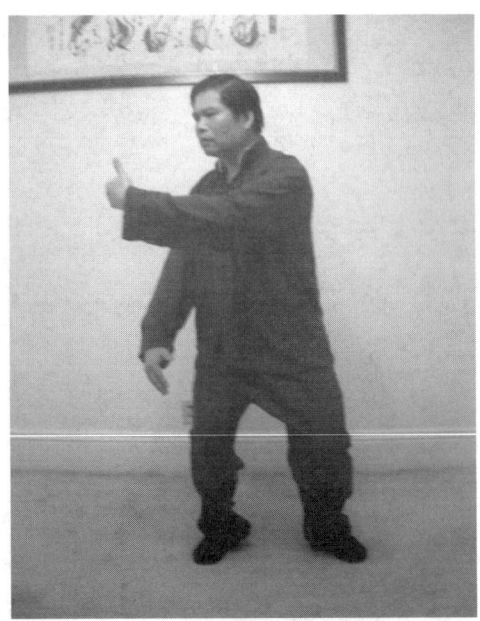

figure 6   *figure 7*

Rotate the hands to the left side of the body with the body's weight shifting onto the left foot *(fig 8)*. Bring the right hand up, and move the left hand down *(fig 9)*. Rotate the hands to the right side of the body again with the hands remaining the same and the weight shifting right. Turn the right foot out 45 degrees. The knees remain bent *(fig 10)*.

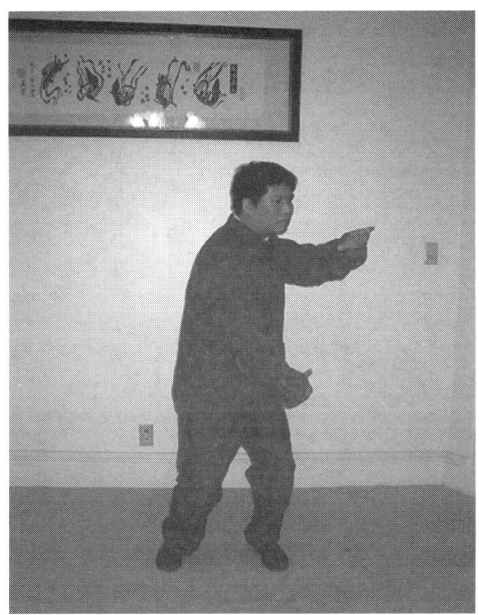

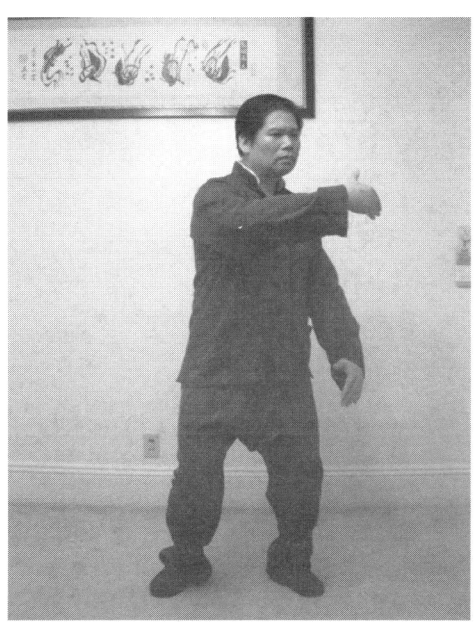

figure 8

figure 9

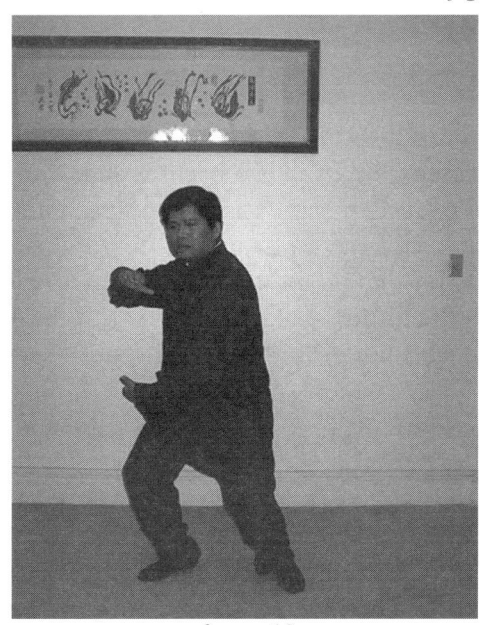

figure 10

2. Grasp the Sparrow's Tail
Part 1: Left Hand Warding Off
From the preceding movement with the body weight on the right foot, pick up the left foot, and step forward *(fig 11)*. As the body's weight shifts forward onto the left foot, separate the hands; the left hand comes up while the right hand goes down to the right side of the hip *(fig 12)*.

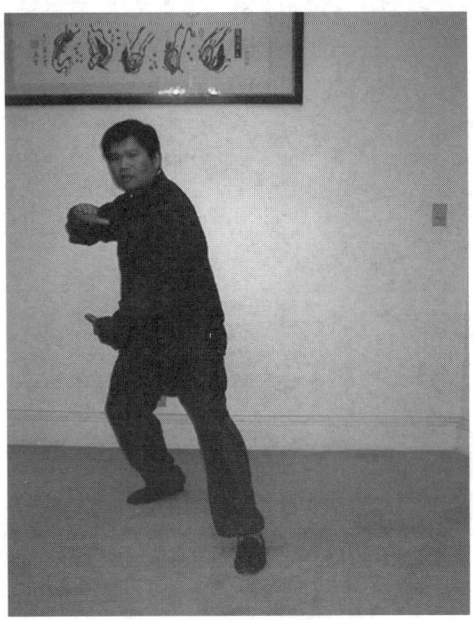

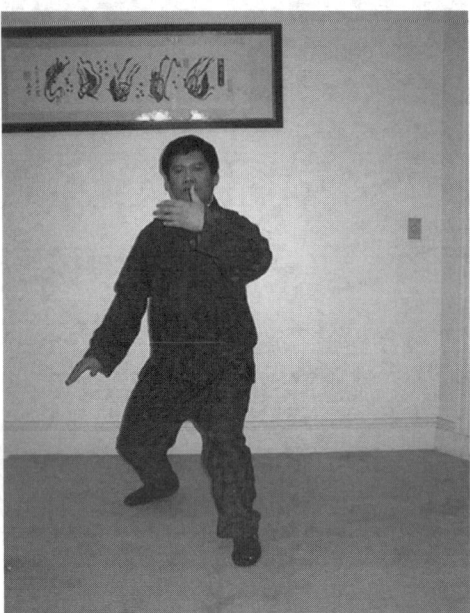

figure 11   *figure 12*

Part 2: Right Hand Warding Off
From the preceding movement with the body weight on the left foot, turn the left foot inward while at the same time the left hand makes a complete clockwise circle to end with the palm facing down at the chest *(fig 13)*. Bring the right hand over the left hand, and make a complete clockwise circle to end just above the left knee with the palm face up. Turn the head to the right, and look out from the right shoulder *(figs 14 - 16)*.

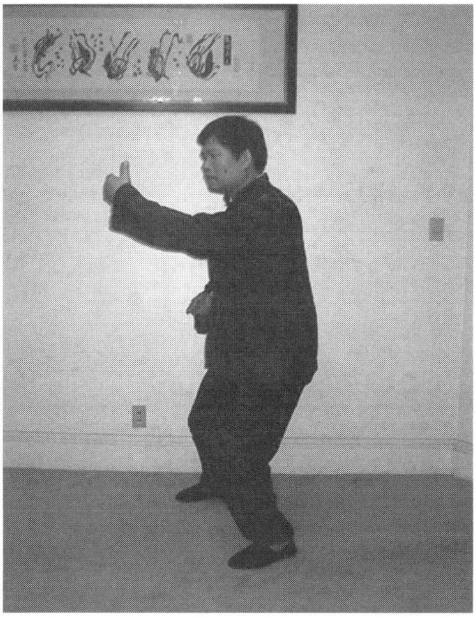

figure 13

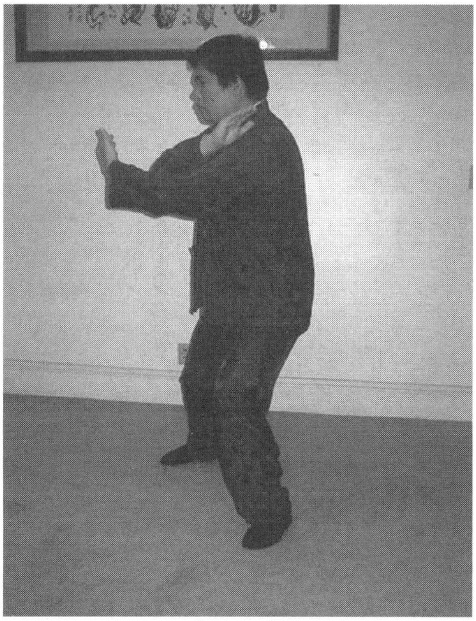

figure 14

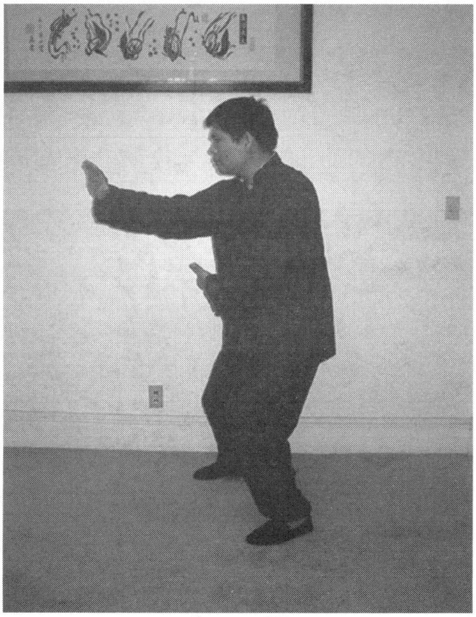

figure 15

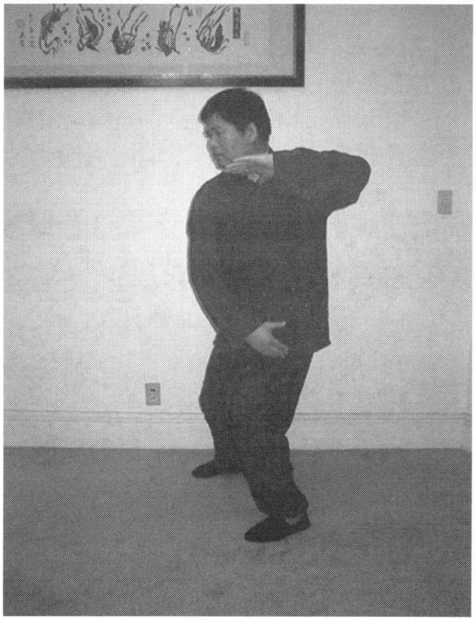

figure 16

Pick up the right foot, and step forward *(fig 17)*. While the body weight is shifting onto the right foot, bring both hands up level with the face *(fig 18)*. The right palm is facing in, and the left palm is facing out.

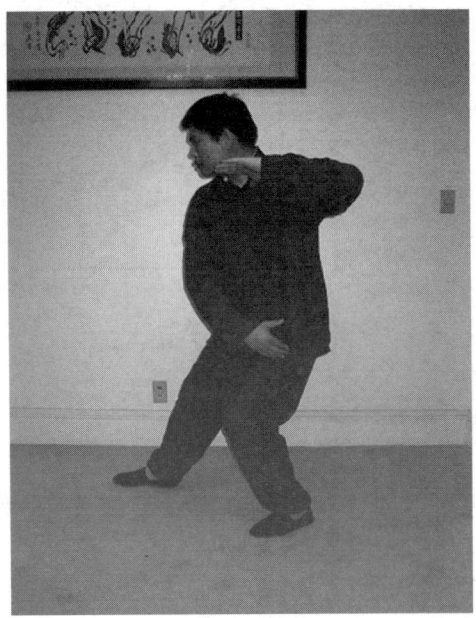

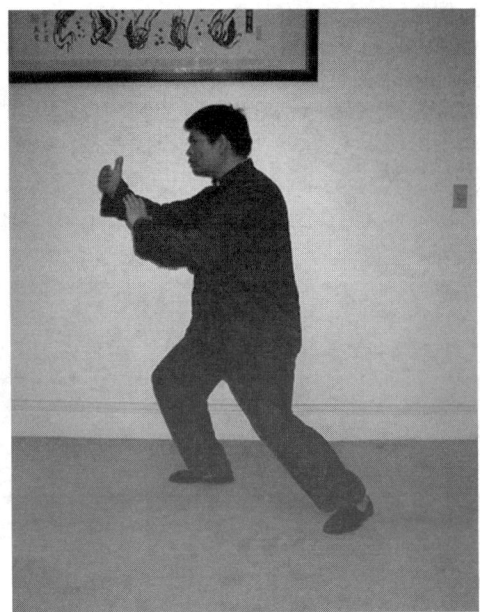

figure 17

figure 18

Part 3: Roll Back
From the preceding movement, turn both palms so the left palm faces up and the right palm faces down *(fig 19)*. Bring the hands back to the left side of the hip, and at the same time, shift the body weight back onto the left foot *(fig 20)*.

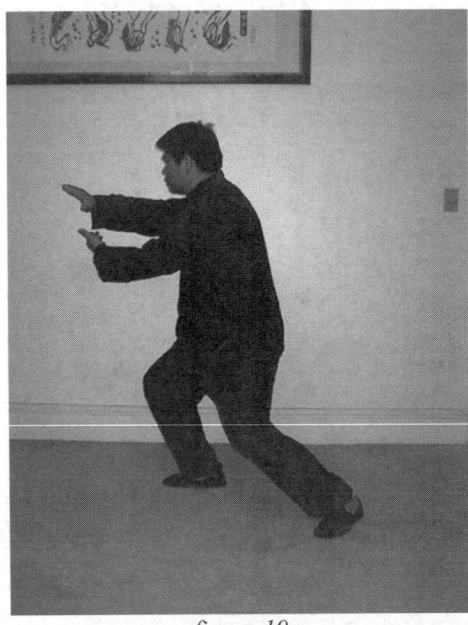

figure 19

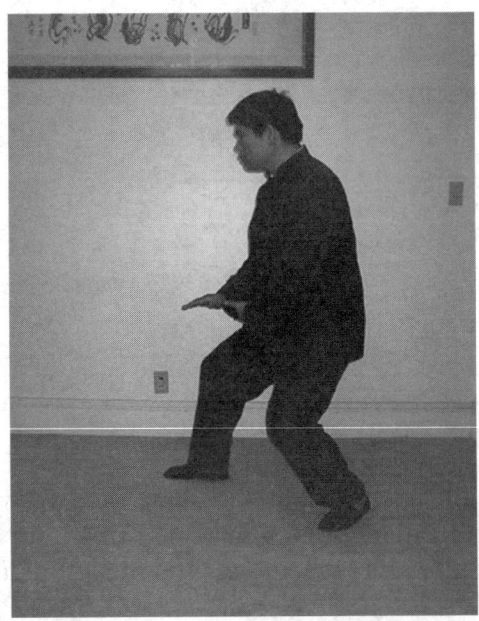

figure 20

THE 43 MOVEMENT LARGE FRAME SOLO FORM

Part 4: Press

From the preceding movement, turn the left palm face down and the right palm face up. The left palm is now above the right. Then adhere the left palm to the right palm/wrist *(fig 21)*. Press the hands forward with the body weight shifting onto the right foot *(fig 22)*.

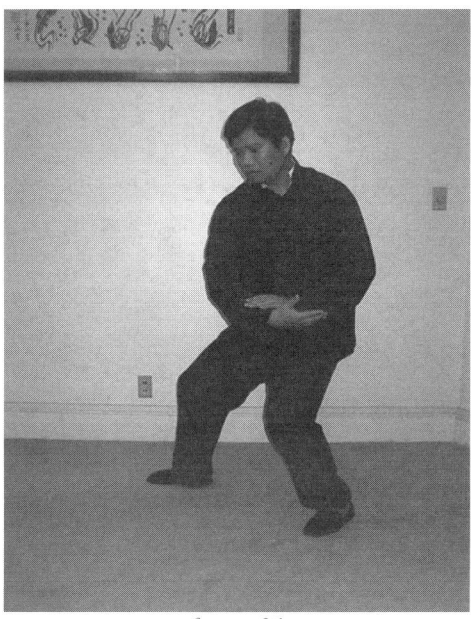

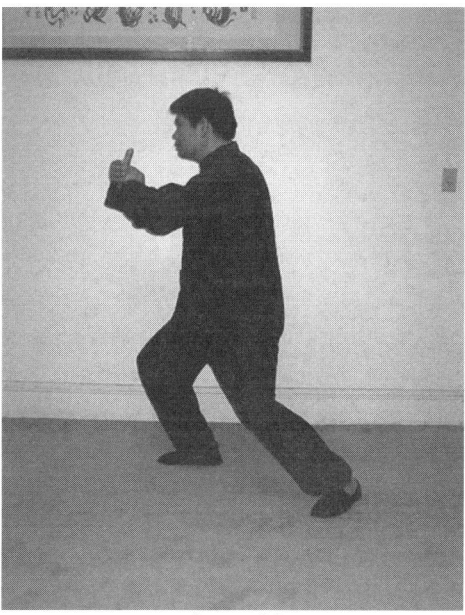

figure 21   *figure 22*

Part 5: Push

From the preceding movement, turn the palms face down, the left palm on top of the right palm *(fig 23)*, and bring the two hands directly back to the chest with the palms still facing down while shifting the weight onto the left foot *(fig 24)*. Separate the hands at the chest with the wrists bent and the palms facing forward *(fig 25)*. Push the hands forward while shifting the body weight onto the right foot *(fig 26)*.

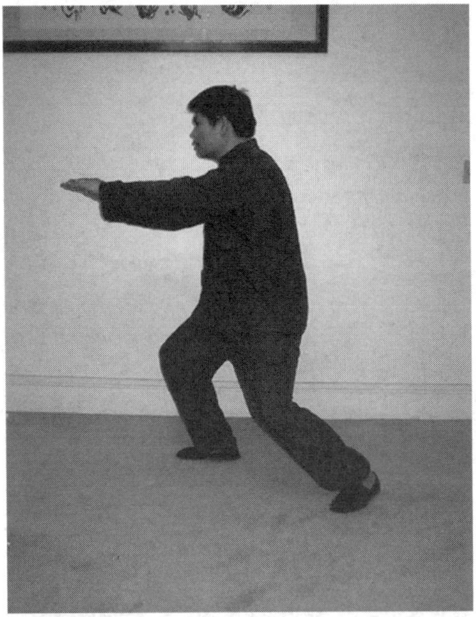

TAI CHI CHUAN – A COMPARATIVE STUDY

figure 23

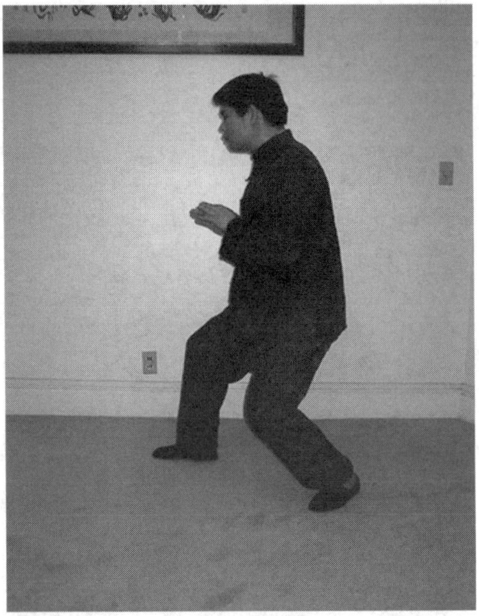

figure 24

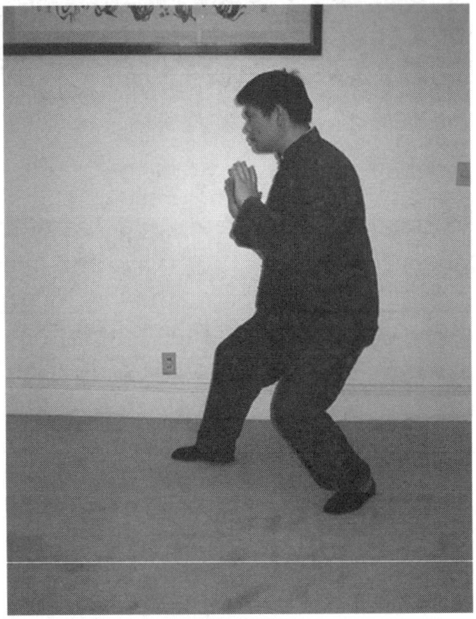

figure 25

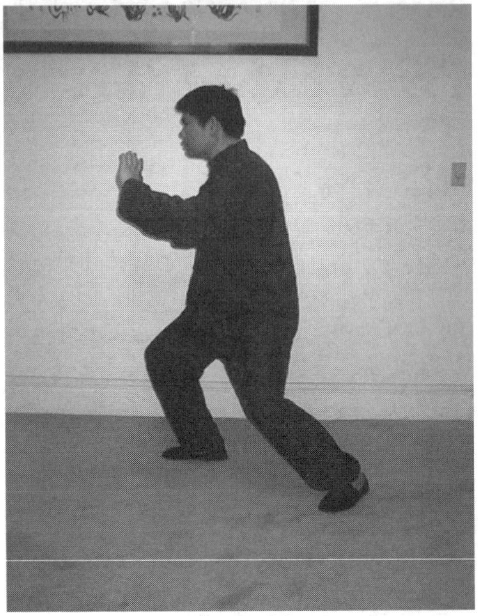

figure 26

3. Single Whip

From the preceding movement, rotate the waist with the hands moving in a complete counter clockwise circle over the head with the body's weight first on the left foot then shifting onto the right foot *(figs 27 - 29)*. Bring the right fingers together to form a beak, and bend the wrist to form the hook; extend the right arm, and set the left hand at the right hip with the palm facing in *(fig 30)*. Turn the head to the left, pick up the left foot, and step to the left *(fig 31)*. With the body weight on the left foot, move the left arm up and out to the left. *(fig 32)*. Turn the left palm forward while the right hook remains the same *(fig 33)*.

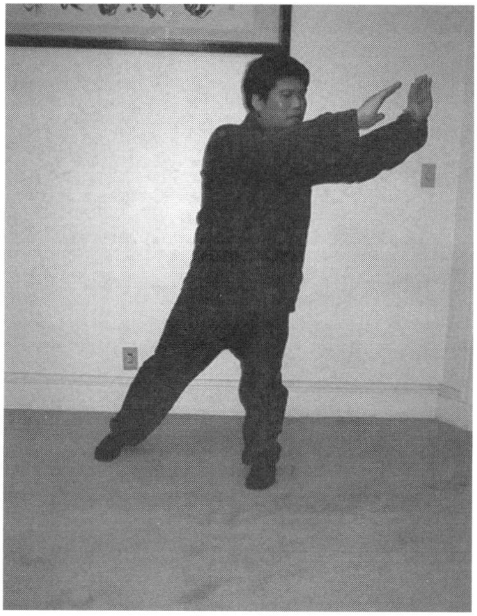

figure 27

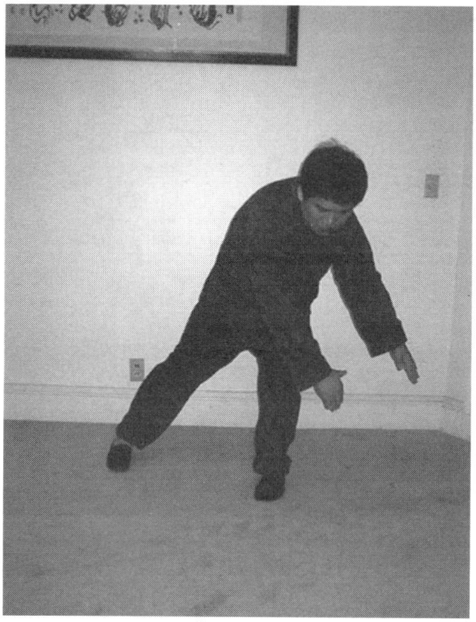

figure 28

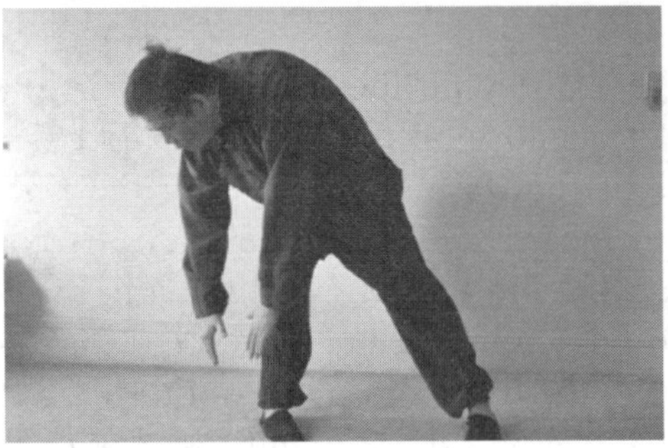

figure 29

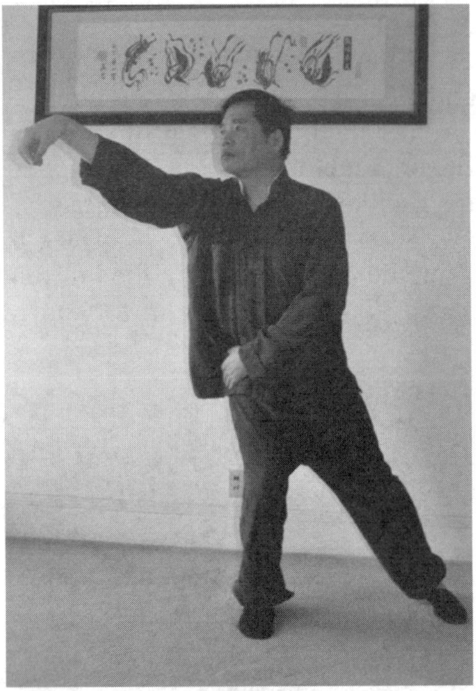

figure 30

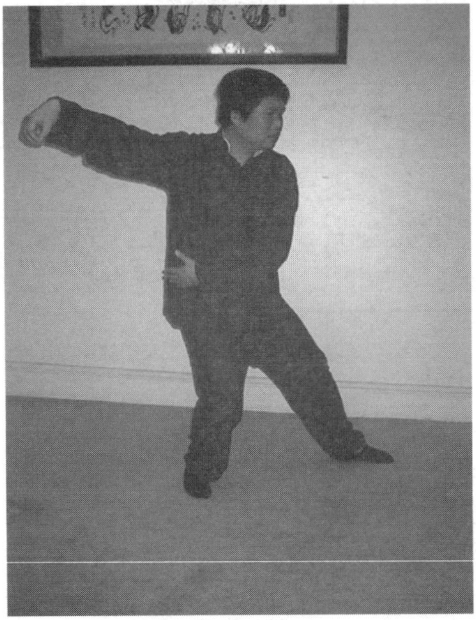

figure 31

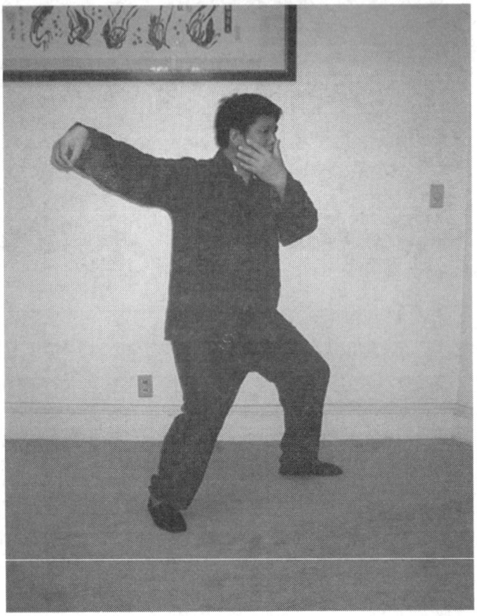

figure 32

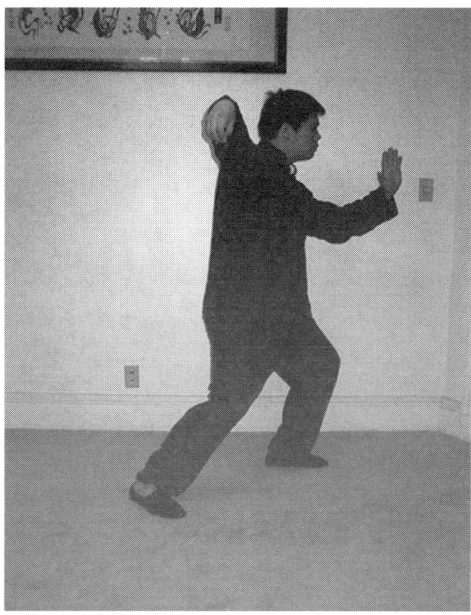

figure 33

4. Play Guitar

From the preceding movement, with the body weight on the left foot, open the right hand's hook, swing the right arm forward; the left hand comes down to the left hip *(fig 34)*. Pick up the right foot, and step nearer to the left foot *(fig 35)*. The right hand comes back in front of the chest, and the left hand goes up and forward to face level so the right palm is next to the left elbow *(figs 36 & 37)*. Pick up the left foot, and land it on the heel *(fig 38)*.

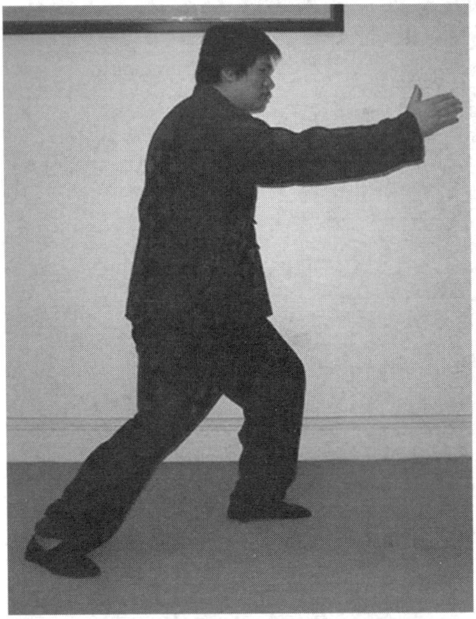

figure 34

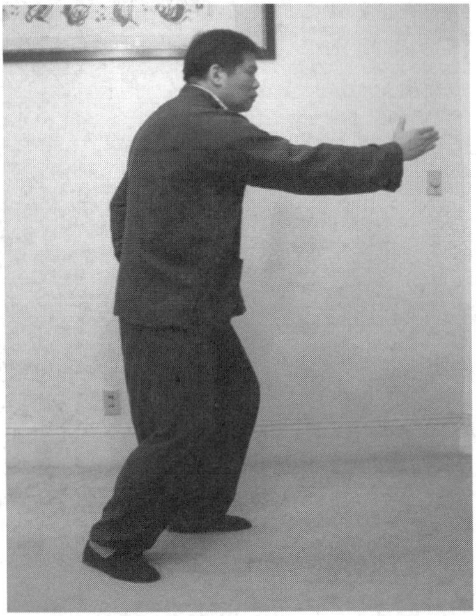

figure 35

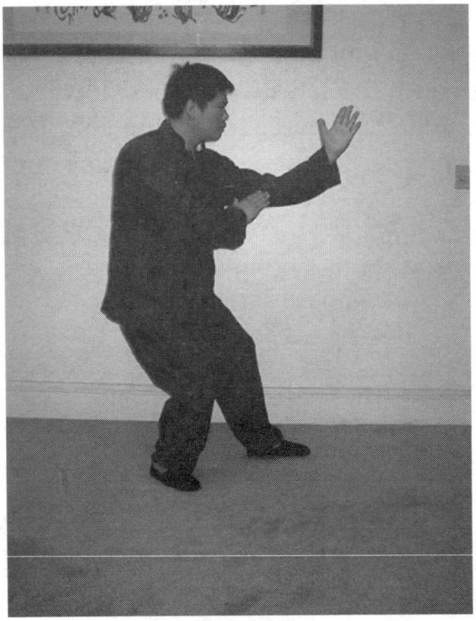

figure 36

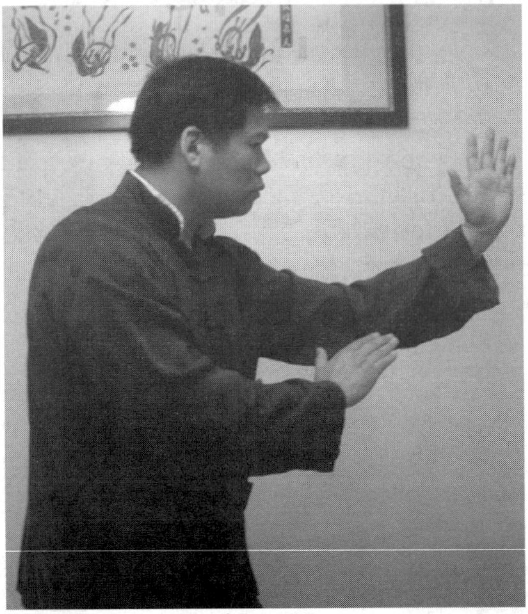

figure 37

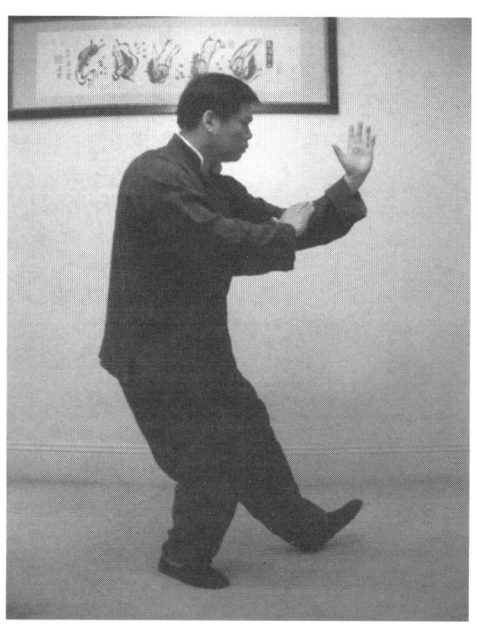

figure 38

5. Step Forward, Parry, Intercept and Punch

From the preceding movement, rotate the left arm until the left palm faces up and the right hand comes up on top of the left arm. The right hand goes forward and closes into a fist; pull the left hand back next to the right elbow and shift the body weight onto the left foot *(figs 39 - 42)*.

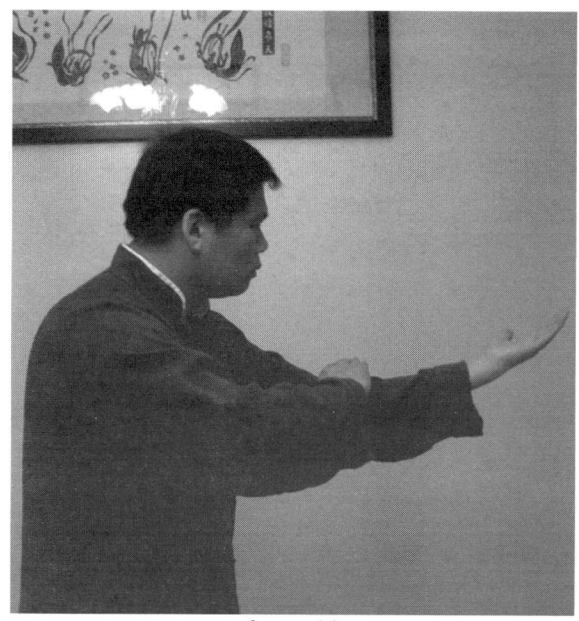

figure 39

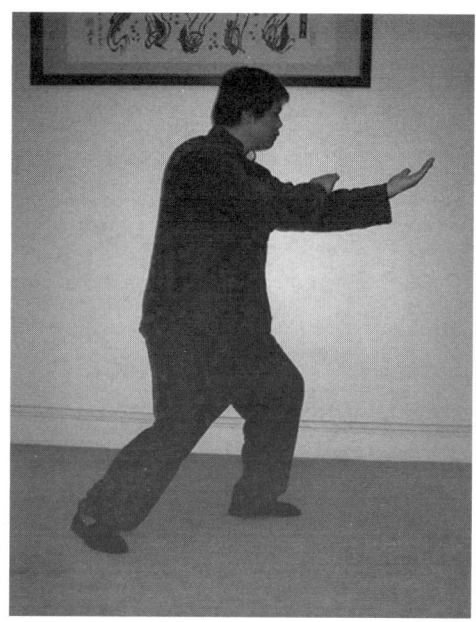

figure 40

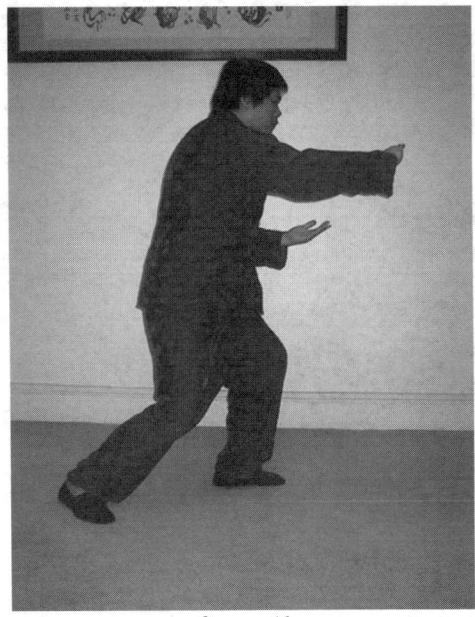

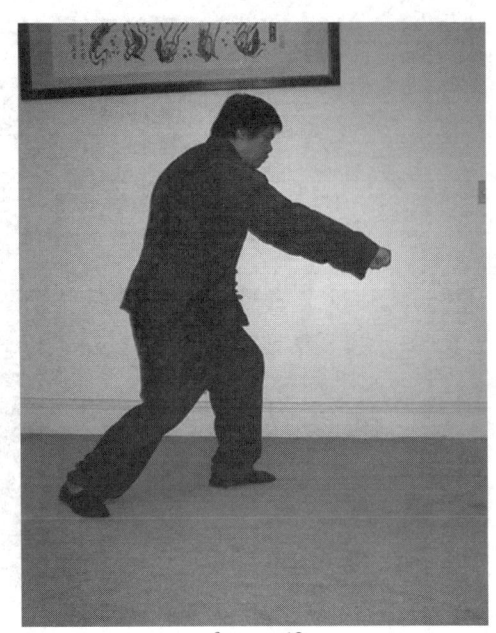

figure 41 *figure 42*

Bring the right fist to the left side of the hip *(fig 43)*. The right foot steps forward with the toes pointing forward *(fig 44)*. The left palm pushes on the right hand's forearm. Push the hands forward with the body weight shifting onto the right foot *(fig 45)*.

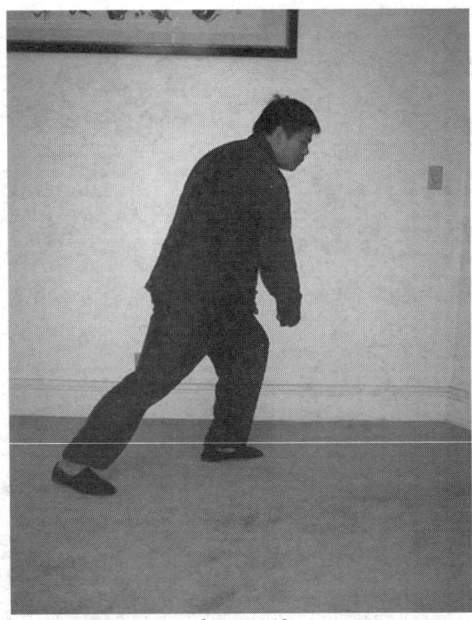

figure 43 *figure 44*

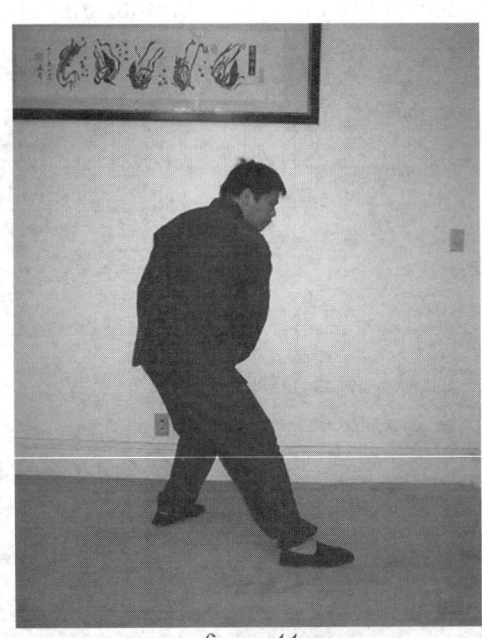

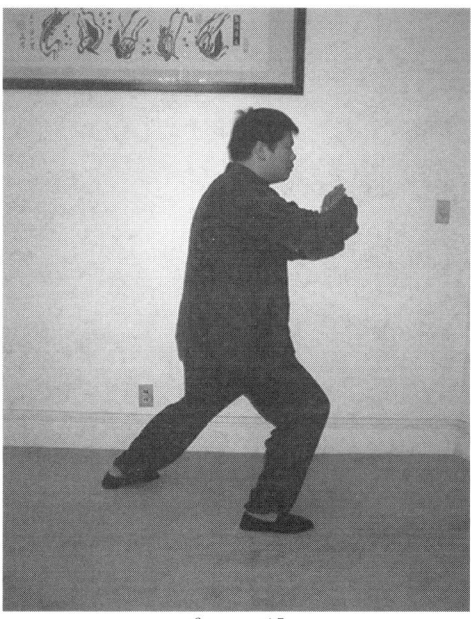

figure 45

Turn the right toes out, and separate the hands with the right fist pulling back to the right hip and the left palm pushing forward *(fig 46)*. With the body weight on the right foot, pick up the left foot, and make a clockwise circle-sweep-and-step forward. At the same time, the left hand makes a horizontal clockwise circle in front of the chest (this should be done in sync with the left foot's circle sweep) *(fig 47)*. While the body weight is shifting onto the left foot, the right fist punches forward, and the left palm comes back next to the right elbow *(fig 48)*.

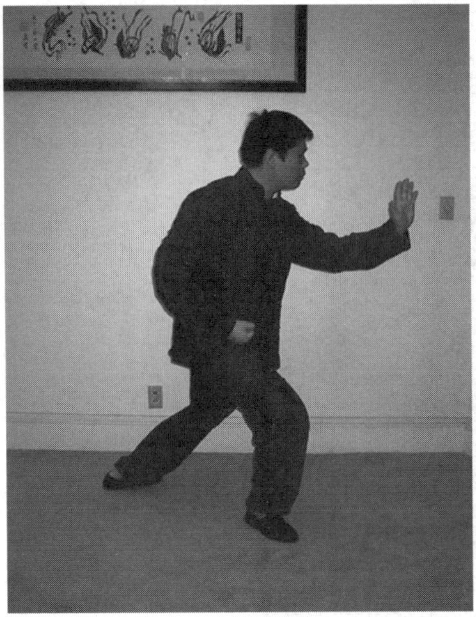

TAI CHI CHUAN – A COMPARATIVE STUDY

figure 46

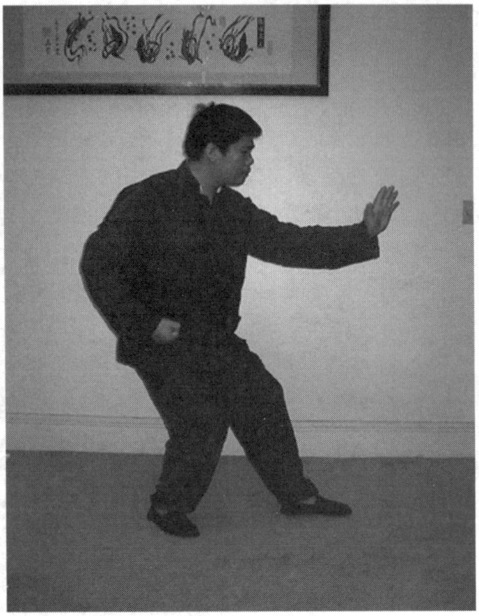

figure 47

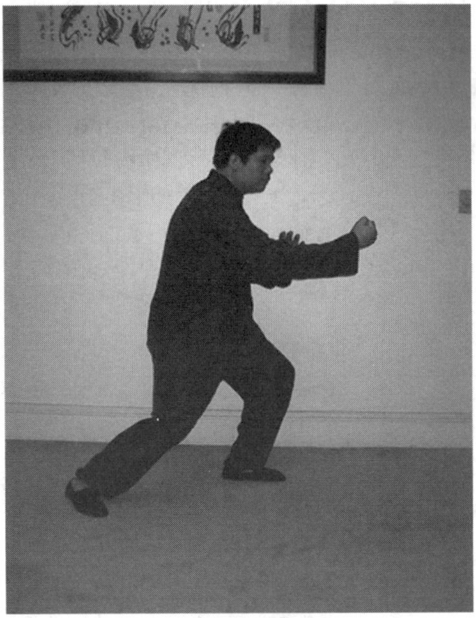

figure 48

6. Seal Tightly
From the preceding movement, put the left hand under the right elbow with the palm facing up *(fig 49)*. Open the right fist, and bring it back to the right side of the hip with the body weight shifting onto the right foot and the left

THE 43 MOVEMENT LARGE FRAME SOLO FORM

arm pushing forward with the palm face up *(figs 50 & 51)*. Circle the hands in front of the chest with the palms facing forward *(fig 52)*. Push the hands forward while shifting the body weight onto the left foot *(fig 53)*.

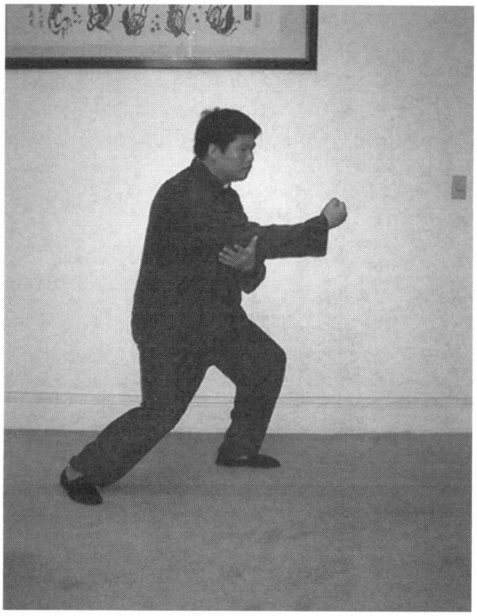

figure 49

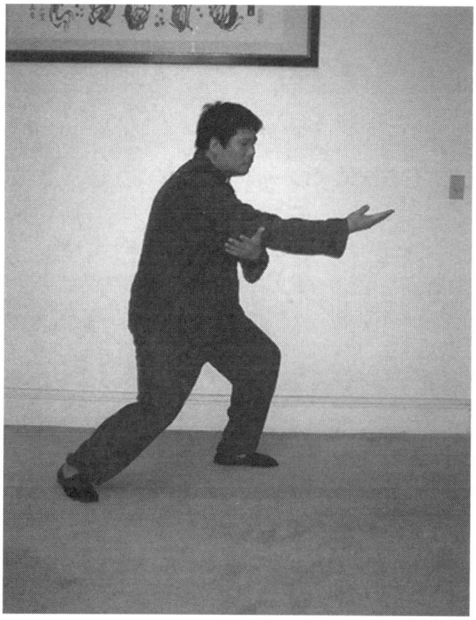

figure 50

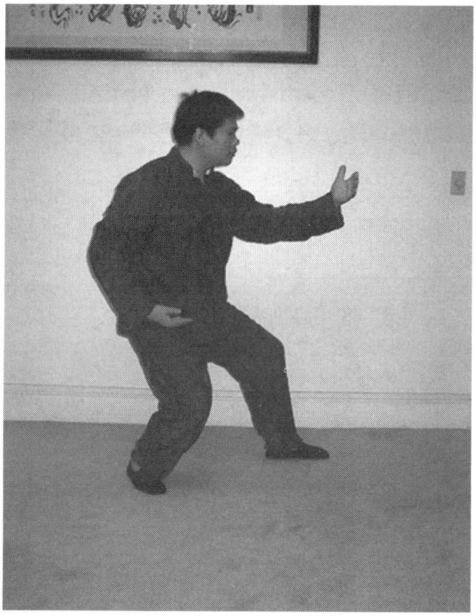

figure 51

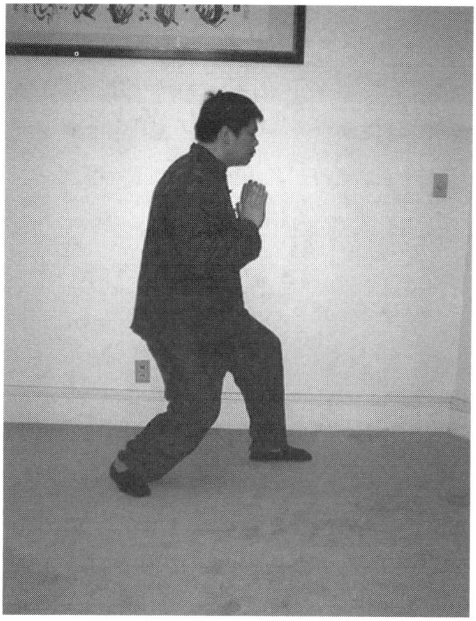

figure 52

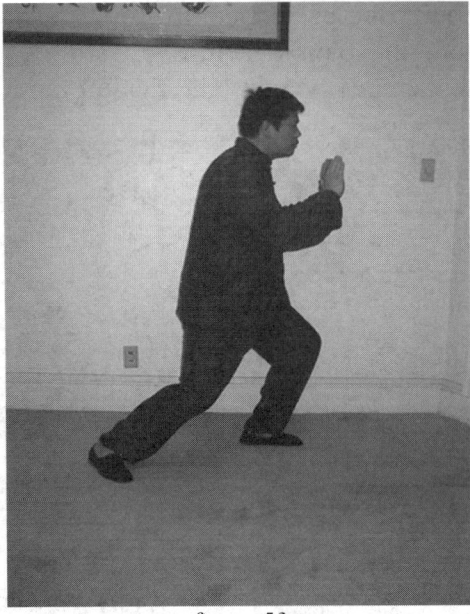

figure 53

7. Cross Hands

From the preceding movement, the left hand does not move while the right hand makes a clockwise circle to the right, and at the same time, the right toes turn out with the body weight shifting onto the right foot *(figs 54 & 55)*. Shift the body's weight onto the left foot, and bring the right hand back, crossing it on the left wrist with the left hand on top and the right hand on bottom *(fig 56)*.

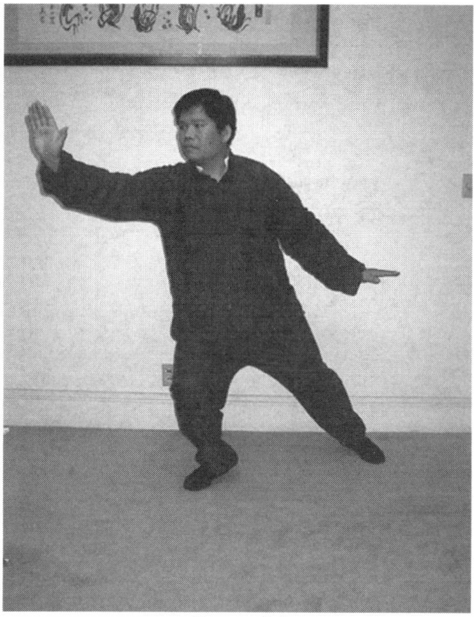

THE 43 MOVEMENT LARGE FRAME SOLO FORM

figure 54

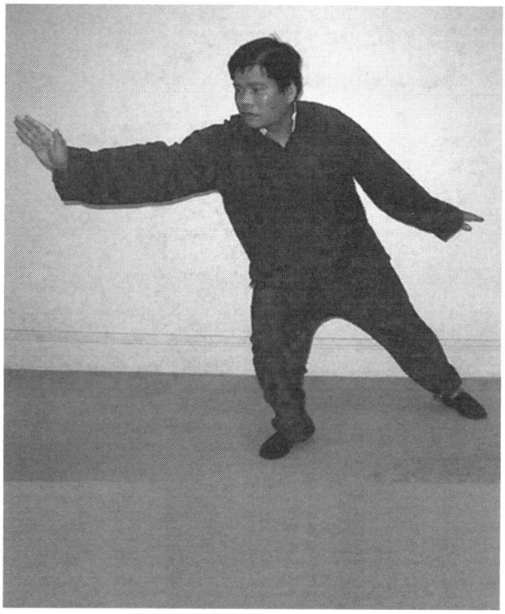

figure 55

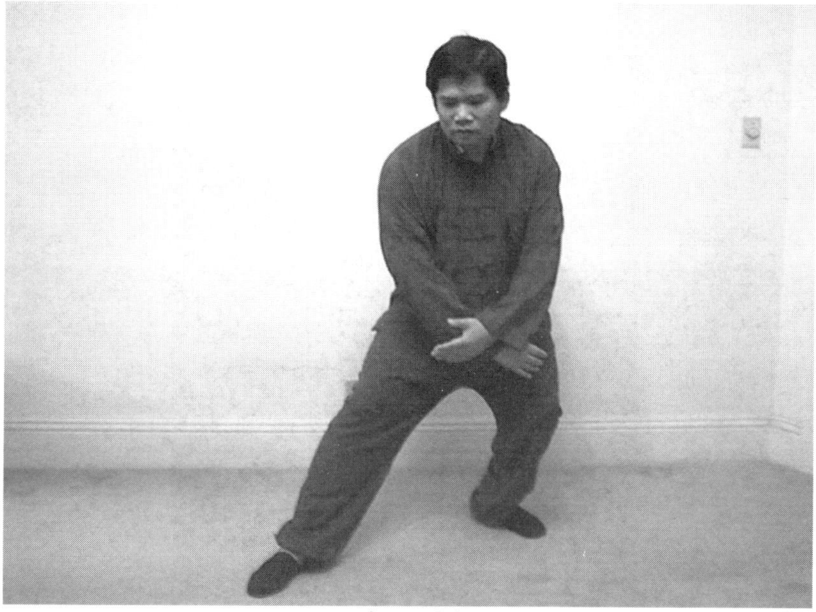

figure 56

Pick up the right foot, and step forward; shift the weight forward and push the hands forward to face level with the left hand inside and right hand outside *(figs 57 & 58)*. Pick up the left foot, and step up next to the right foot with the knees bent. The wrists are crossed and the elbows point down *(fig 59)*.

TAI CHI CHUAN – A COMPARATIVE STUDY

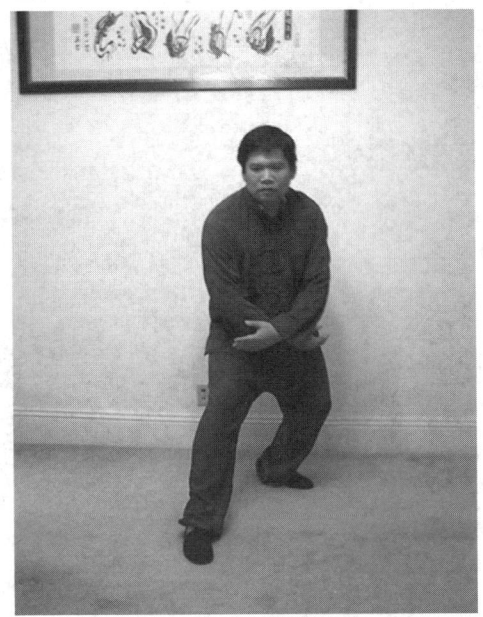

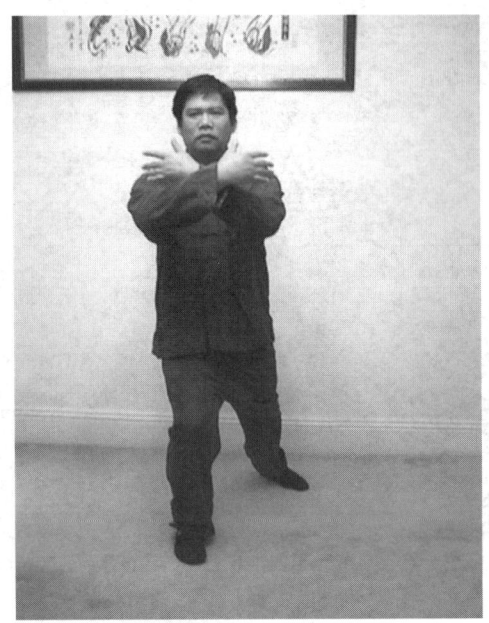

figure 57

figure 58

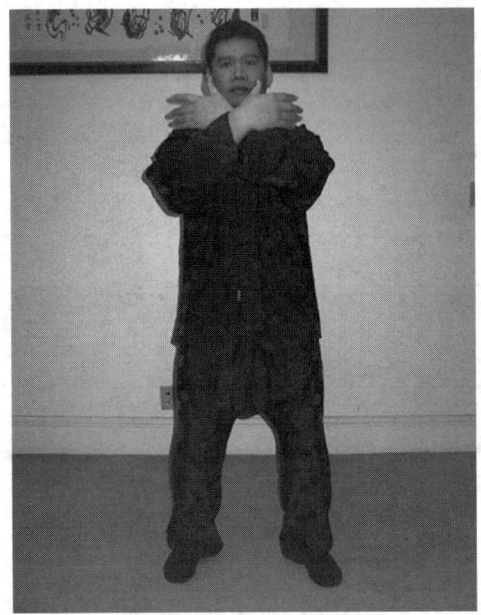

figure 59

8. Embrace Tiger Return to the Mountain
From the preceding movement, turn the palms so that they face out *(fig 60)*. Turn the head to the right corner. With the body weight on the left foot, pick up the right foot, and step forward *(figs 61 & 62 show the same move from different angles)*. While shifting the body weight onto the right foot, the right hand goes

down to the right side of the right knee, and left hand pushes forward from the left shoulder *(figs 63 & 64 show the same move from different angles)*.

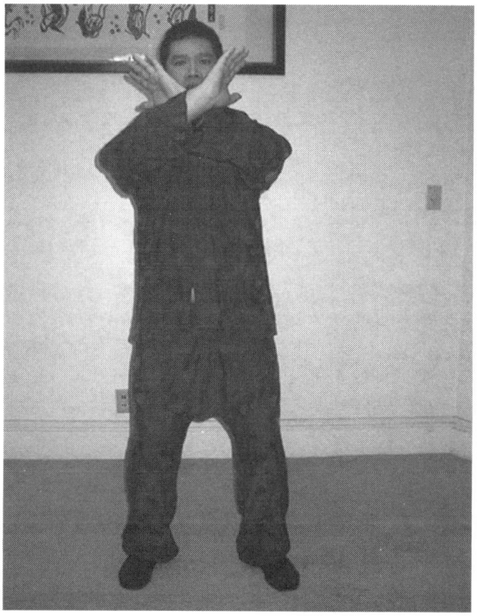

figure 60

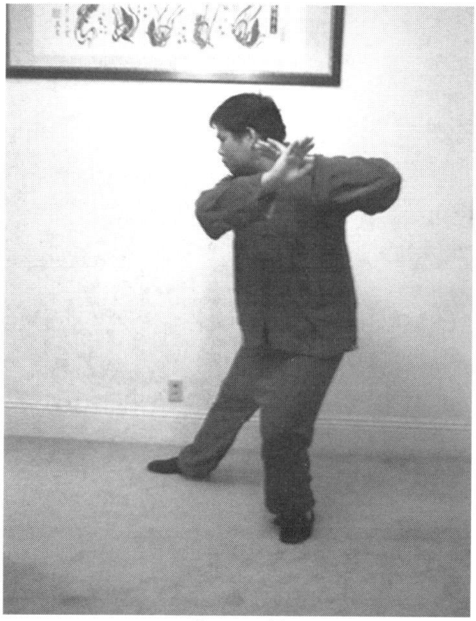

figure 61

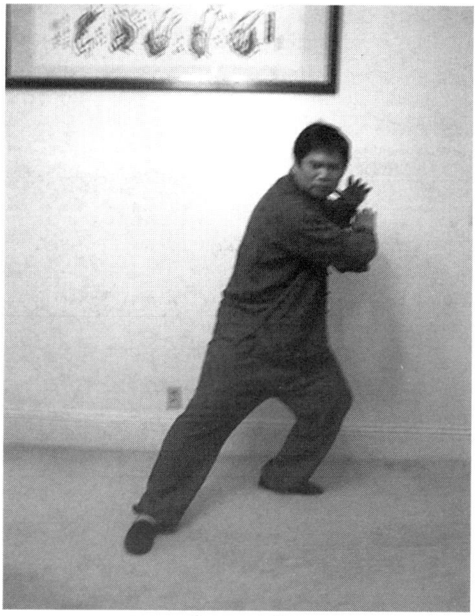

figure 62

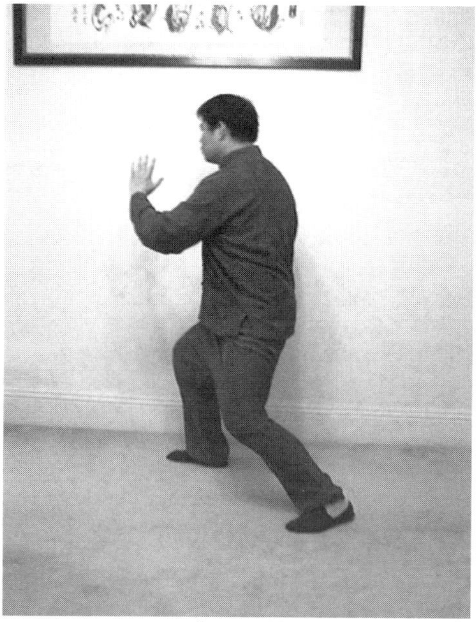

figure 63

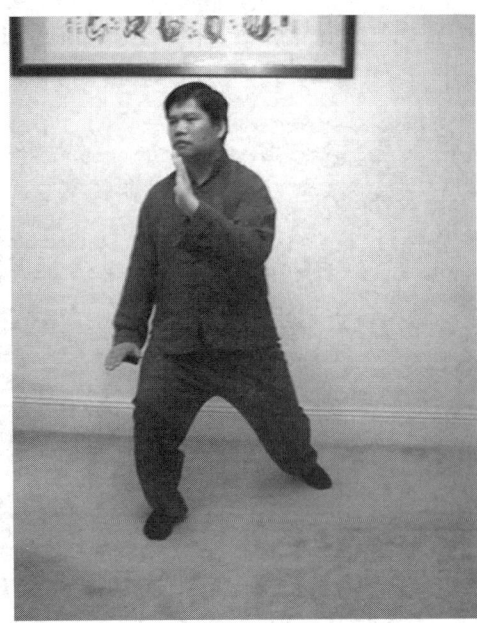

figure 64

9. Grasp Sparrow's Tail
Part 1: Roll Back
From the preceding movement, the right hand moves backward making a counter clockwise circle and ending with the palm next to the right ear *(figs 65 & 66 show the same move from different angles; figs 67 & 68 same move, different angles).*

figure 65

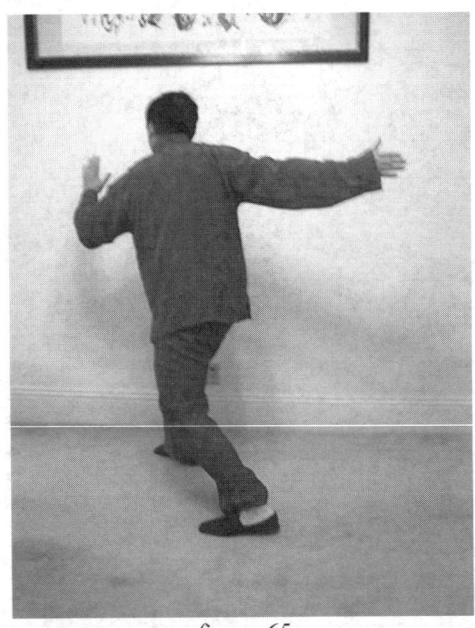

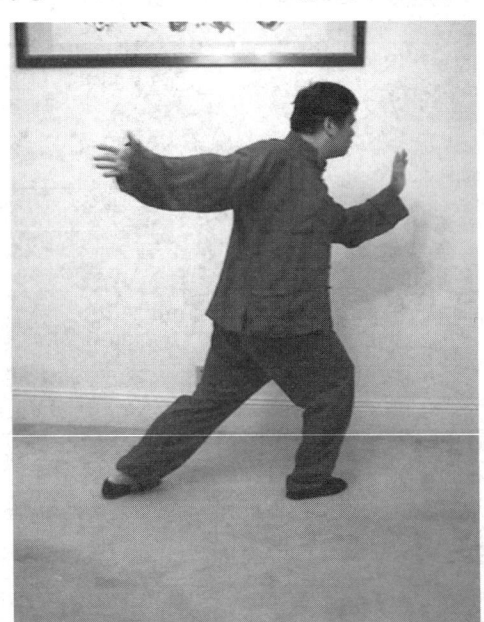

figure 66

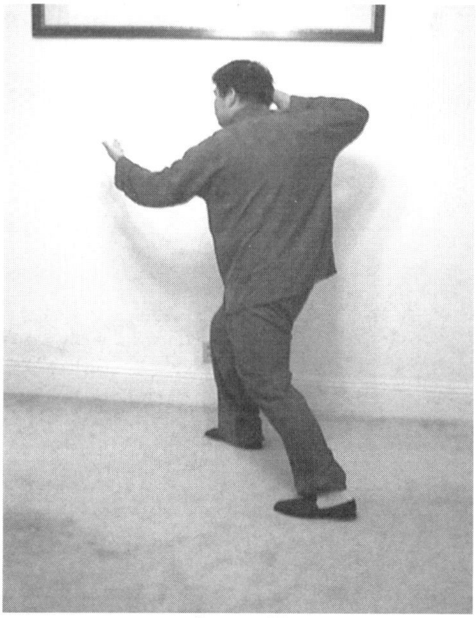

THE 43 MOVEMENT LARGE FRAME SOLO FORM

figure 67

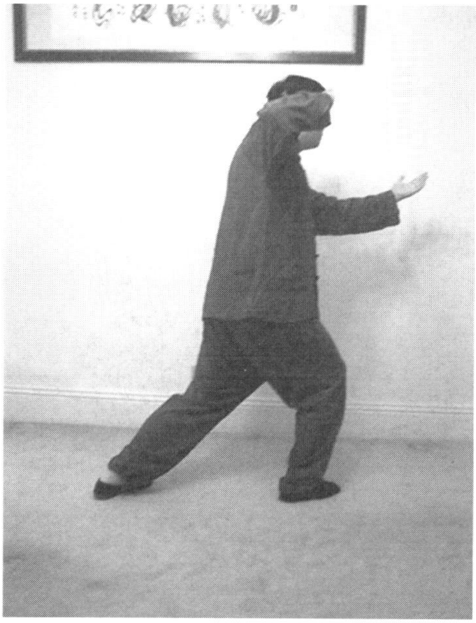

figure 68

Turn the left palm to face up; then move the right hand forward until it is over the left hand with the palm facing down *(figs 69 & 70 same move, different angles)*. Bring the hands back to the left side of the hip, and at the same time, shift the body weight onto the left foot *(figs 71 & 72 same move, different angles)*.

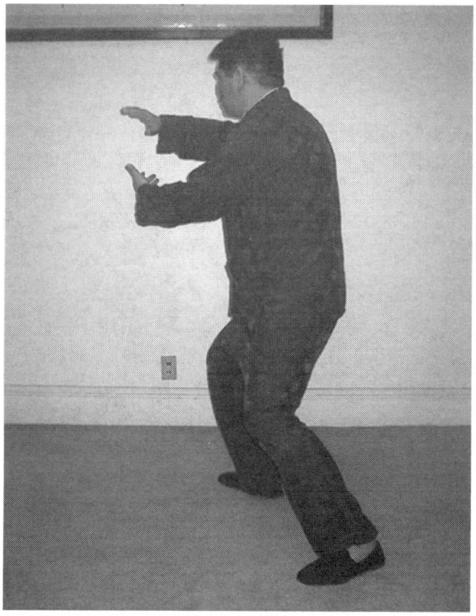

figure 69

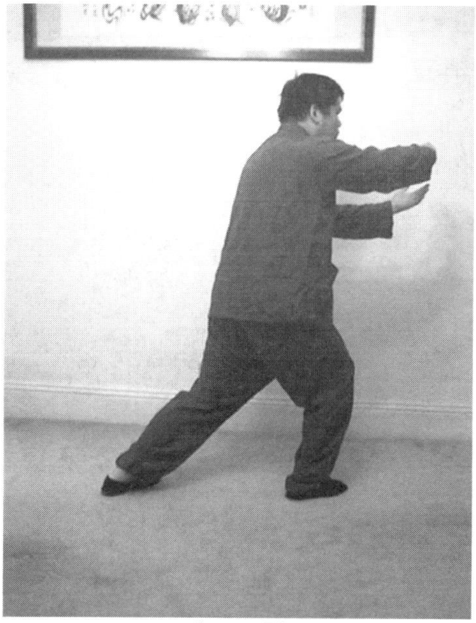

figure 70

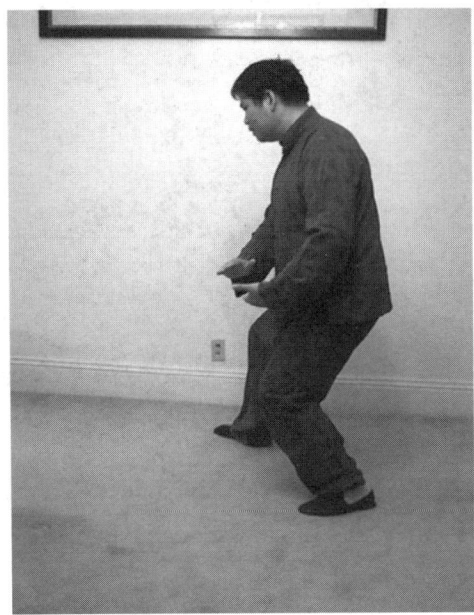

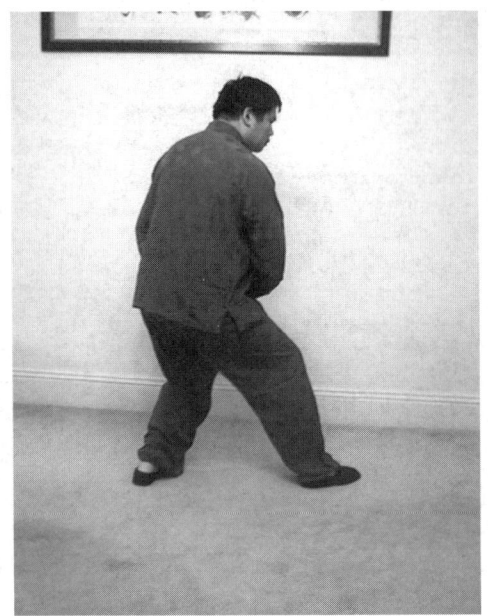

figure 71

figure 72

Part 2: Press

From the preceding movement, turn the left palm face down and the right palm face up, bringing the left above the right *(fig 73)*. The left hand sticks to the right hand *(fig 74)*. Press the hands forward with the body weight shifting onto the right foot *(fig 75)*.

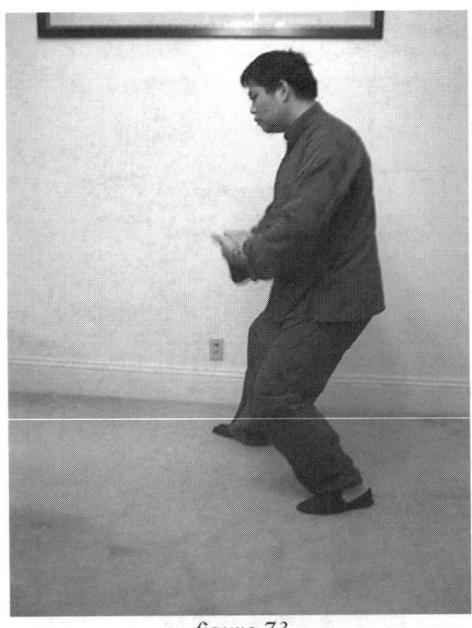

figure 73

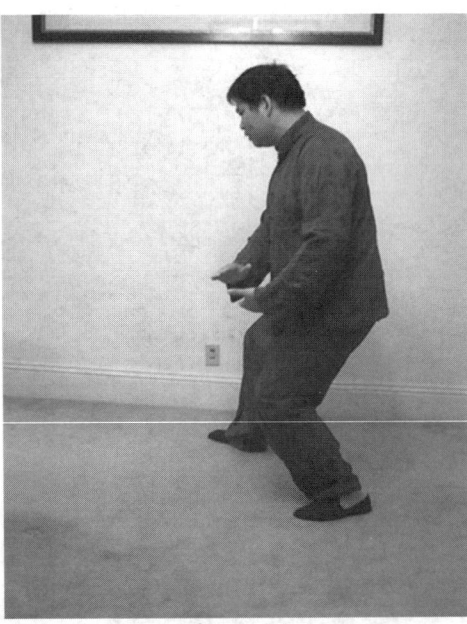

figure 74

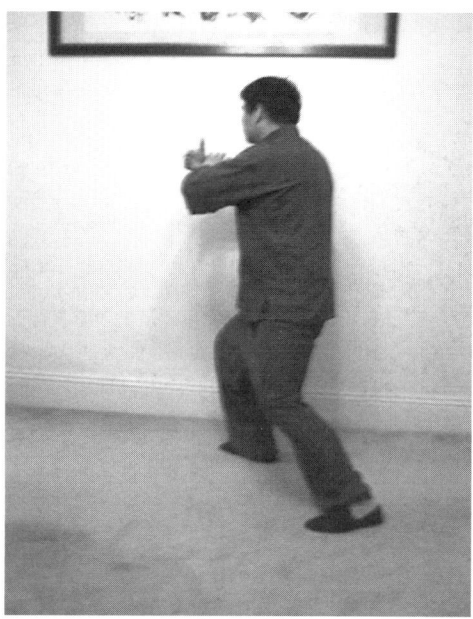

figure 75

Part 3: Push

From the preceding movement, turn the palms face down, the left palm on top of the right palm, and bring the hands back to the chest with the palms face down while shifting the weight back *(figs 76 & 77)*. Separate the hands as the body weight shifts onto the left foot *(fig 78)*. The hands separate with the wrists bent and the palms facing forward. Push the hands forward with the body weight shifting onto the right foot *(fig 79)*.

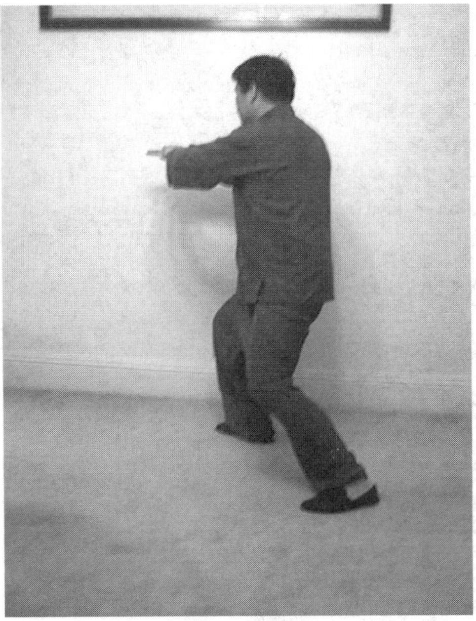

figure 76

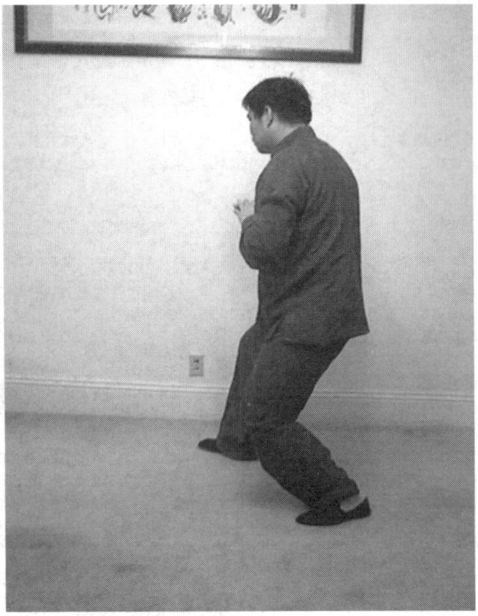

figure 77

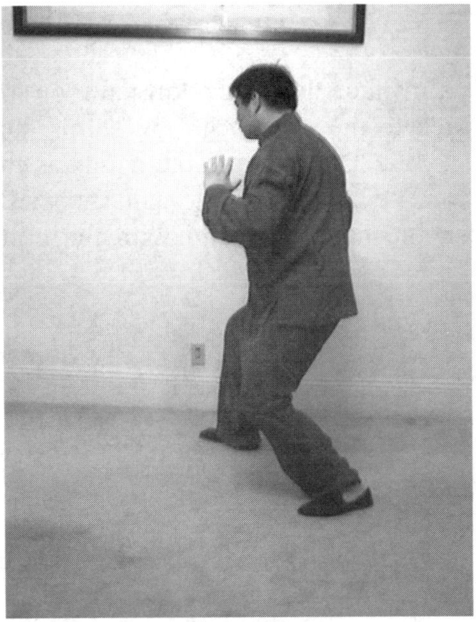

figure 78

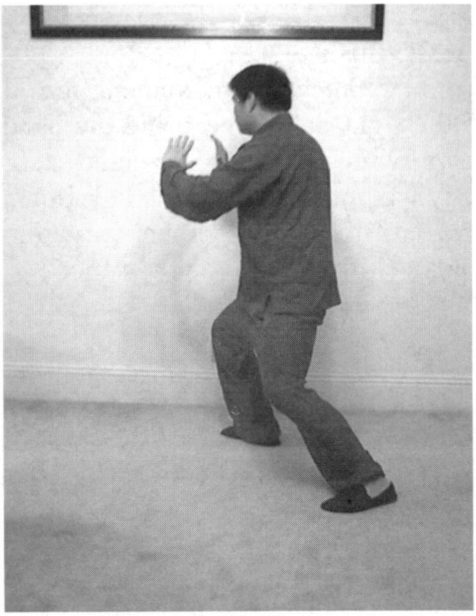

figure 79

10. Diagonal Single Whip
From the preceding movement, rotate the waist as the hands move in a complete counter clockwise circle over the head with the body weight shifting first onto the left foot then back onto the right foot *(figs 80, 81, 82)*.

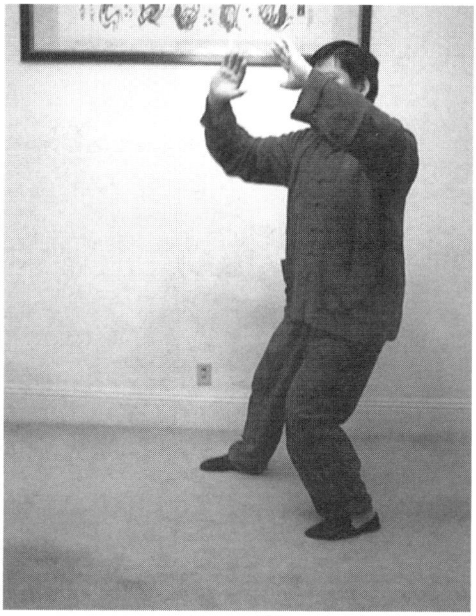

THE 43 MOVEMENT LARGE FRAME SOLO FORM

figure 80

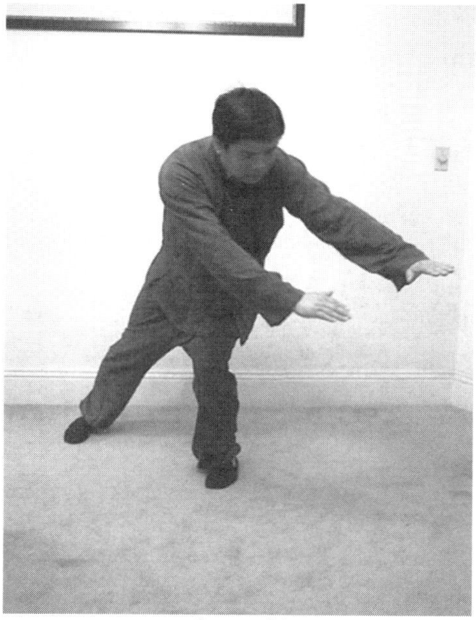

figure 81

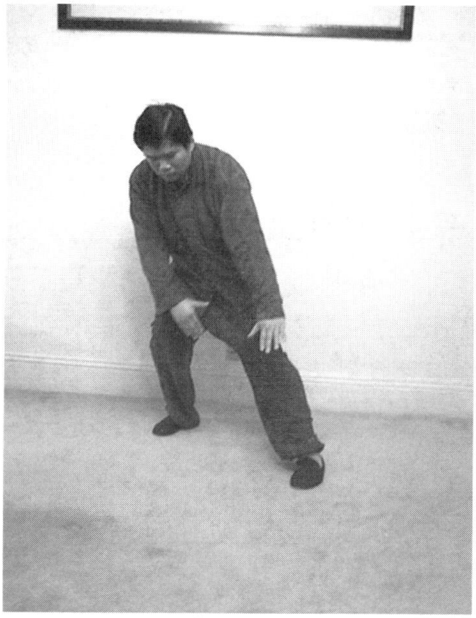

figure 82

Bring the right hand's fingers together to form a beak, and bend the wrist to form a hook; extend the right arm, and set the left hand at the right hip with the palm facing in *(fig 83)*. Move the left arm up and out to the left. Turn the

TAI CHI CHUAN – A COMPARATIVE STUDY

head to the left, pick up the left foot, and step forward to the left *(fig 84)*. With the body weight on the left foot, move the left palm upward, and face forward while the right hand hook remains the same *(fig 85)*.

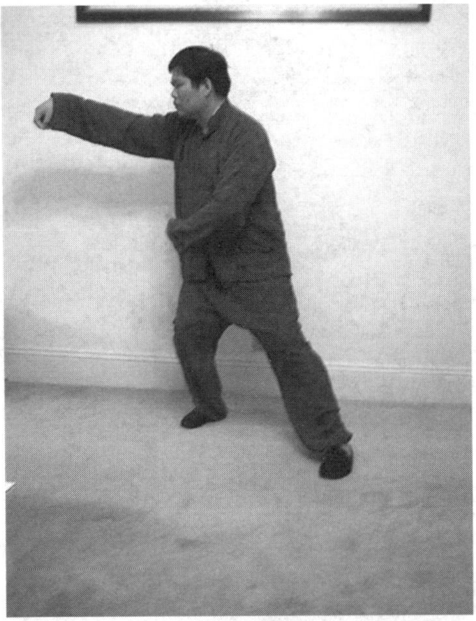

figure 83

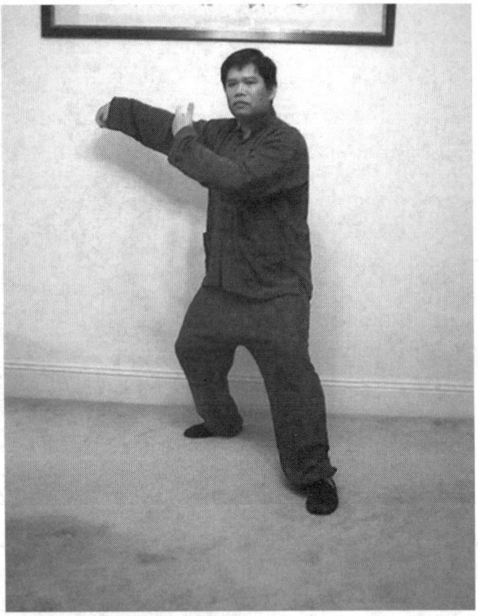

figure 84

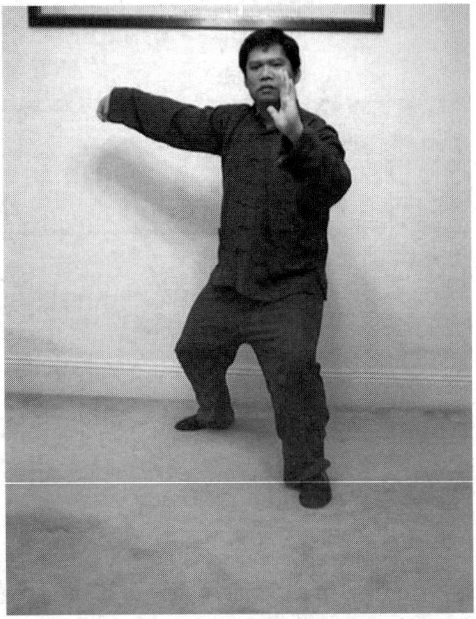

figure 85

11. Fist under Elbow

From the preceding movement, turn the left foot and the body to the left, bringing the right hand in front and the left hand in back of the body *(fig 86)*. With the body weight on the left foot, pick up the right foot, and step next to the left foot with the toes pointing to the corner *(fig 87)*. The right hand then closes into a fist. Shift the body weight onto the right foot, and bring the left hand up by the left hip *(fig 88)*. Look to the left with the body weight on the right foot; place the left foot on the heel; the left hand goes up with the fingers pointing up as the right fist is brought under the left elbow *(fig 89)*.

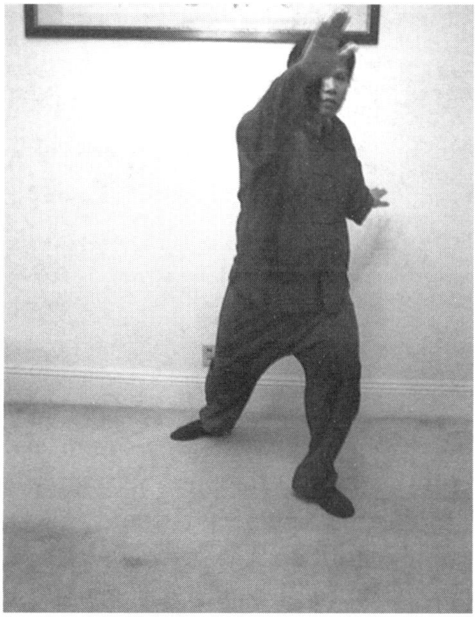

figure 86

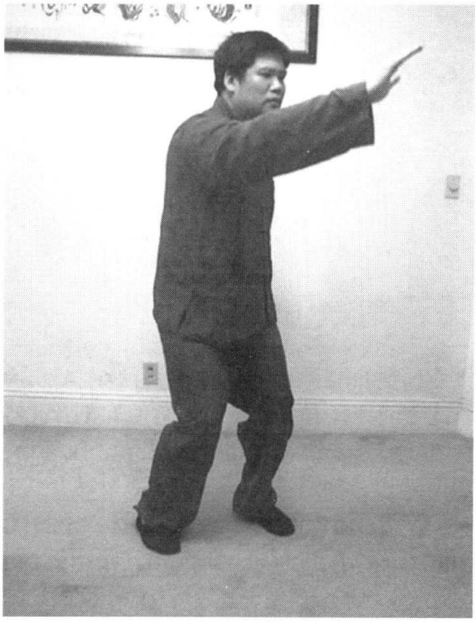

figure 87

TAI CHI CHUAN – A COMPARATIVE STUDY

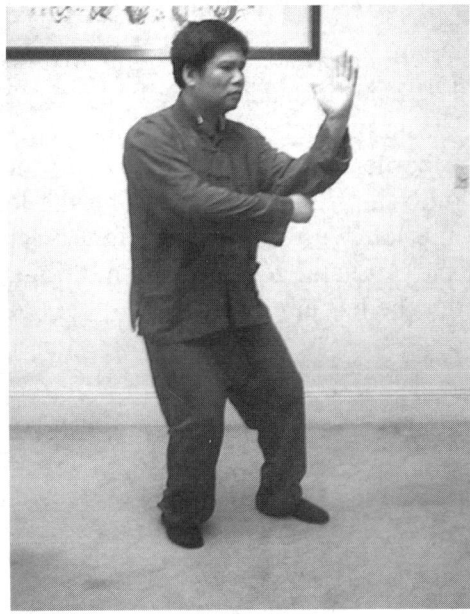

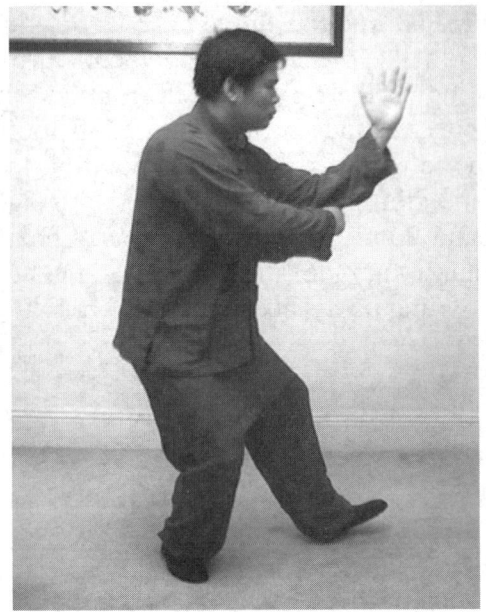

figure 88 *figure 89*

12. Step Backward and Drive Away Monkey (three times)
Part 1: Left Foot Steps Backward

From the preceding movement, open the right fist, swing the right hand behind the body, and extend the left hand forward with the palm facing up *(fig 90)*. With the body weight on the right foot, pick up the left foot, and step backward *(fig 91)*. Bring the right hand up next to the right ear *(fig 92)*. While shifting the weight back to the left foot, push the right hand forward with the palm face forward, and at the same time, bring the left hand back to the left side of the hip with the palm facing up *(fig 93)*.

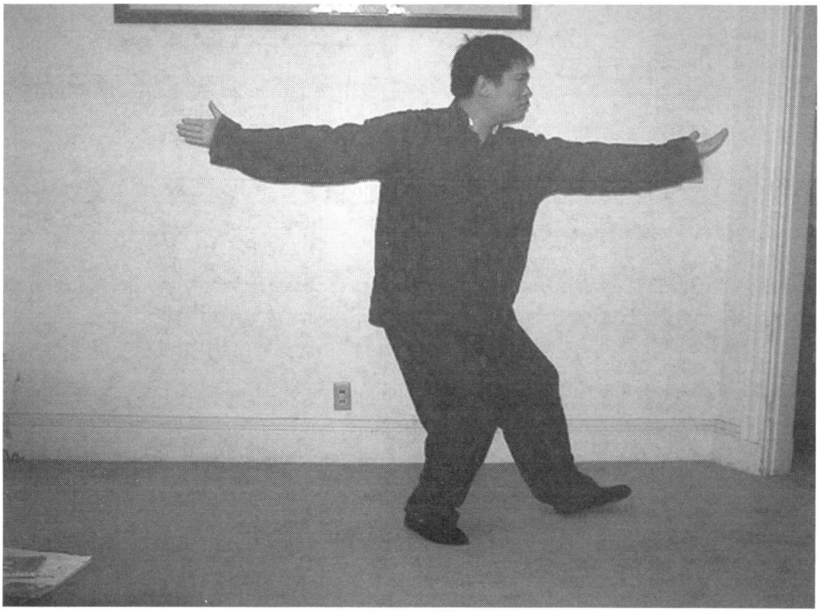

figure 90

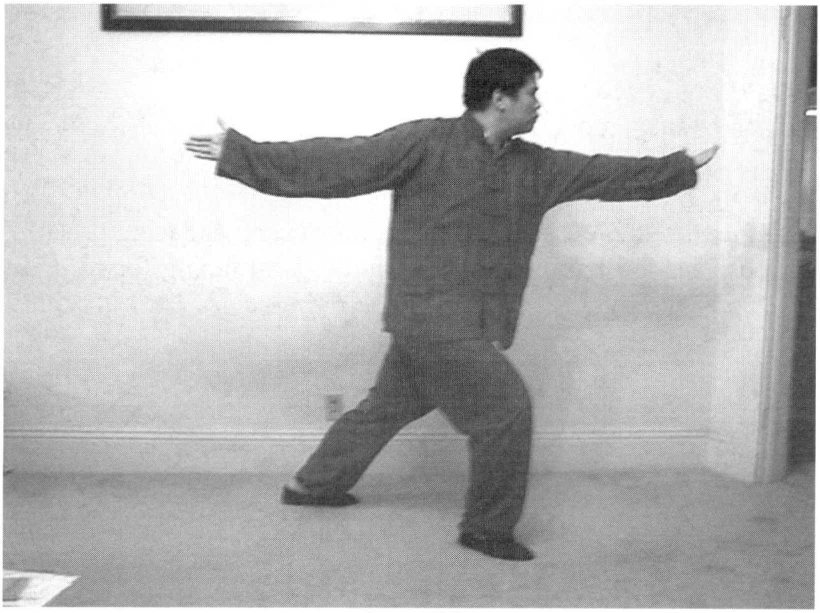

figure 91

figure 92 *figure 93*

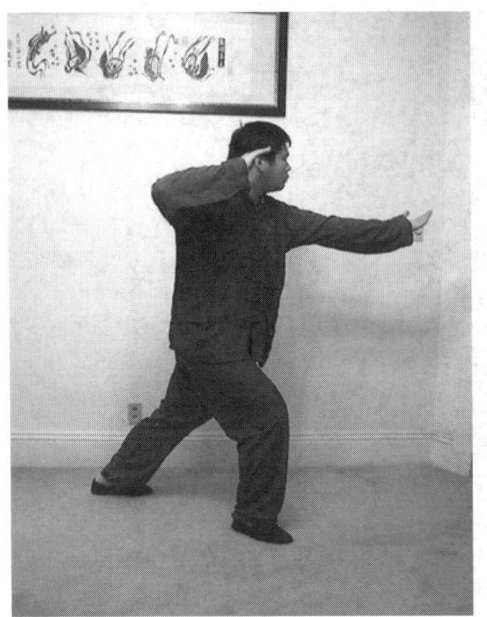

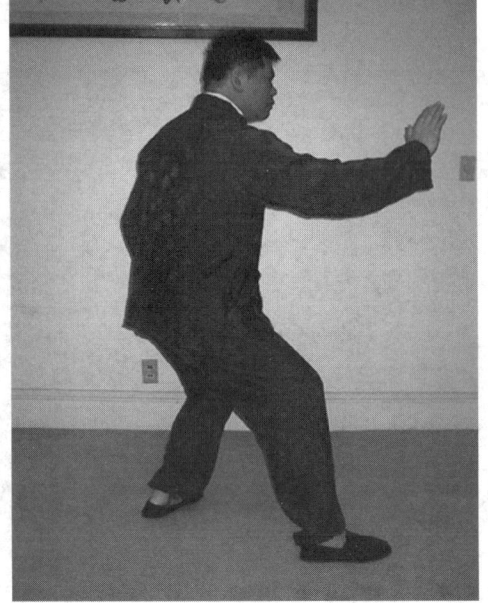

Part 2: Right Foot Steps Backward

From the preceding movement, the left hand swings behind the body. Straighten the right arm with the palm facing up *(fig 94)*. With the body weight on the left foot, pick up the right foot and step it backward *(fig 95)*. Bring the left hand up next to the left ear *(fig 96)*. While shifting the weight back onto the right foot, push the left hand forward with the palm facing forward, and at the same time, bring the right hand back to the right side of the hip with the palm facing up *(fig 97)*.

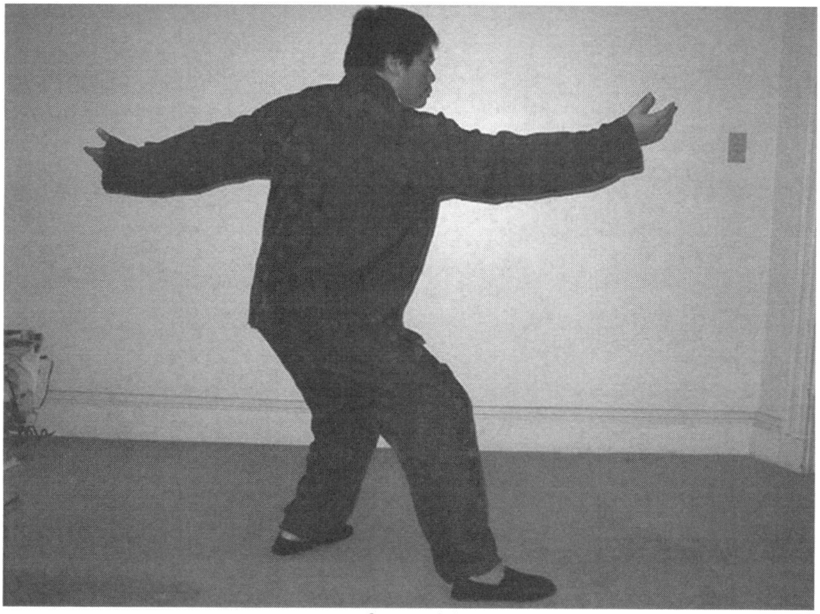

THE 43 MOVEMENT LARGE FRAME SOLO FORM

figure 94

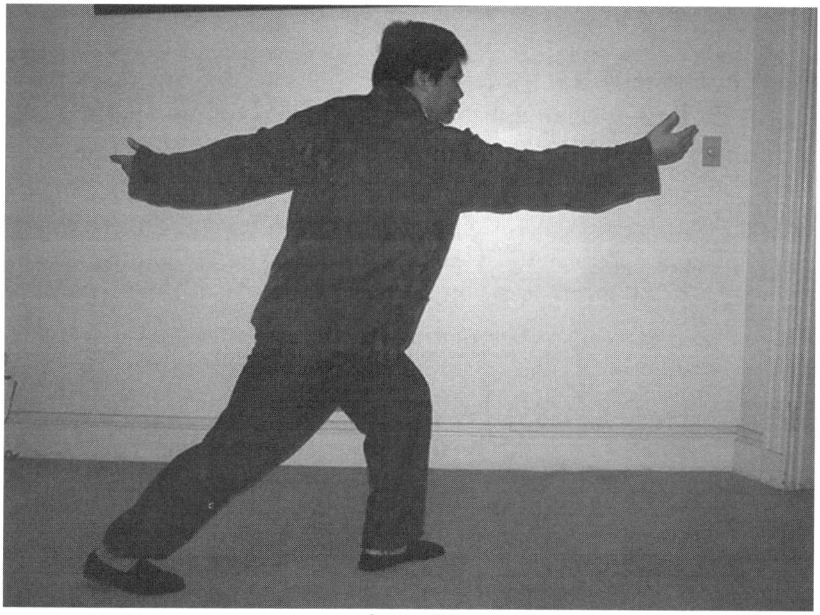

figure 95

figure 96   *figure 97*

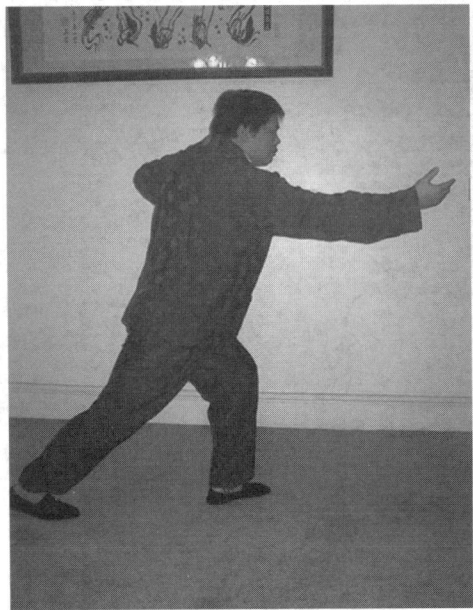

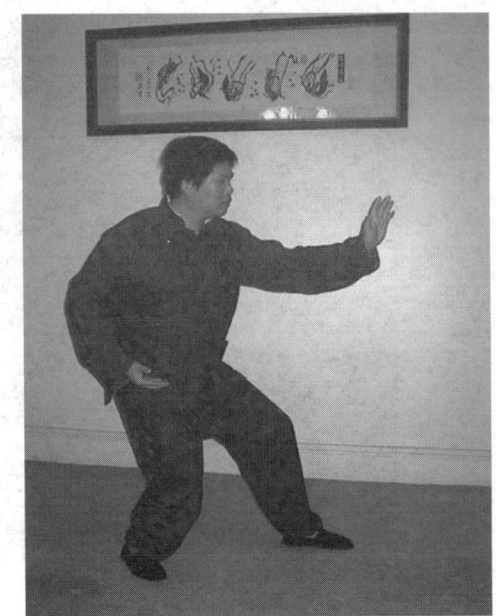

Part 3: Left Foot Steps Backward
From the preceding movement, the right hand swings behind the body. Straighten the left arm with the palm facing up *(fig 98)*. With the body weight on the right foot, pick up the left foot, and step backward *(fig 99)*. Bring the right hand up next to the right ear *(fig 100)*. While shifting the weight back onto the left foot, push the right hand forward with the palm facing forward, and at the same time, bring the left hand back to the left side of the hip with the palm facing up *(fig 101)*.

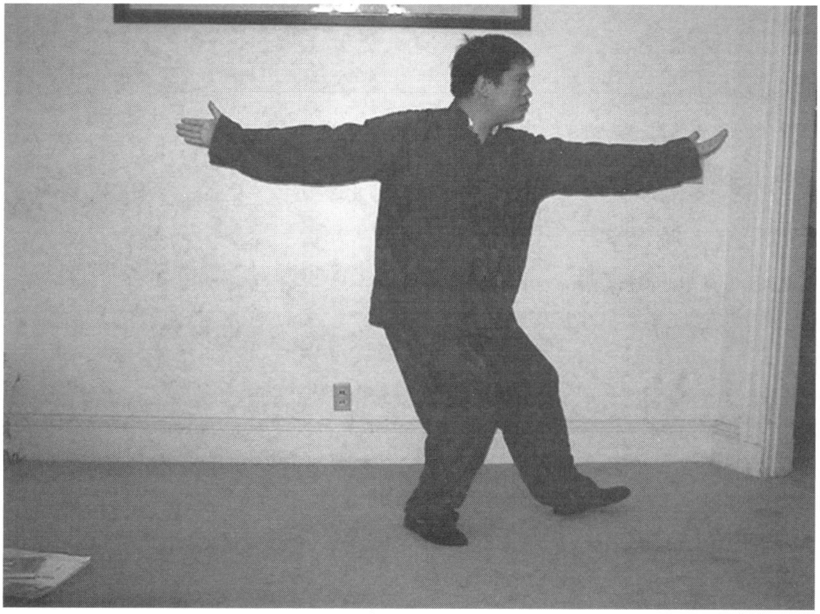

THE 43 MOVEMENT LARGE FRAME SOLO FORM

figure 98

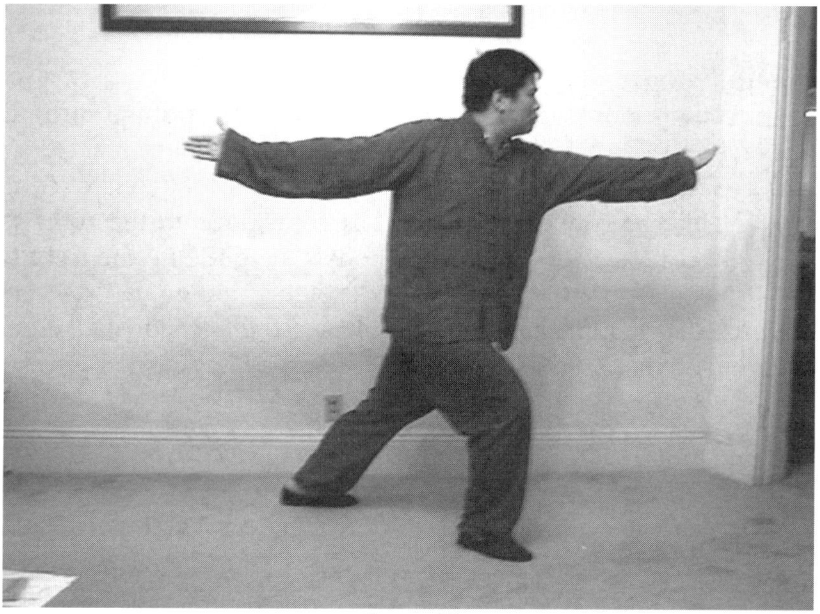

figure 99

figure 100 *figure 101*

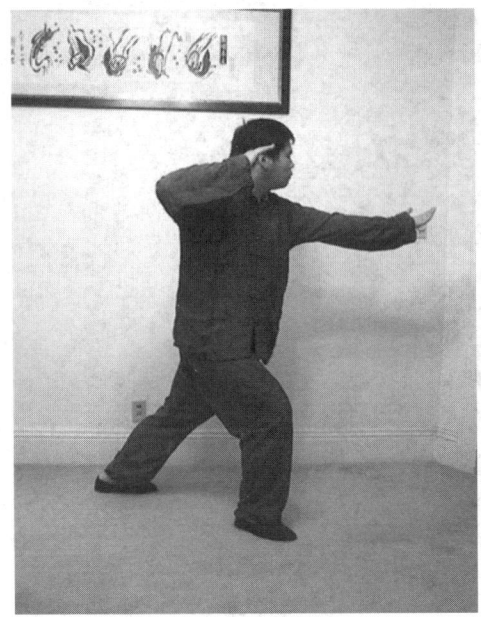

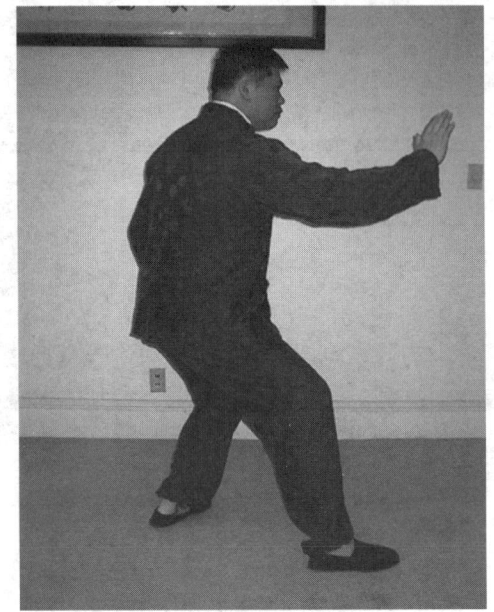

13. Diagonal Flying

From the preceding movement, turn the right toes inward and bring the right hand under the left hand with the palms facing each other *(figs 102 & 103 show the same move at different angles)*. Turn the head, and look out over the right shoulder. With the body weight on the left foot, pick up the right foot, and step to the right corner *(fig 104)*. Shift the body's weight onto the right foot, and at the same time, separate the hands with the right hand going up to face level, palm facing up and the left hand going down to the left side of the body with the palm facing down *(fig 105)*.

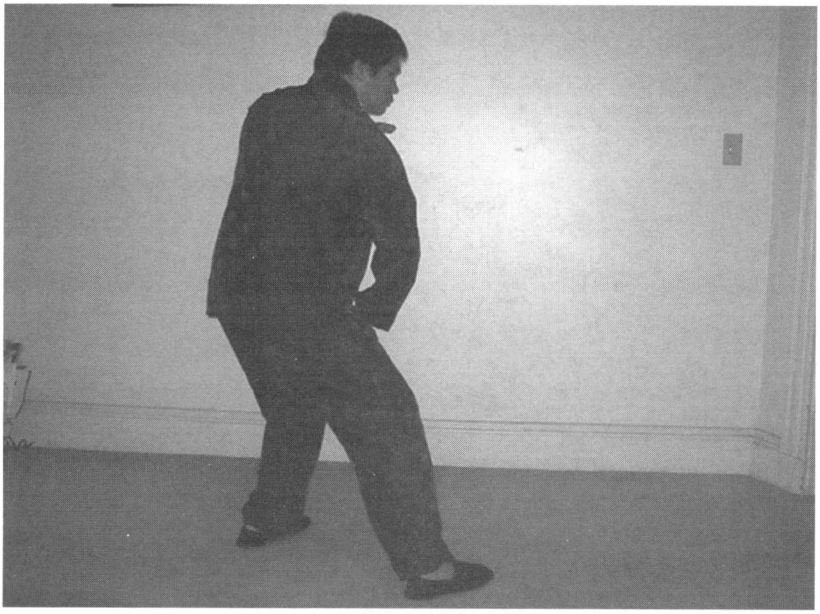

THE 43 MOVEMENT LARGE FRAME SOLO FORM

figure 102

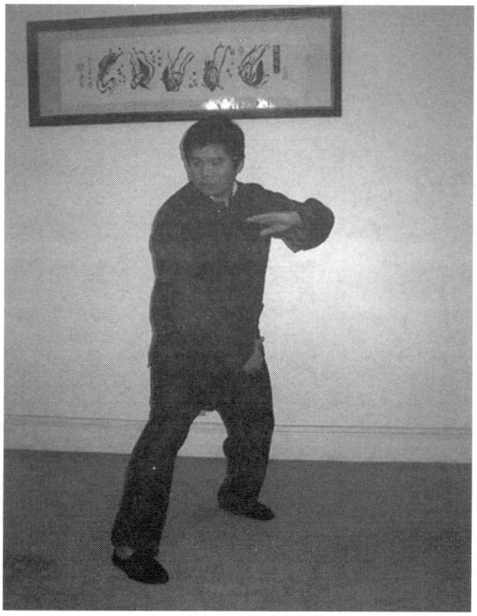

figure 103

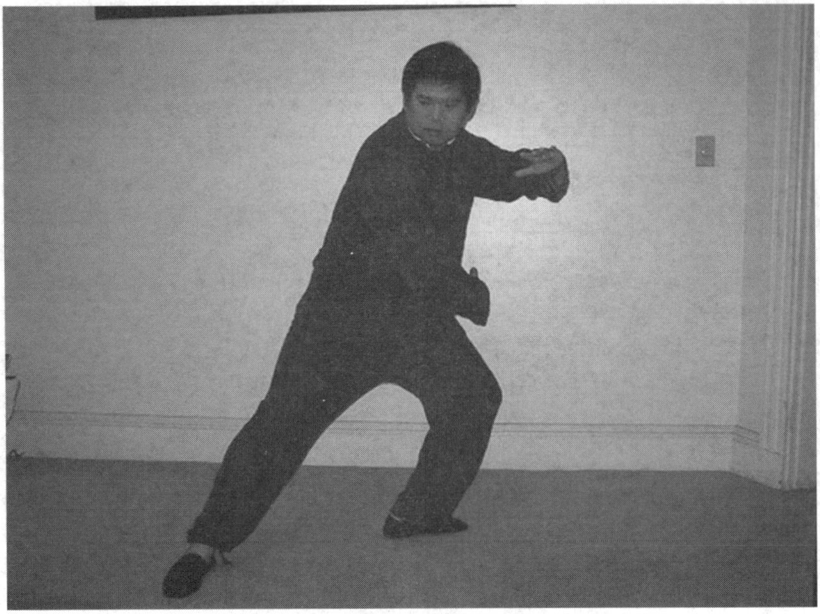

TAI CHI CHUAN – A COMPARATIVE STUDY

figure 104

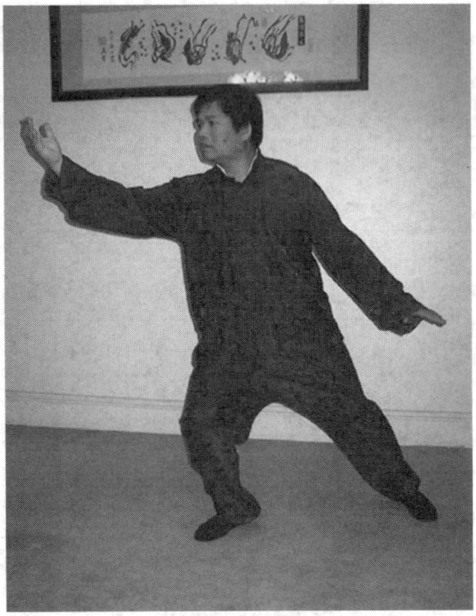

figure 105

14. Lift Hands

From the preceding movement, turn the left foot out. Shift the body weight onto the left foot. Circle the right hand back clockwise to the chest with the left hand coming up behind the right hand *(fig 106)*. With the body weight on the left foot, pick up the right foot, and place it to the front with the right heel on the ground. Push the hands forward together with the palms facing forward *(fig 107)*.

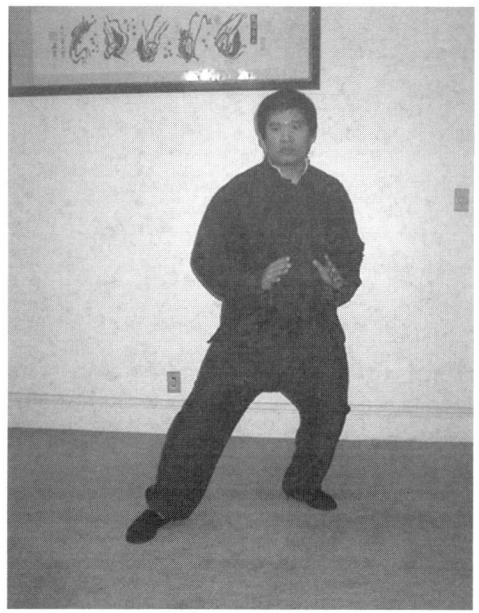

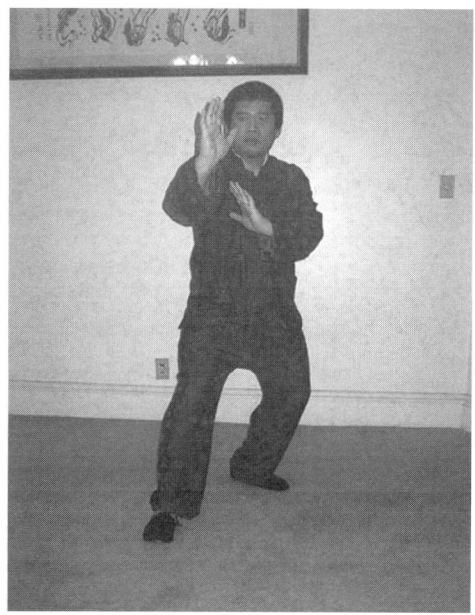

figure 106   *figure 107*

15. White Crane Spreads Its Wings
From the preceding movement, turn the left palm up and the right palm down. Pull the hands down to the left side of the body. Pick up the right foot, and step forward *(fig 108)*. With the left palm brought near the right arm, shift the body weight onto the right foot *(fig 109)*; then separate the hands with the right hand going up and the left hand coming down *(fig 110)*. With the body weight on the right foot, look out to the left, and pick up the left foot; then place it down on its toes. Turn the right palm face out, and bring it up in front of the forehead with the thumb pointing down, and at the same time, rotate the waist to the left. The left hand remains on the left side of the body *(fig 111)*.

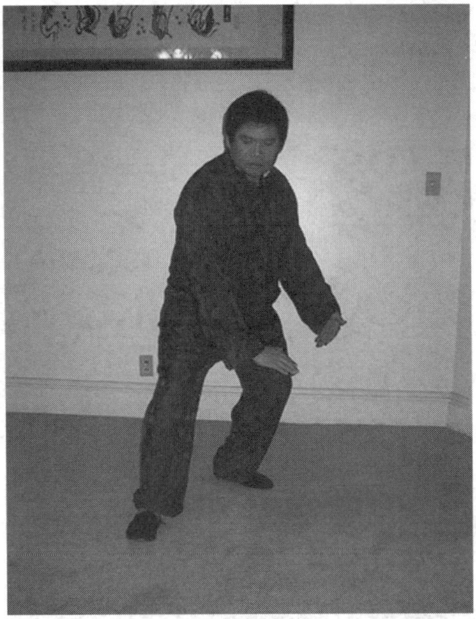

TAI CHI CHUAN – A COMPARATIVE STUDY

figure 108

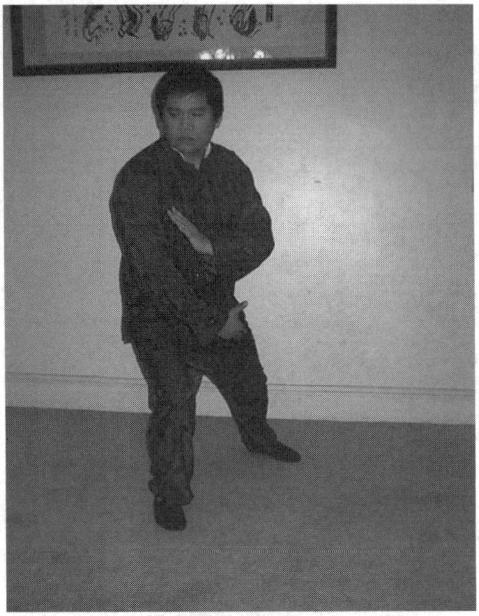

figure 109

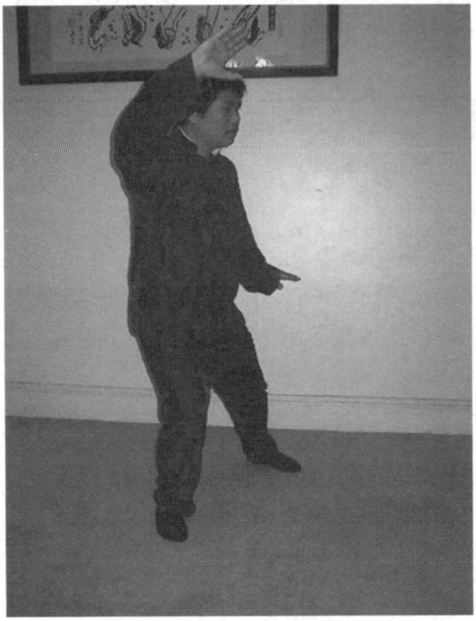

figure 110

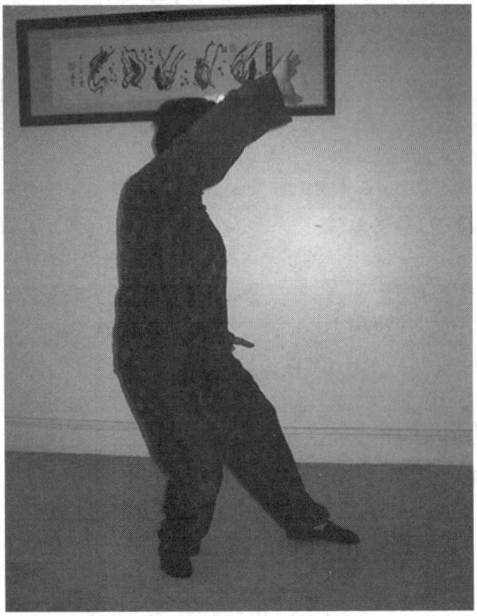

figure 111

16. Brush Knee, Twist Step and Push the Right Hand Forward

From the preceding movement, the right arm makes a counter clockwise motion coming down to chest level with the palm facing up *(fig 112)*. The left hand makes a clockwise motion coming up to chest level with the palm facing in; the right hand arrives near the right hip *(fig 113)*. Continuing, the right hand makes another counter clockwise motion and ends up next to the right ear. The left hand makes a clockwise motion and stops at the right side of the waist. With the body weight still remaining on the right foot, pick up the left foot, and step forward *(fig 114)*. Shift the body weight forward onto the left foot as the left hand goes down to the left side of the left knee with the palm facing down, and the right hand pushes forward to the center of the chest from the right ear with the palm facing forward *(fig 115)*.

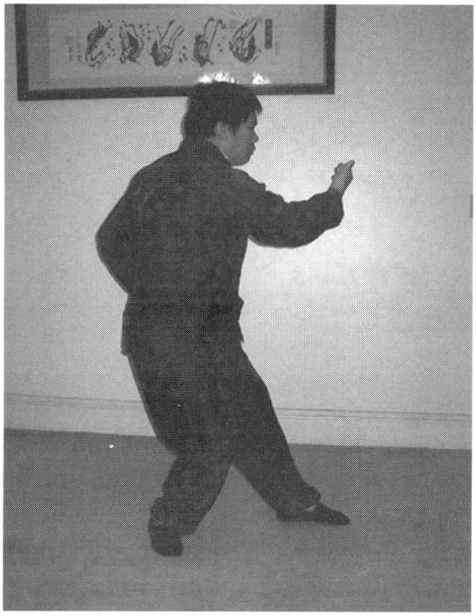

figure 112

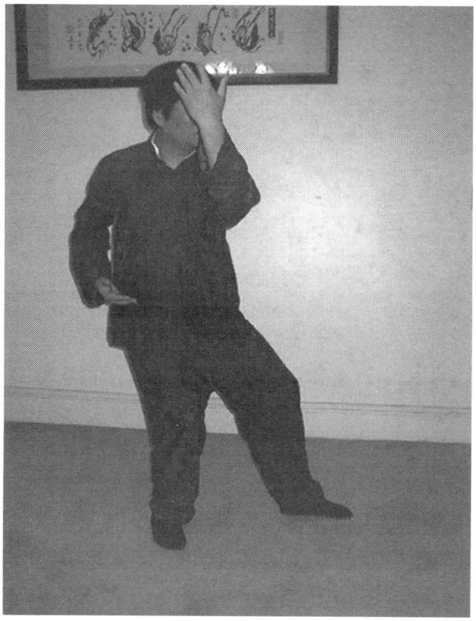

figure 113

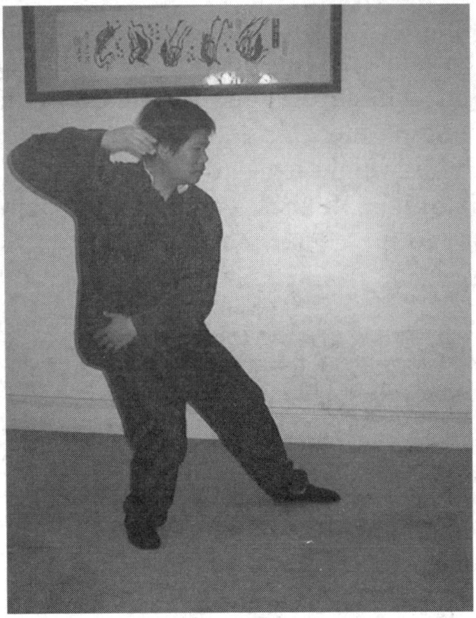

figure 114

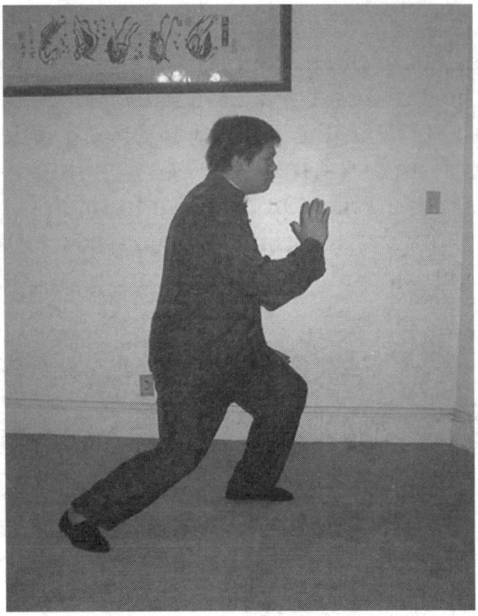

figure 115

17. Pick Up Needle in Sea Bottom

From the preceding movement, the right foot steps up beside the left foot. Bring the right hand back in front of the chest with the body weight still on the left foot *(fig 116)*. Retract the right foot and put it down on the ground, shifting the weight onto it, then bring the left foot back; the hands come back to the chest *(figs 117 & 118)*. Set the right fingers pointing down next to the left palm. Then bend down in front of the body with the body weight remaining on the right foot. While bending, the left hand pushes down to the left side of the left leg with the palm face down, and the right palm reaches down at the center of the body; the eyes are looking forward *(fig 119)*.

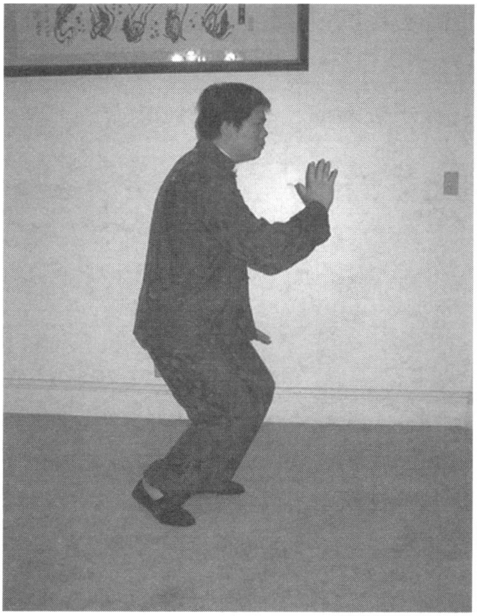

figure 116

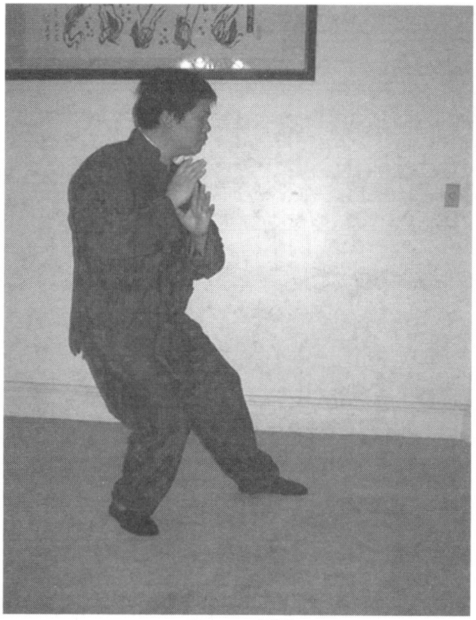

figure 117

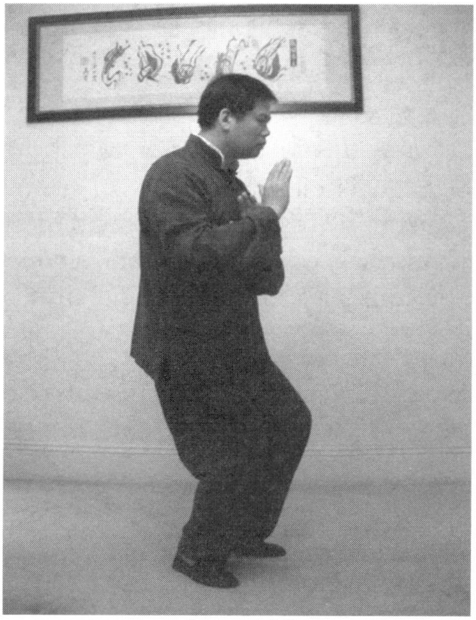

figure 118

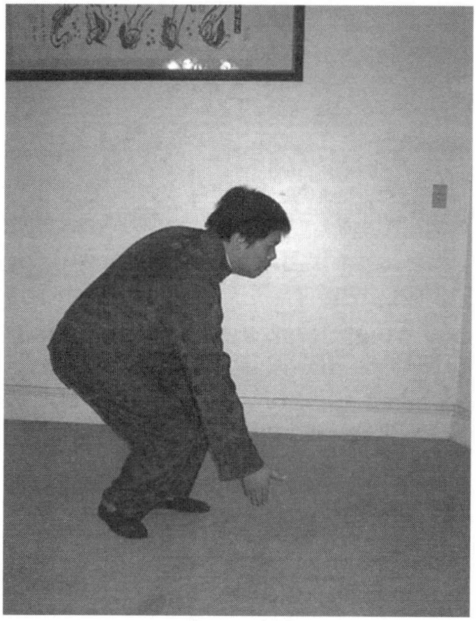

figure 119

18. Fan Back

From the preceding movement, the body weight remains on the right foot. The body and both hands come up together with the hands in front of the chest *(fig 120)*. Turn the right palm so that it faces out, pick up the left foot, and step forward. Set the right hand next to the right ear. The left hand pushes forward from the chest, and the body weight shifts onto the left foot *(fig 121)*.

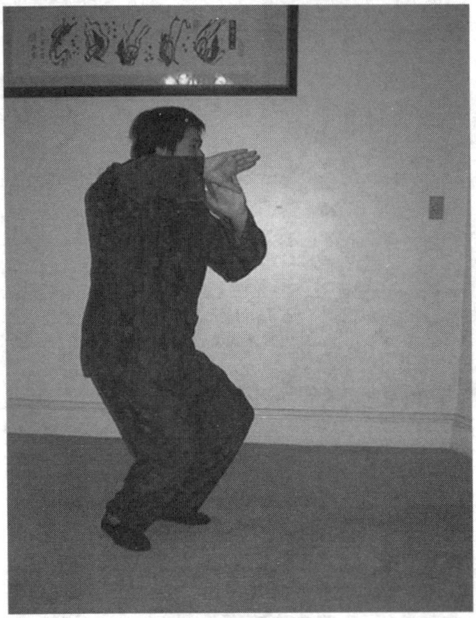

figure 120

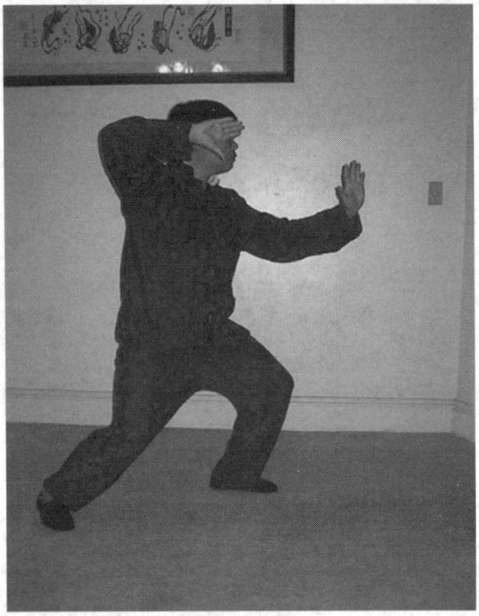

figure 121

19. Turn Around and Punch

From the preceding movement, the right hand is closed into a fist; bring it down to the right hip *(fig 122)*. Rotate the waist to the right; the left hand moves to the right with the palm facing away from the body, and the body weight shifts onto the right foot *(fig 123)*. Bring the left hand to the left, and shift the body weight onto the left foot again *(fig 124)*.

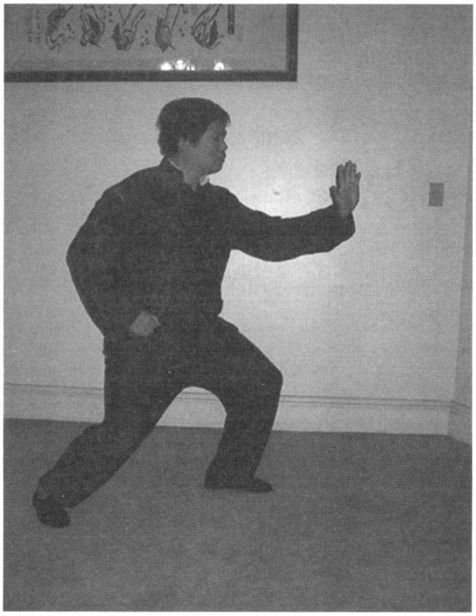

THE 43 MOVEMENT LARGE FRAME SOLO FORM

figure 122

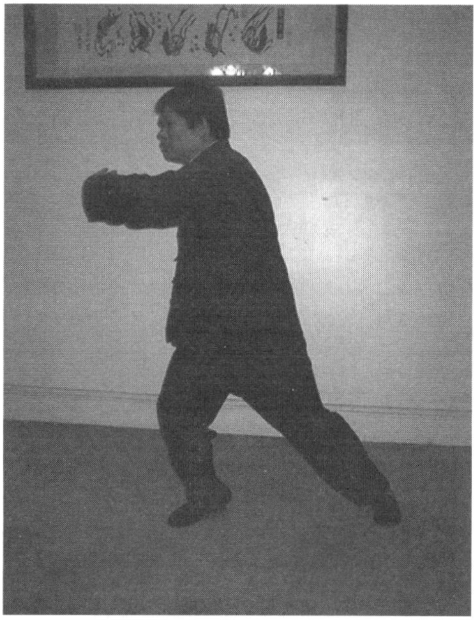

figure 123

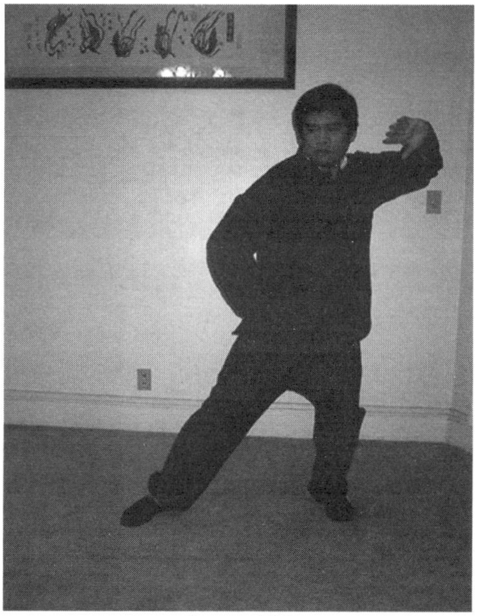

figure 124

Turn the head to the right, pick up the right foot, and step forward; then the right fist comes up, the left hand goes down *(fig 125)*. Shift the body weight onto the right foot as the right hand comes up to the chest and sweeps forward in a back fist while the left hand moves in front of the left shoulder *(fig 126)*.

With the body weight on the right foot, pull the right fist back onto the right side of the hip, and push the left palm forward *(fig 127)*.

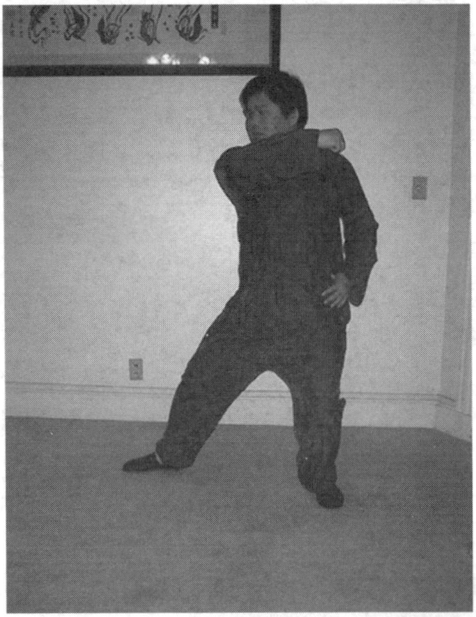

figure 125

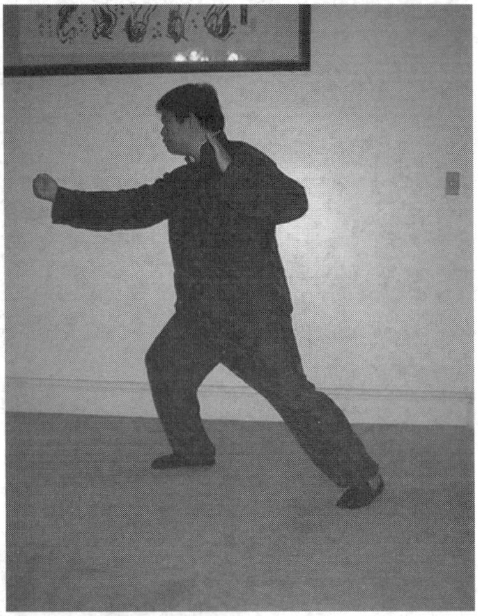

figure 126

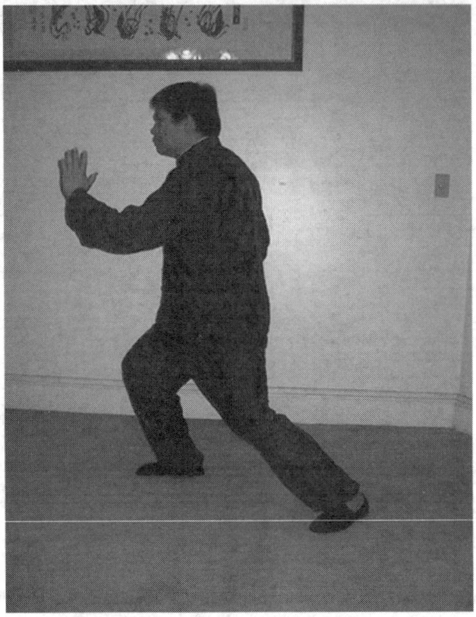

figure 127

20. Part the Wild Horse's Mane (right)

From the preceding movement, turn the left palm face up, and reach the right fist out over of the left palm *(fig 128)*. Shift the body's weight onto the left foot. Open and pull the right hand back under the left hand with the palms facing each other as if they were holding a ball *(fig 129)*. Pick up the right foot, and step to the right corner. Shift the body weight onto the right foot, and separate the hands by lifting the right hand up to face level while the left hand goes down to the left side of the body with the palm facing down *(fig 130)*.

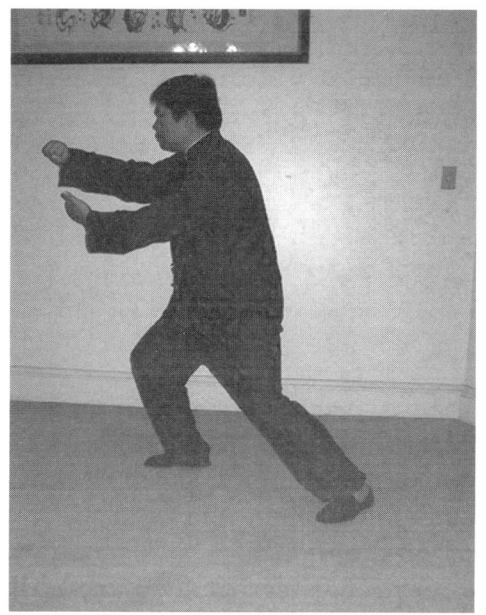

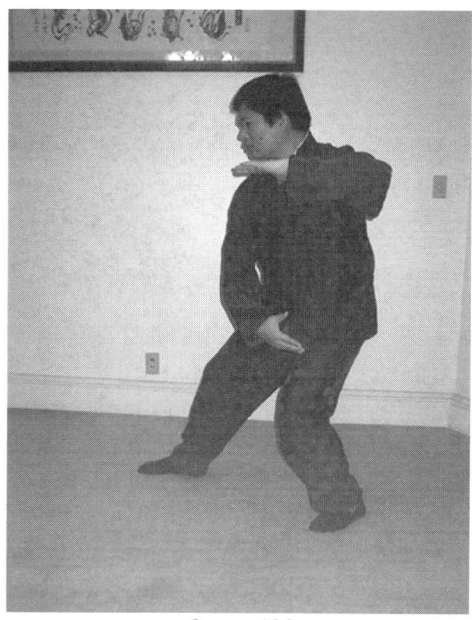

figure 128

figure 129

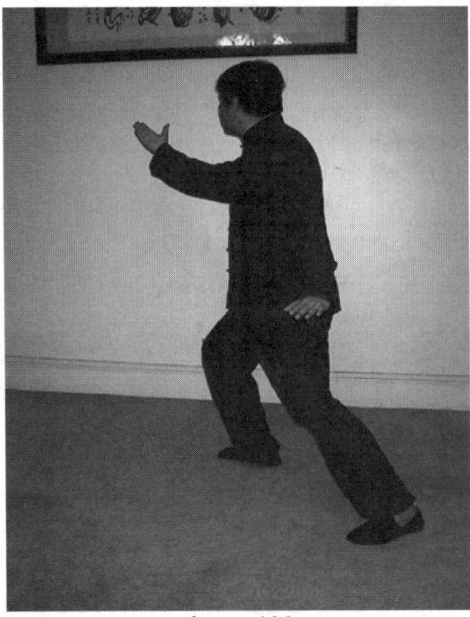

figure 130

21. Left Hand Warding Off

From the preceding movement, shift the body weight onto the left foot while the right hand makes a complete counter clockwise circle and ends at the chest with the palm face down. The left hand also moves in a counter clockwise circle, stopping above the right knee as the body weight returns to the right foot *(figs 131 - 133)*. With the body weight on the right foot, pick up the left foot, and step forward. Shift the body weight onto the left foot, and at the same time, separate the hands with the left hand coming up to face level and the right hand going down to the right side of the body with the palm facing down *(fig 134)*.

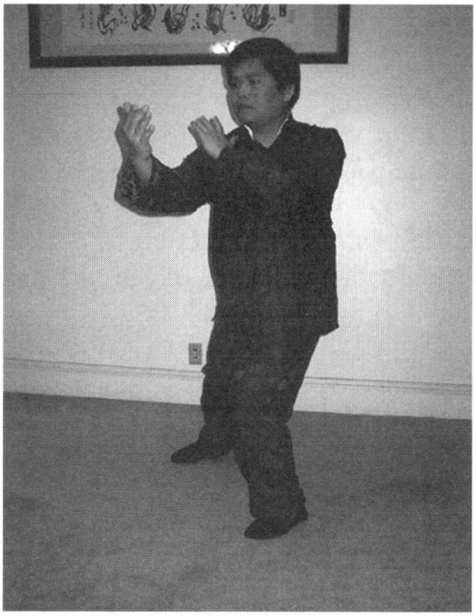

THE 43 MOVEMENT LARGE FRAME SOLO FORM

figure 131

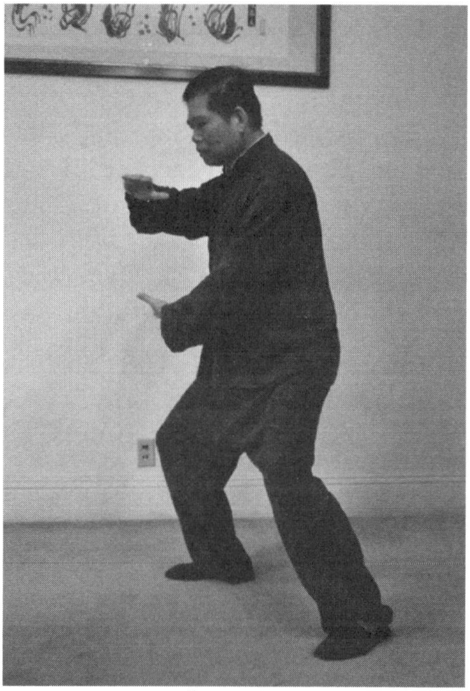

figure 132

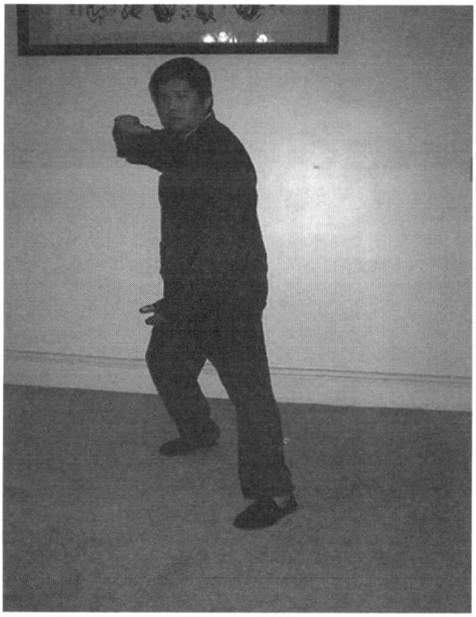

figure 133

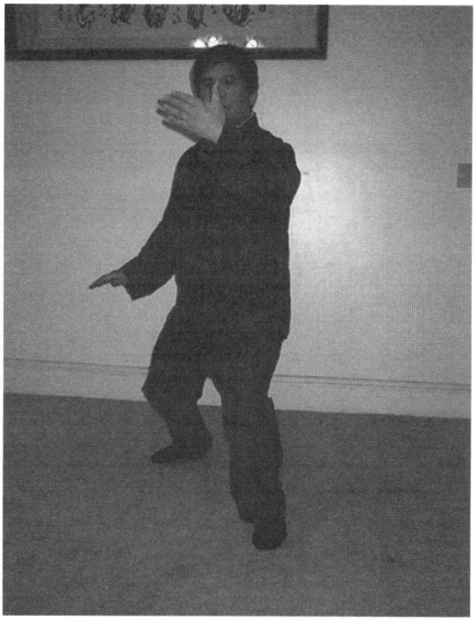

figure 134

22. Waving Hands Like Clouds (7 times)
Part 1: Left Hand Waving Like Clouds

From the preceding movement, with the body weight on the left foot, turn the left foot inward. Simultaneously, the left hand makes a complete clockwise circle and ends at the chest level with the palm facing down. The right hand also moves in a clockwise circle, arriving above the left knee with the palm facing up *(figs 135 -137)*. The right foot then steps up next to the left foot. Bring the right hand up to face level with the palm facing in. Push the left hand down above the left knee with the palm facing down *(figs 138 & 139)*.

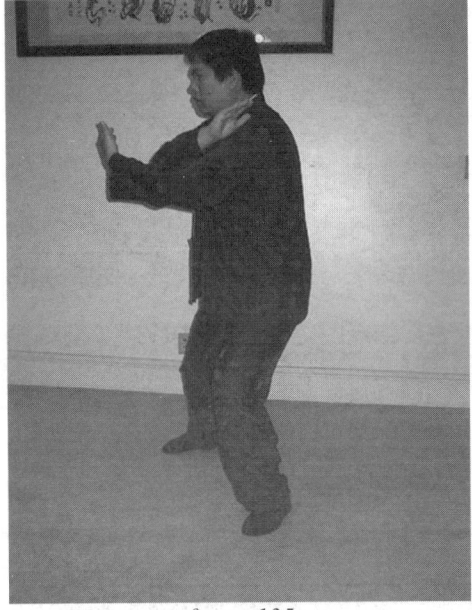

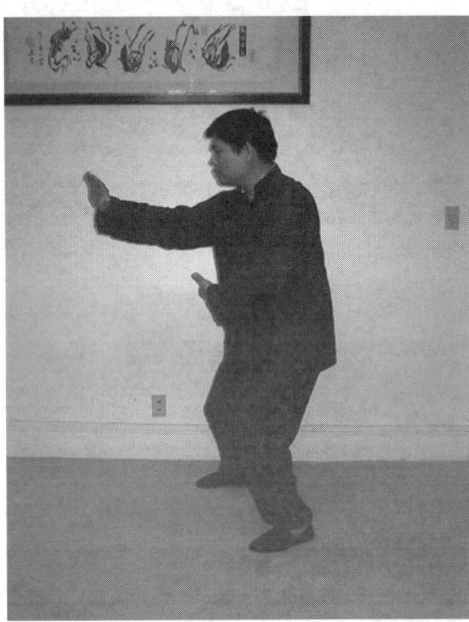

figure 135

figure 136

THE 43 MOVEMENT LARGE FRAME SOLO FORM

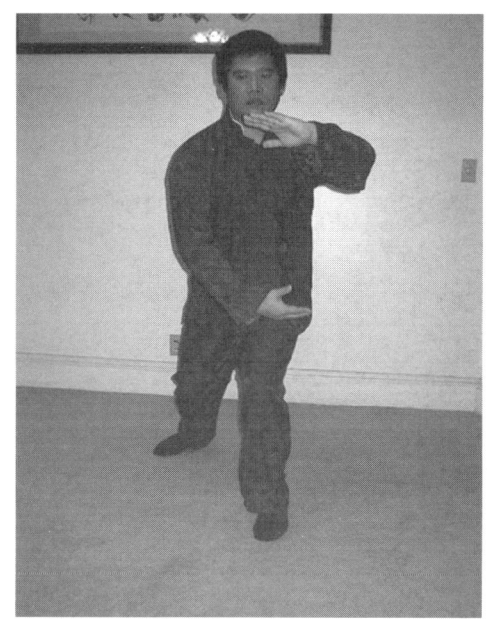

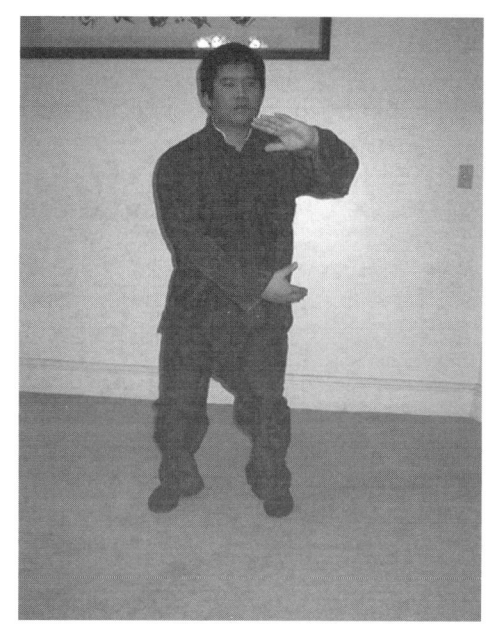

figure 137

figure 138

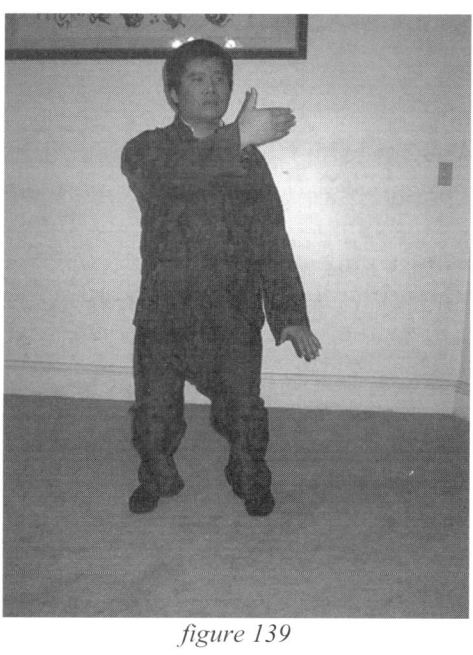

figure 139

Part 2: Right Hand Waving Like Clouds

From the preceding movement, rotate the hip to the right. The body weight and the hands follow the waist to the right *(fig 140)*.

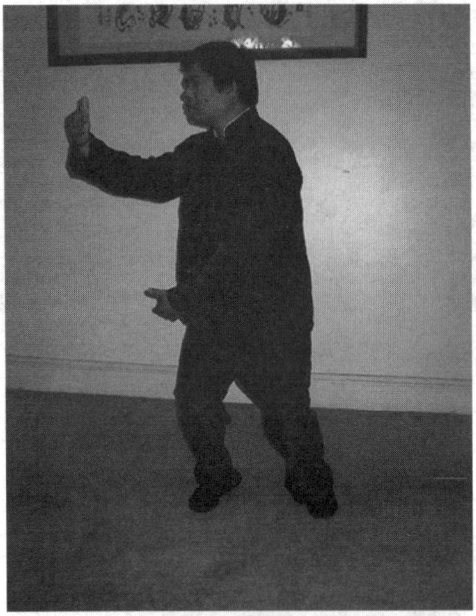

figure 140

Part 3: Left Hand Waving Like Clouds

From the preceding movement, change hands by bringing the left hand up to face level with the palm facing in and pushing the right hand down above the right knee with the palm facing in as well *(fig 141)*. Pick up the left foot, and step out to the left. Rotate the hip to the left, shifting the body weight to the left foot. The hands follow the waist to the left *(figs 142 & 143)*.

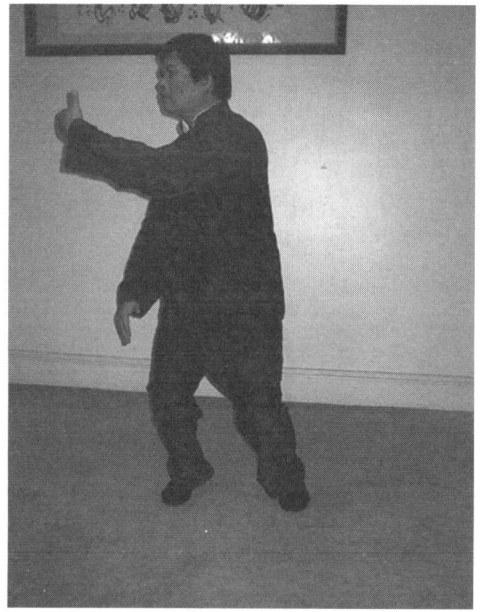

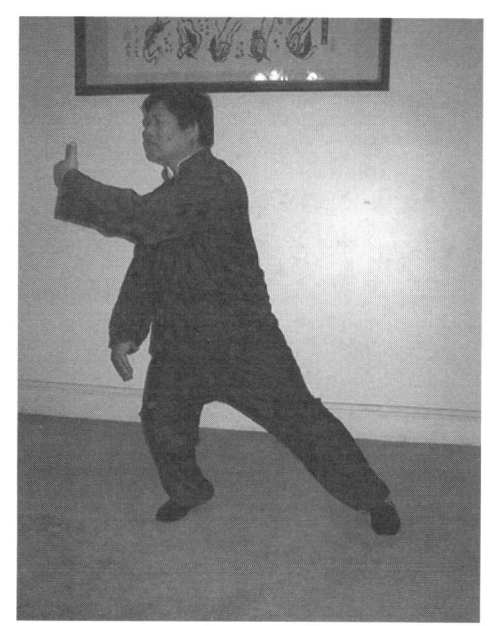

figure 141

figure 142

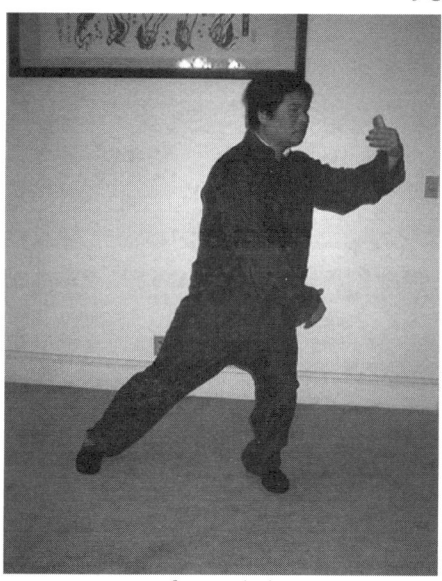

figure 143

Part 4: Right Hand Waving Like Clouds

From the preceding movement, change hands by bringing the right hand up to face level and pushing the left hand down above the left knee with the palm facing in *(fig 144)*. Pick up the right foot, and step next to the left foot *(fig 145)*; then rotate the hip to the right shifting the body weight to the right foot. The hands follow the waist to the right *(fig 146)*.

TAI CHI CHUAN – A COMPARATIVE STUDY

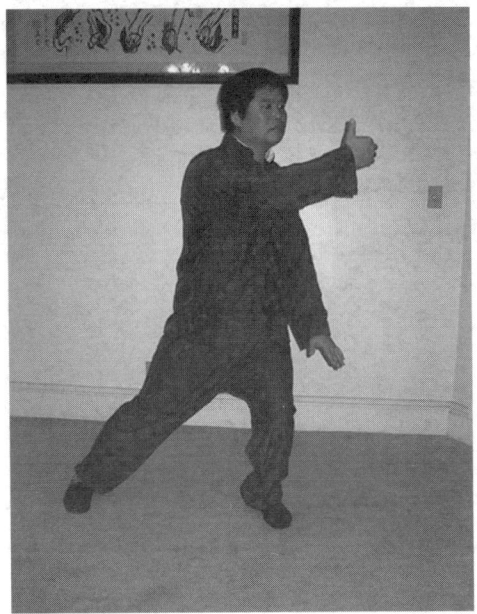

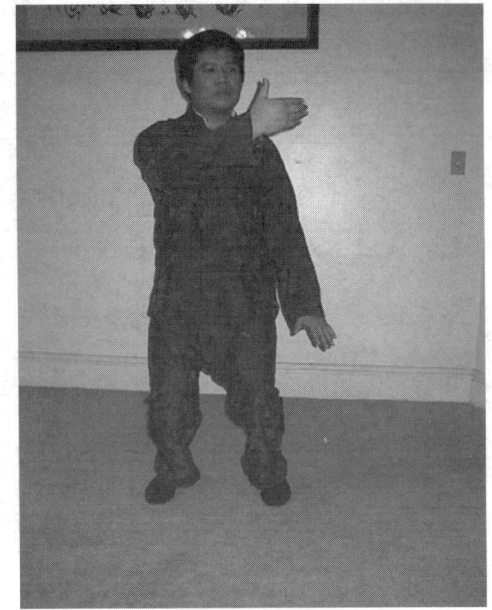

figure 144

figure 145

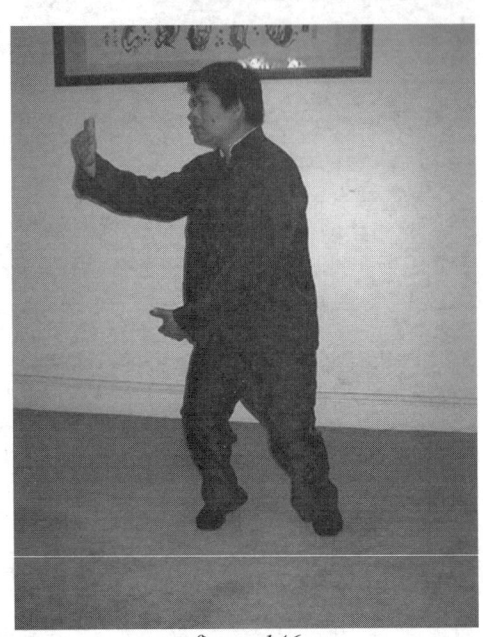

figure 146

Part 5: Left Hand Waving Like Clouds

From the preceding movement, change hands by bringing the left hand up to face level with the palm facing in and pushing the right hand down above the right knee with the palm facing in *(fig 147)*. Pick up the left foot, and step out to the left *(fig 148)*. Rotate the hip to the left. The body weight and the hands follow the waist to the left *(fig 149)*.

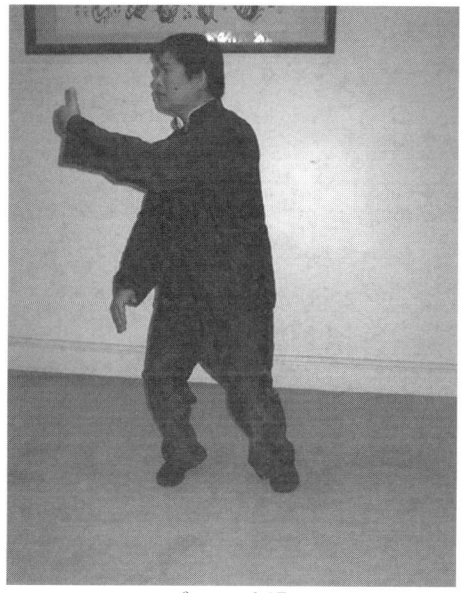

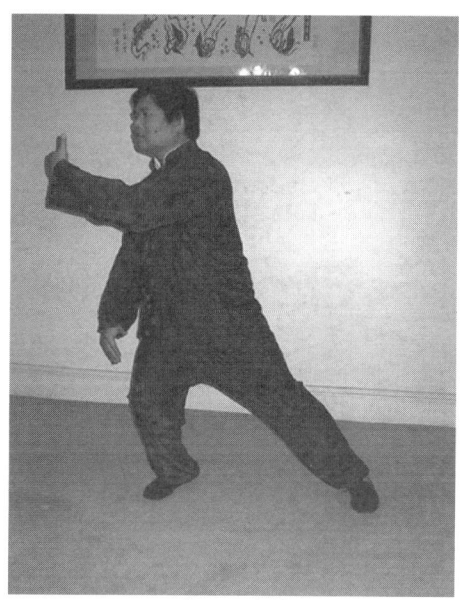

figure 147

figure 148

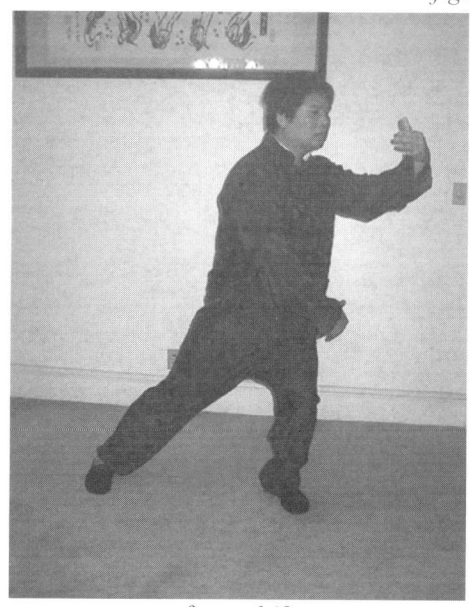

figure 149

Part 6: Right Hand Waving Like Clouds
From the preceding movement, change hands by bringing the right hand up to face level with the palm facing in and pushing the left hand down above the left knee with the palm facing in *(fig 150)*. Pick up the right foot, and step next to the left foot *(fig 151)*; then rotate the hip to the right with the body weight. The hands follow the waist to the right *(fig 152)*.

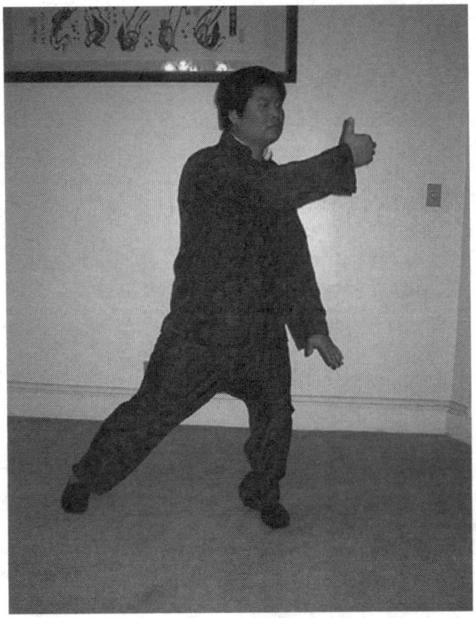

figure 150

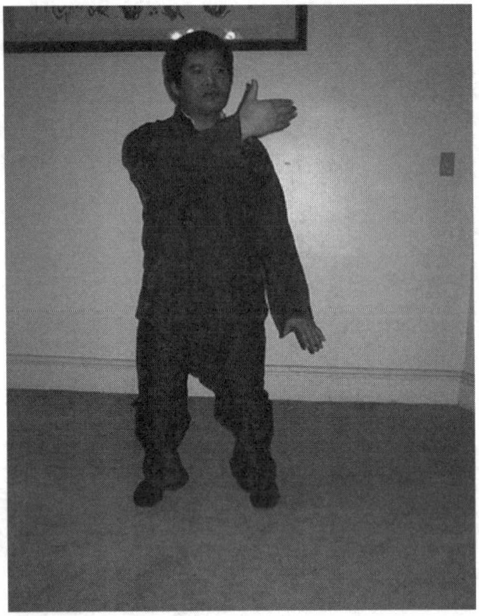

figure 151

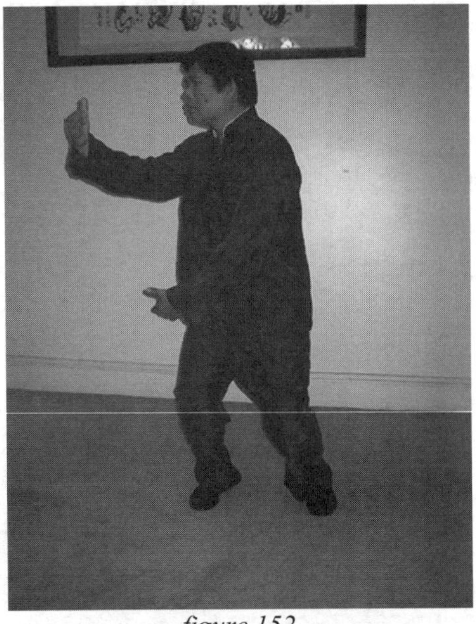

figure 152

Part 7: Left Hand Waving Like Clouds

From the preceding movement, change hands by bringing the left hand up to face level with the palm facing in and pushing the right hand down above the right knee with the palm facing in *(fig 153)*. Pick up the left foot, and step out to the left *(fig 154)*. Rotate the hip to the left. The body weight and the hands follow the waist to the left *(fig 155)*.

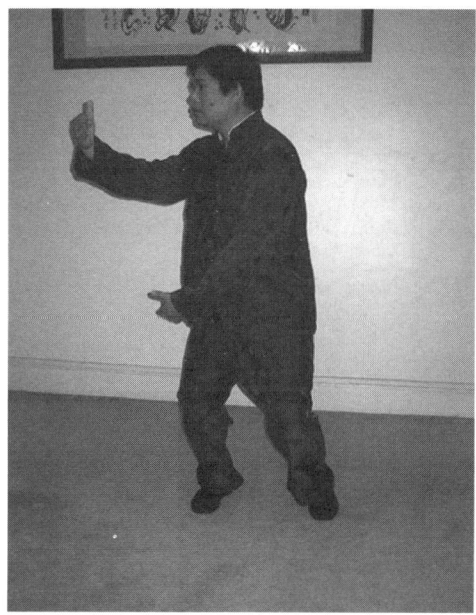

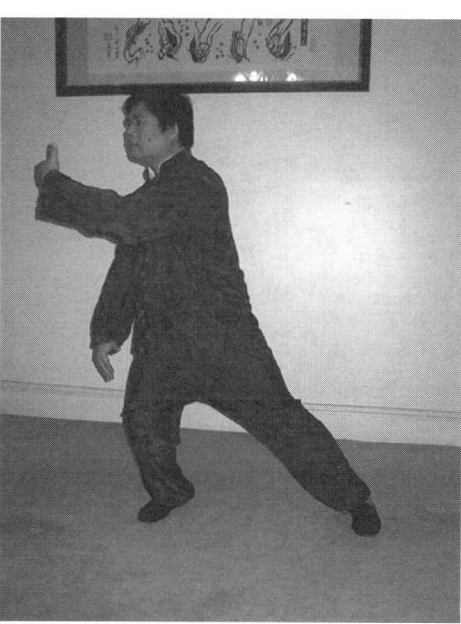

figure 153

figure 154

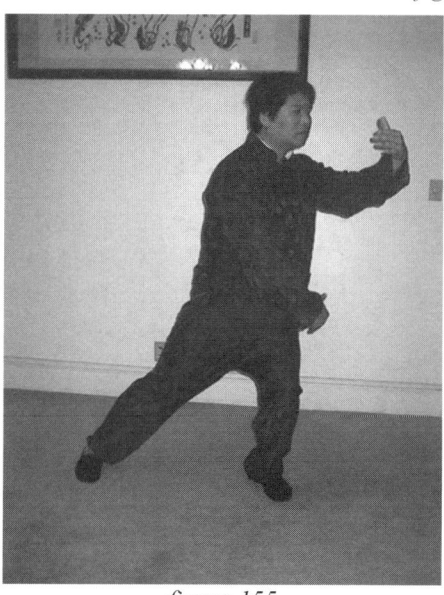

figure 155

TAI CHI CHUAN – A COMPARATIVE STUDY

Part 8: Right Hand Waving Like Clouds

From the preceding movement, change hands by bringing the right hand up to face level with the palm facing in and pushing the left hand down above the left knee with the palm facing in *(fig 156)*. Pick up the right foot, and step next to the left foot *(fig 157)*; then rotate the hip to the right. The body weight and the hands follow the waist to the right *(fig 158)*.

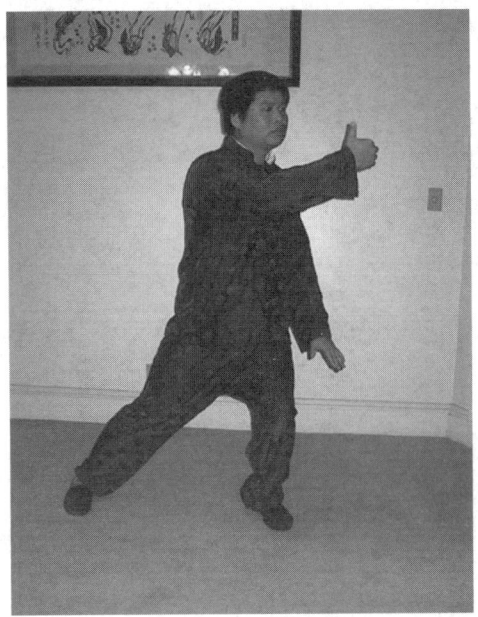

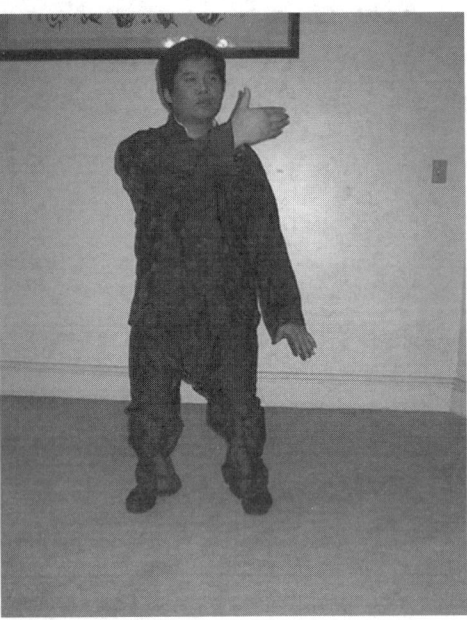

figure 156

figure 157

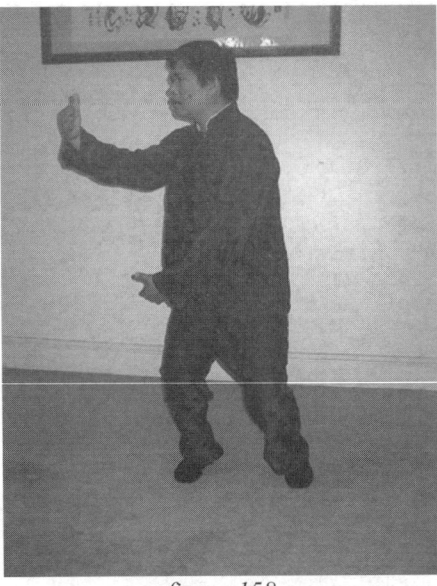

figure 158

23. Single Whip

From the preceding movement, extend the right arm outward, bringing the right fingers together to form a beak and then bending the wrist to form a hook *(fig 159)*. Turn the head, look to the left, pick up the left foot, and step to the left *(fig 160)*. Shift the body weight forward onto the left foot as the left arm moves in an arc from the right hip to the left side of the body ending at shoulder height. The palm ends up facing out. The right hook remains the same *(figs 161 & 162)*.

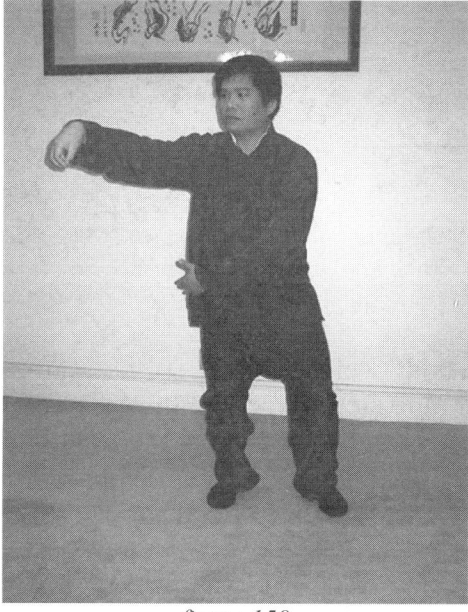

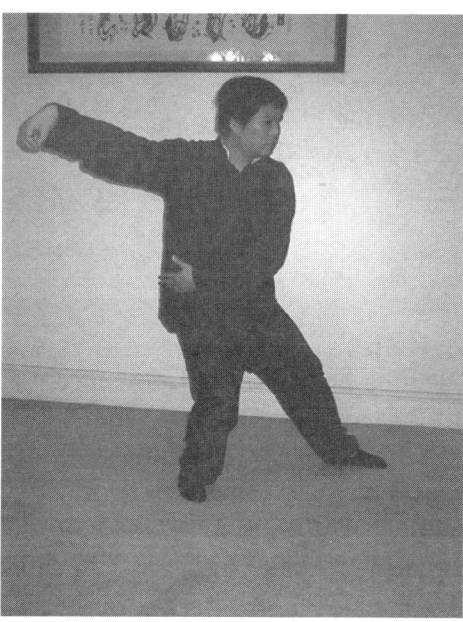

figure 159

figure 160

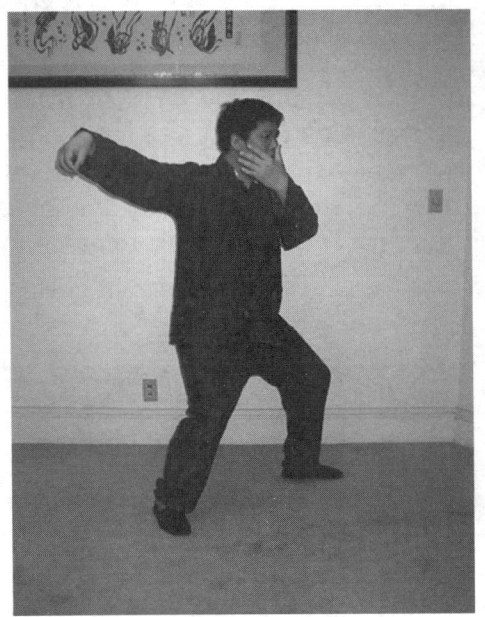

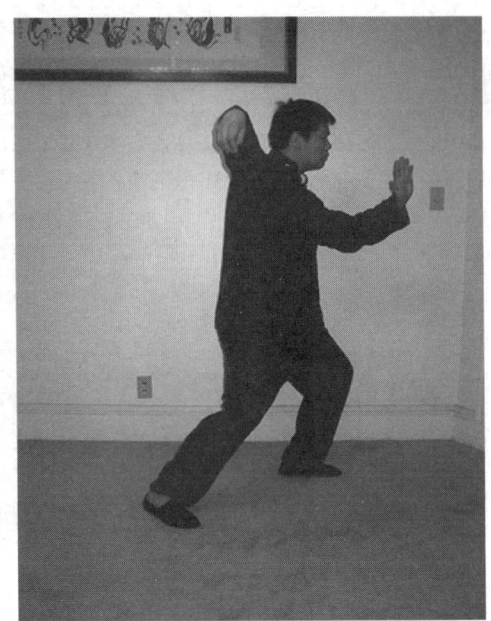

figure 161 *figure 162*

24. High Pat the Horse

From the preceding movement, with the body weight on the left foot, turn the left palm face up, pick up the right foot, and step up behind the left foot *(fig 163)*. With the body weight shifting onto the right foot, open the right hand, and bring it next to the right ear *(fig 164)*. Place the left foot on the toes. Push the right palm forward. The palm faces forward and down. At the same time, bring the left hand back onto the left side of the waist *(fig 165)*.

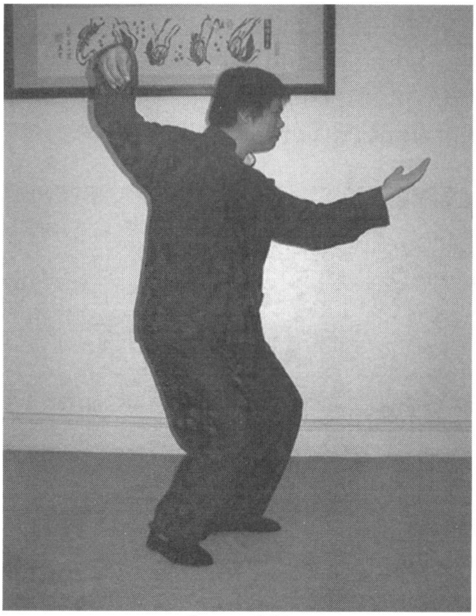

THE 43 MOVEMENT LARGE FRAME SOLO FORM

figure 163

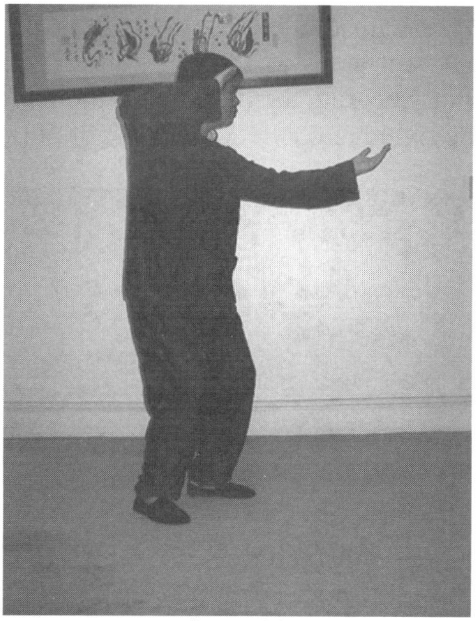

figure 164

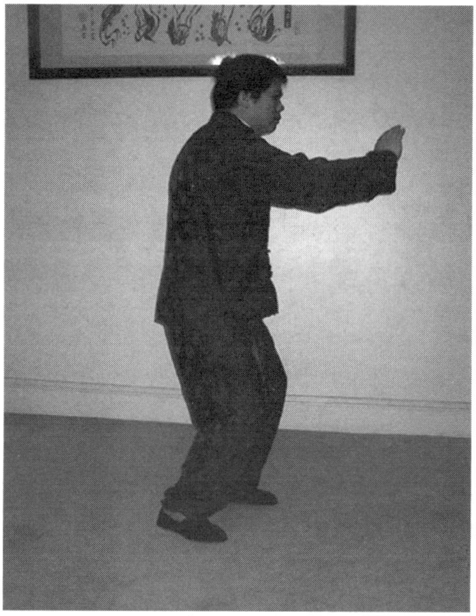

figure 165

25. Side Kicks
Part 1: Right Foot Kick
From the preceding movement, the right hand makes a clockwise circle and stops in front of the chest while the left hand makes a clockwise circle and

TAI CHI CHUAN – A COMPARATIVE STUDY

stops with the left elbow in front of the right hand palm *(figs 166 & 167)*. The left foot steps to the left corner with the body weight shifting onto the left foot. Separate the hands with the left hand coming back next to the left ear and the right hand extending straight out to the right corner *(figs 168 & 169)*.

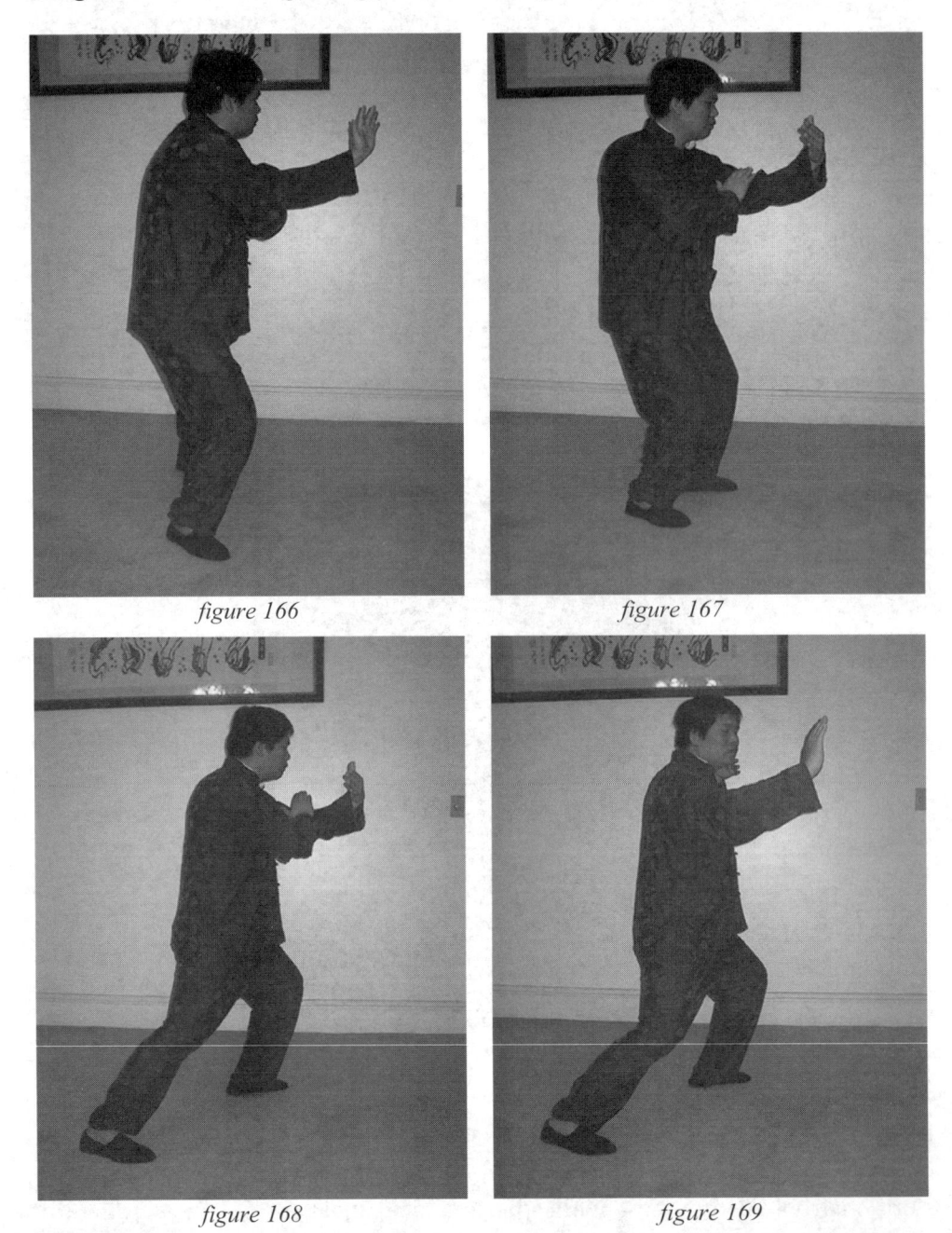

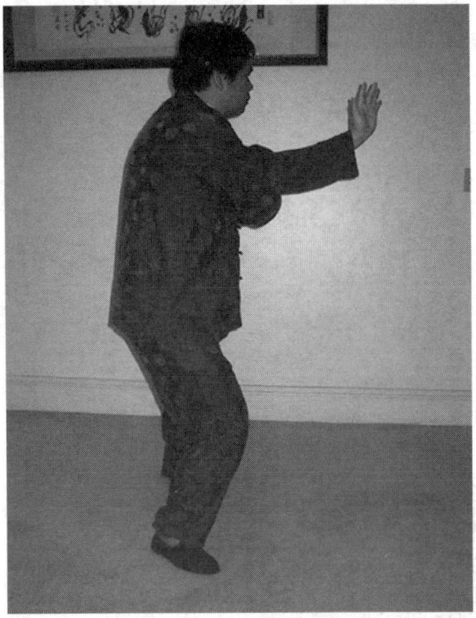

figure 166

figure 167

figure 168

figure 169

The left hand then comes under the right elbow *(fig 170)*. Separate the hands out to the sides and rejoin them in front of the right foot which steps up and lands with the toes on the ground pointing to the right corner *(fig 171)*. Rotate the arms up and out. Separate the hands with the right hand going to the right corner and the left hand going to the left corner *(figs 172 & 173)*. The body remains facing the left corner. With the body weight remaining on the left foot, raise the right leg up, and kick with the side of the foot to the right corner *(fig 174)*.

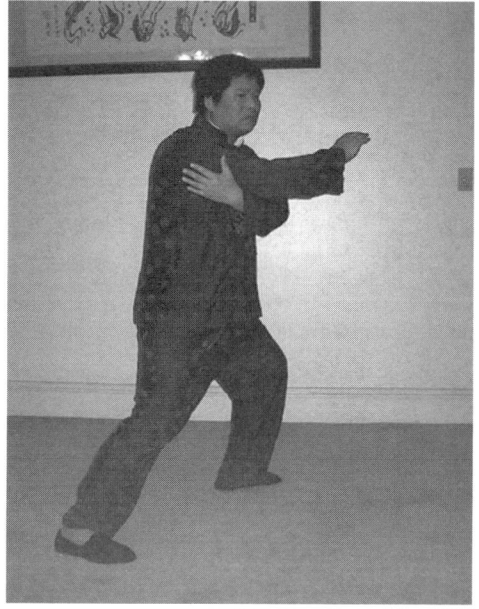

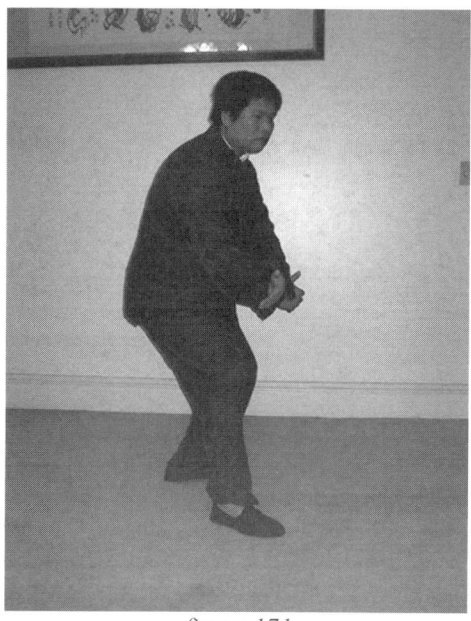

figure 170

figure 171

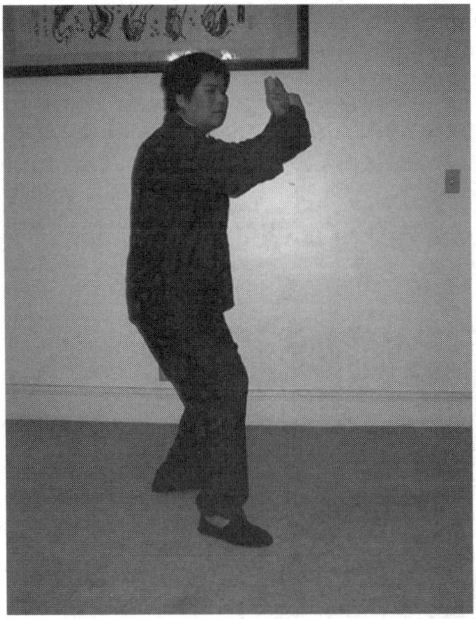

TAI CHI CHUAN – A COMPARATIVE STUDY

figure 172

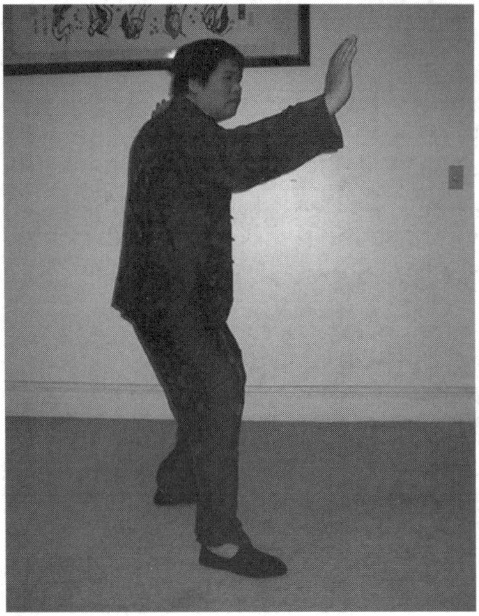

figure 173

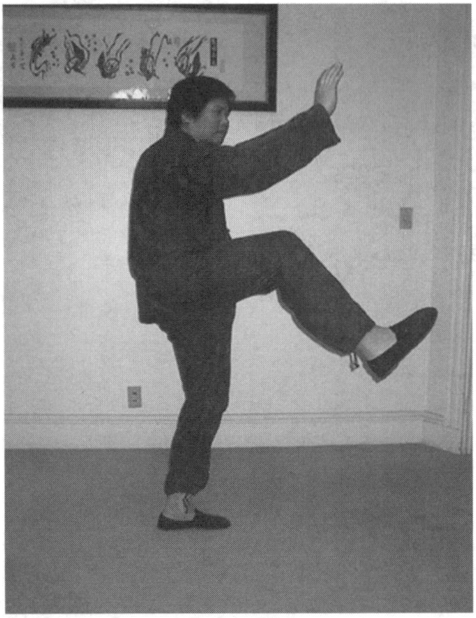

figure 174

Part 2: Left Foot Kick
From the preceding movement, bring the right foot back, suspending it next to the left foot. The body remains balanced by the left foot. Turn the body to the left while the right hand comes in front of the chest with the palm facing in *(fig

175). The right foot steps down to the right corner. Bring the left hand next to the right elbow *(fig 176)*. With the body weight shifting onto the right foot, separate the hands with the right hand going next to the right ear and the left hand going straight to the left corner *(fig 177)*. The right hand then comes under the left elbow *(fig 178)*.

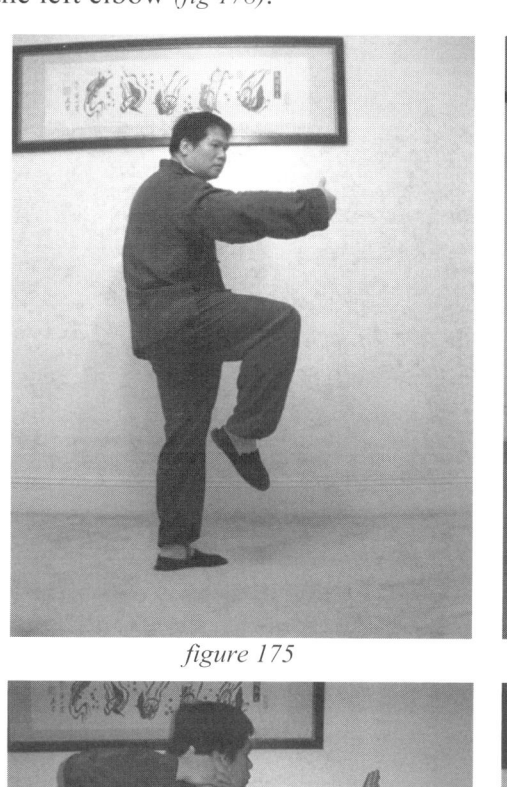

figure 175

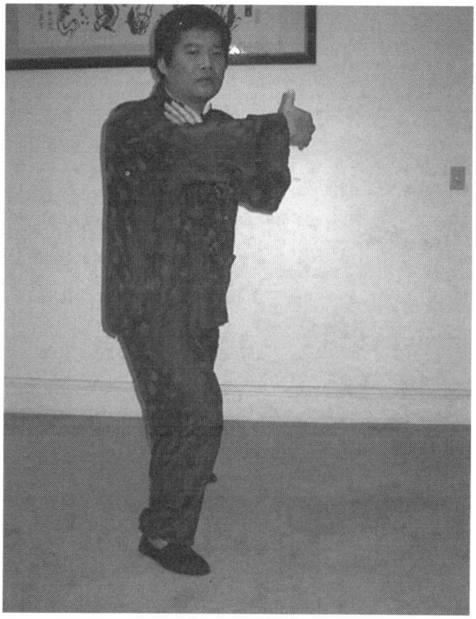

figure 176

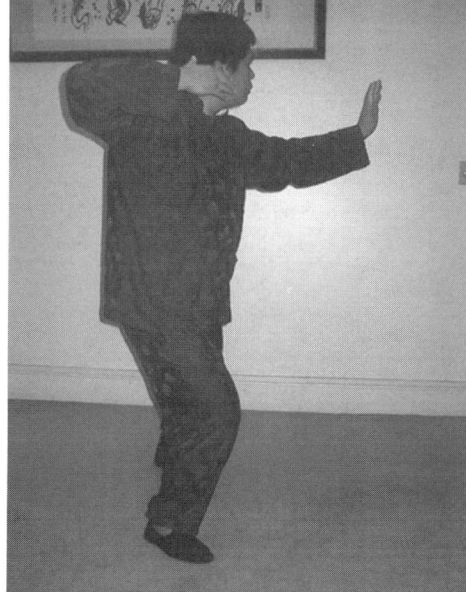

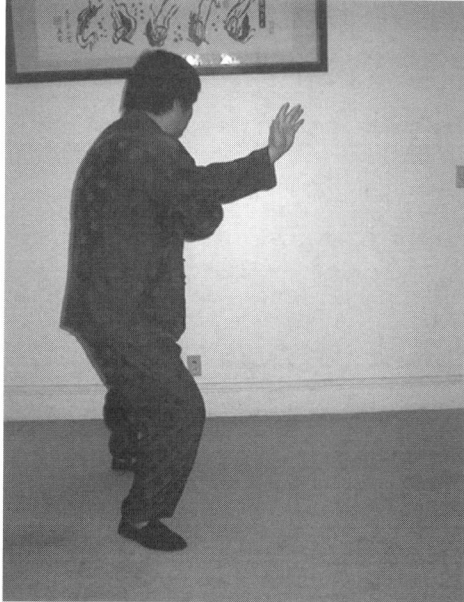

figure 177

figure 178

Separate the hands to the sides in a downward arc, and rejoin them in front of the left foot which steps up and lands with the toes on the ground pointing to the left corner *(fig 179)*. Bring the hands up, and separate them to both sides with the left hand going to the left corner and the right hand to the right *(fig 180)*. The body remains facing to the right corner. With the body weight on the right foot, raise the left leg up, and kick with the side of the foot to the left corner *(fig 181)*.

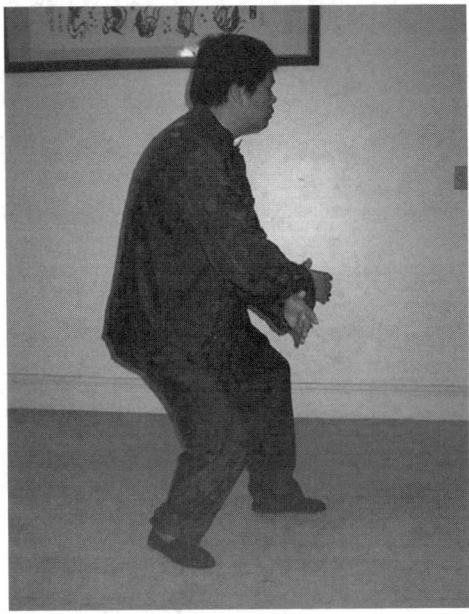

figure 179

figure 180

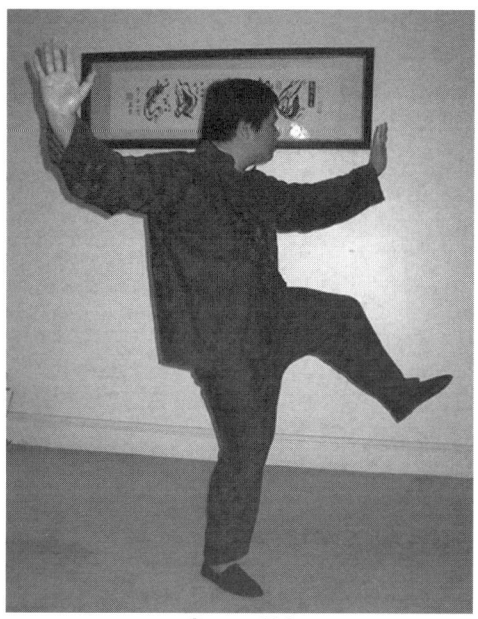

figure 181

26. Fair Lady Works on Shuttles (2 times)
Part 1: Left Corner Shuttle
From the preceding movement, the left foot comes back down next to the right leg. Turn the body to the left with the right hand crossing in front of the chest, palm facing up, and the left hand coming down to the left hip *(fig 182)*. Turn the body to the right. Simultaneously, the left hand crosses in front of the chest with the palm facing up to the right, and the right hand comes down to the right hip *(fig 183)*. The left foot steps to the left corner *(fig 184)*.

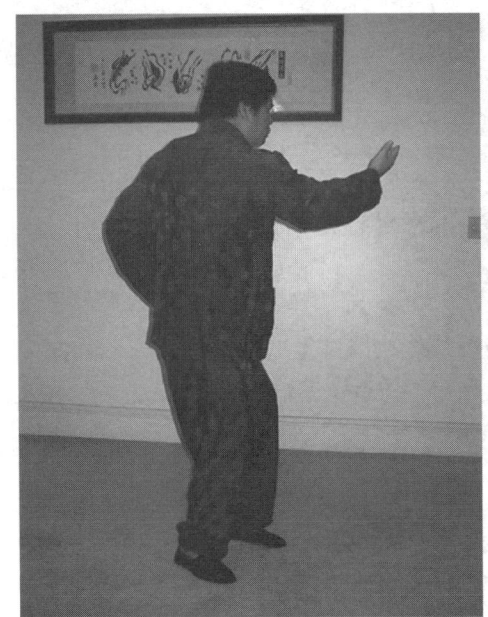

figure 182

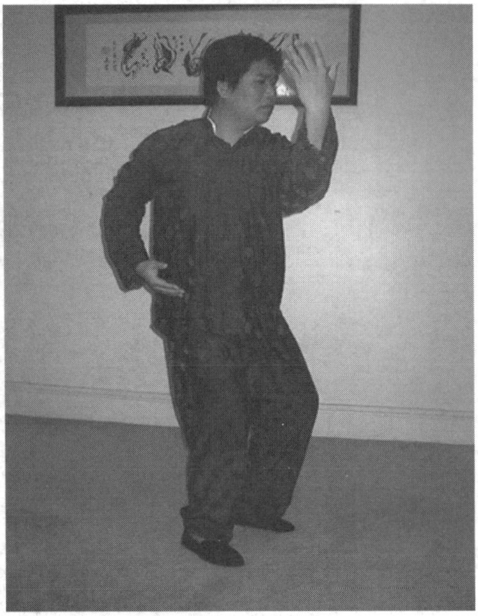

figure 183

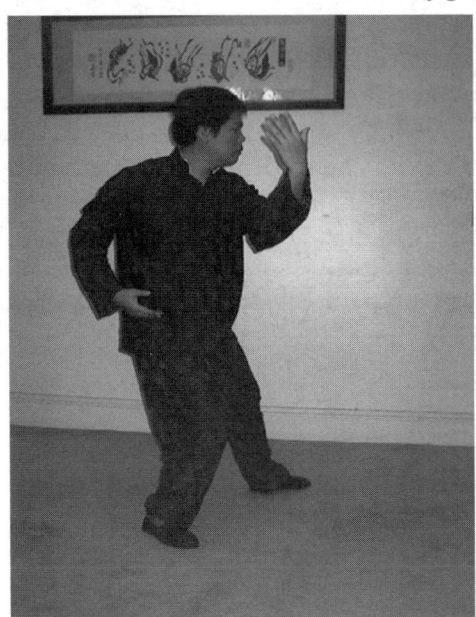

figure 184

Shift the body weight onto the left foot with the hands going forward to Ward-off *(fig 185)*. Turn the right palm face up and the left palm face down; then pull the hands down to the hip *(fig 186)*. Lift the left hand up above the head with the palm facing up and out, and push the right hand forward from the right shoulder with the body weight shifting onto the left foot *(fig 187)*.

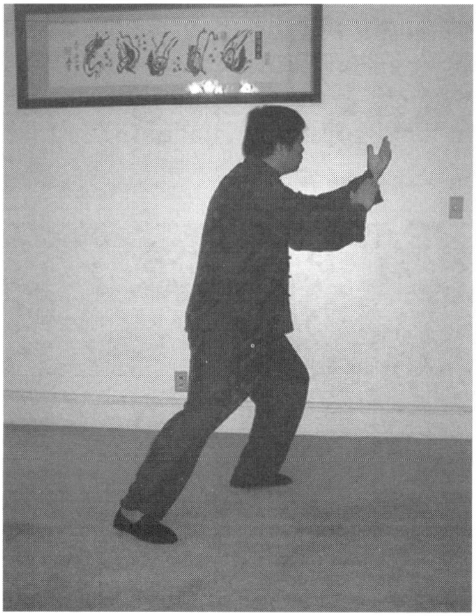

figure 185

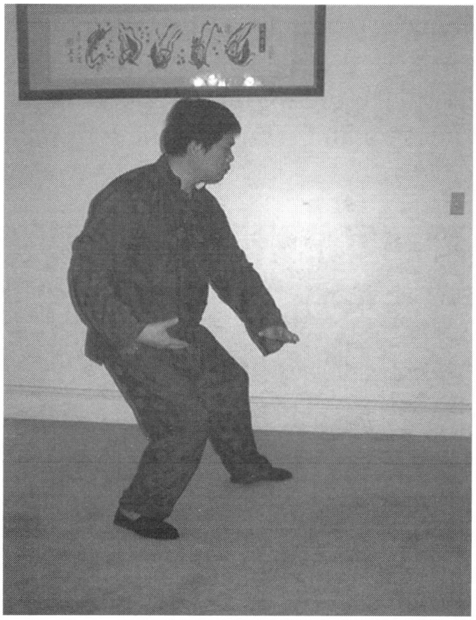

figure 186

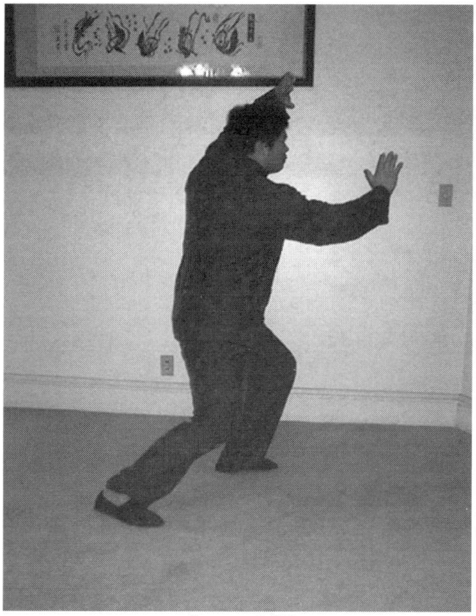

figure 187

Part 2: Right Corner Shuttle

From the preceding movement, shift the body weight backward onto the right foot, and move the hands back to the chest with the right palm next to the left elbow *(fig 188)*. Turn the left foot inward, and bring the right hand back and across to the right. At the same time, the left hand lowers and arrives under the right hand *(fig 189)*. Return the body weight to the left foot. The left hand comes up and returns to the left; the right hand goes down under the left hand *(fig 190)*.

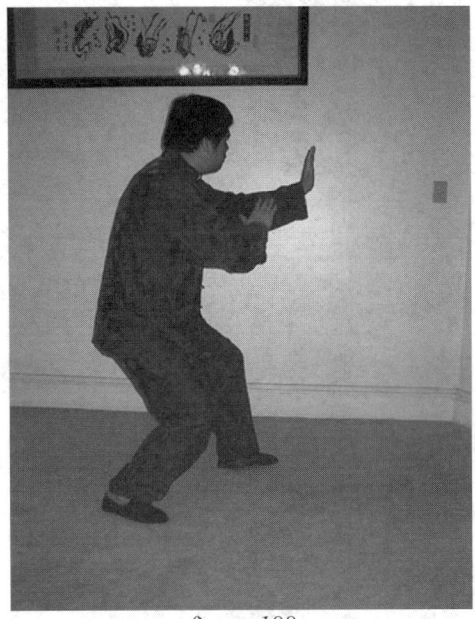

figure 188

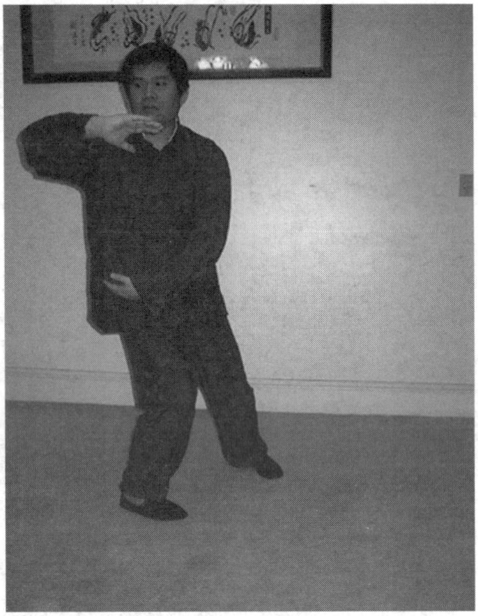

figure 189

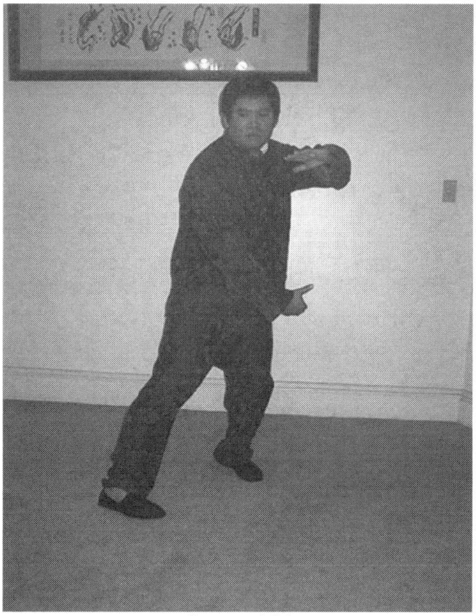

figure 190

With the body weight remaining on the left foot, turn the head, and look out to the right corner. Pick up the right foot, and step forward to the right corner while at the same time the hands are warding off forward with the right hand outside and the left hand inside *(figs 191 & 192)*. Next, turn the hands so the left palm faces up and the right palm faces down. Pull the hands down to the hip as the body weight shifts onto the left foot *(fig 193)*. Lift the right hand up above the head with the palm facing up and out while the left hand pushes forward from the left shoulder and the body weight shifts forward onto the right foot *(fig 194)*.

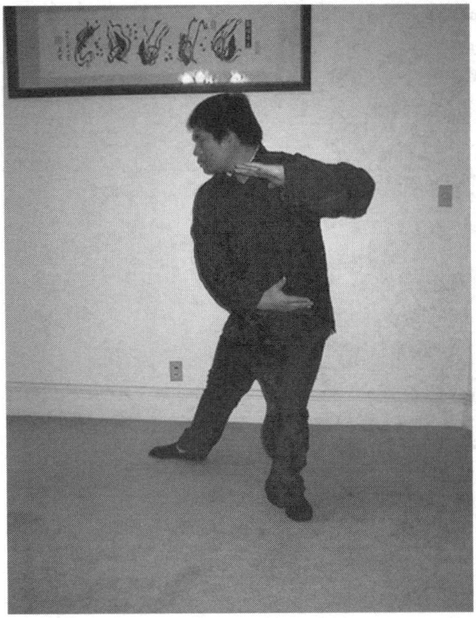

figure 191

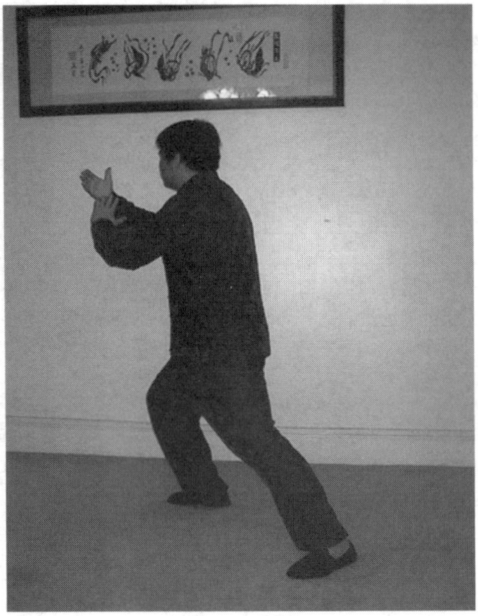

figure 192

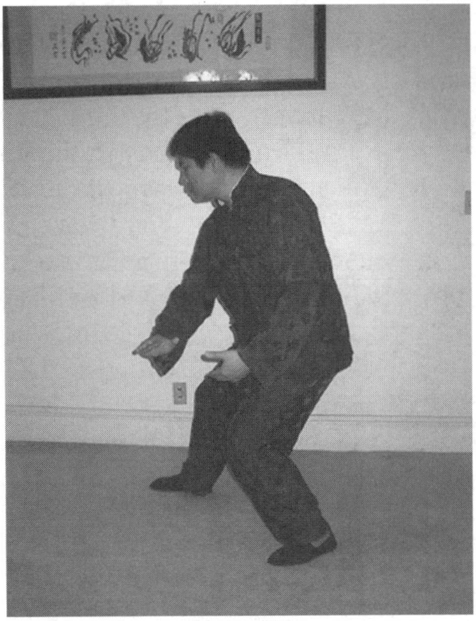

figure 193

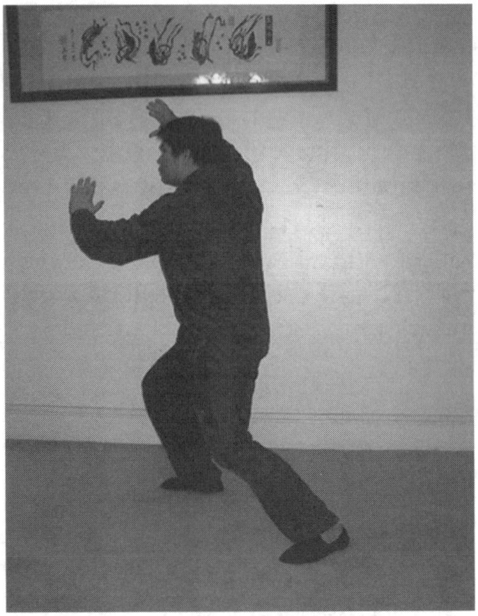

figure 194

27. Left Hand Warding Off

From the preceding movement, bring the right hand down in front of the body with the left hand coming back next to the right elbow and the body weight shifting back onto the left foot *(fig 195)*. Rotate the waist to the left with the hands facing down and the body weight remaining on the left foot *(fig 196)*. Shift the body weight onto the right foot, and separate the hands with the right hand coming up to the chest and the left hand going down above the right knee *(fig 197)*. With the body weight on the right foot, pick up the left foot, and step forward. Then shift the body weight forward onto the left foot, and at the same time, separate the hands, with the left hand coming up to face level and the right hand going down to the right side of the body with the palm facing down *(fig 198)*.

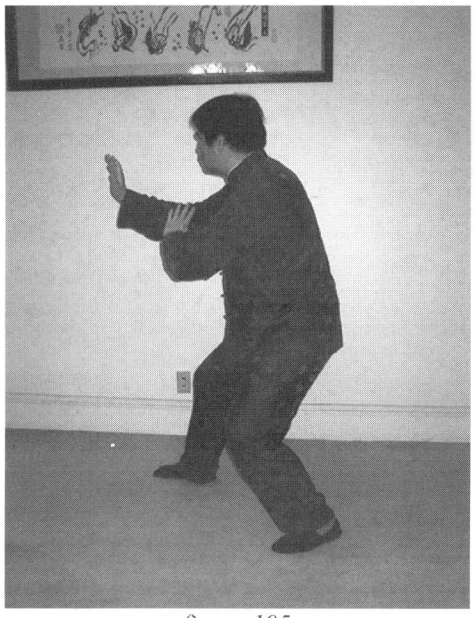

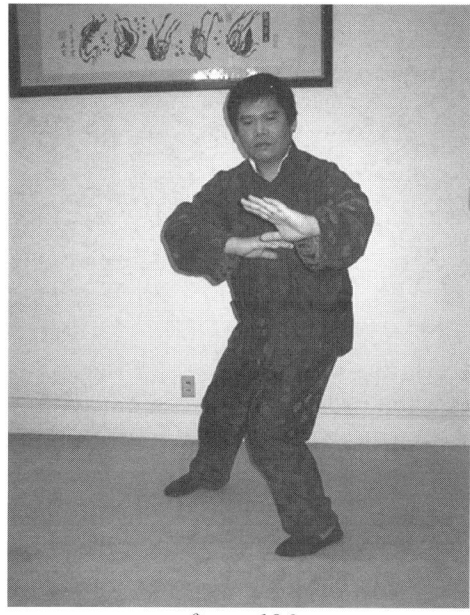

figure 195

figure 196

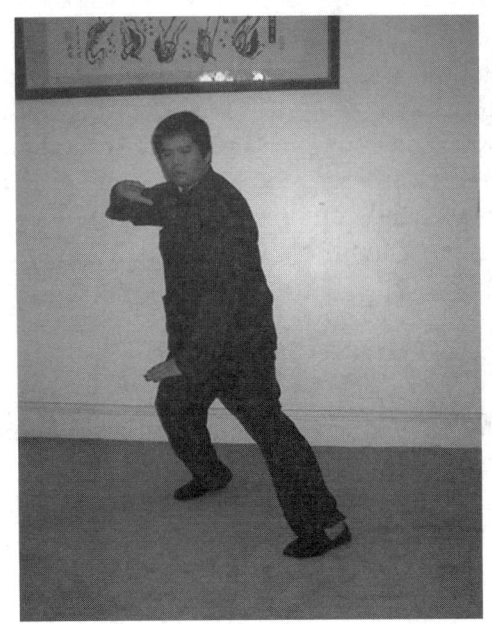

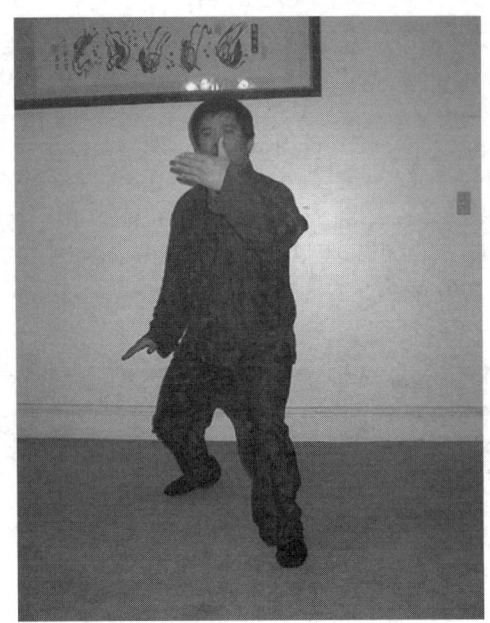

figure 197 *figure 198*

28. Right Foot Kick

From the preceding movement with the body weight on the left foot, turn the left foot inward; at the same time, the left hand makes a complete clockwise circle and ends with the palm face down *(fig 199)*. Bring the right hand over the left hand; then make a complete counter clockwise circle and end with the right wrist under the left. Move the right foot forward. The right foot lands with the toes on the ground *(figs 200 & 201)*. Separate the hands with the right hand going to the front and the left hand going to the back *(fig 202)*. With the body weight on the left foot, pick up the right foot and kick forward with the heel *(fig 203)*.

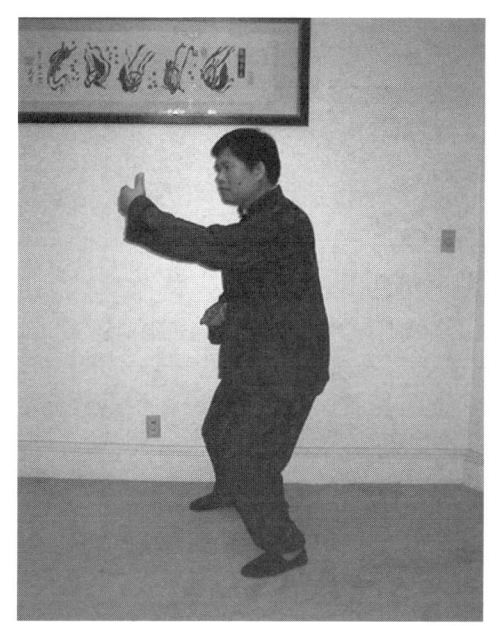

figure 199

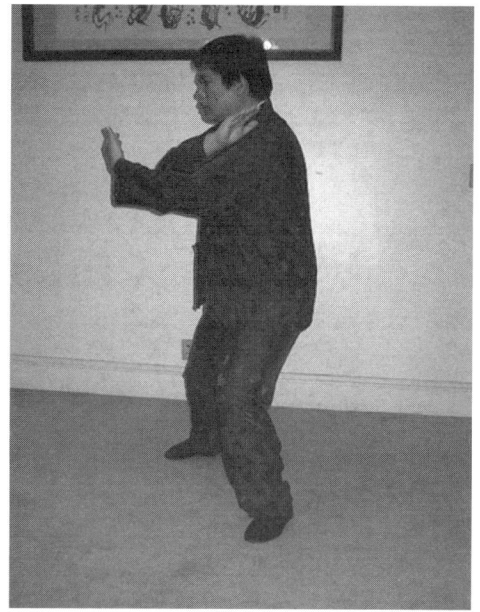

figure 200

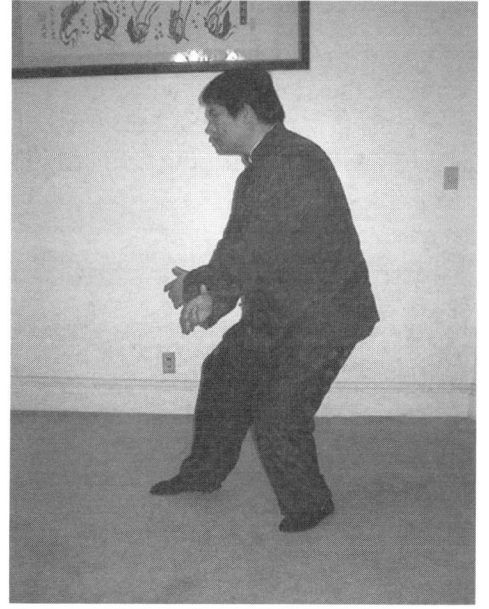

figure 201

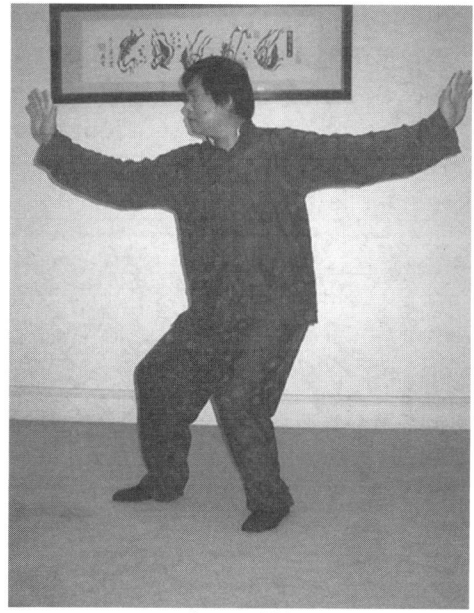

figure 202

TAI CHI CHUAN – A COMPARATIVE STUDY

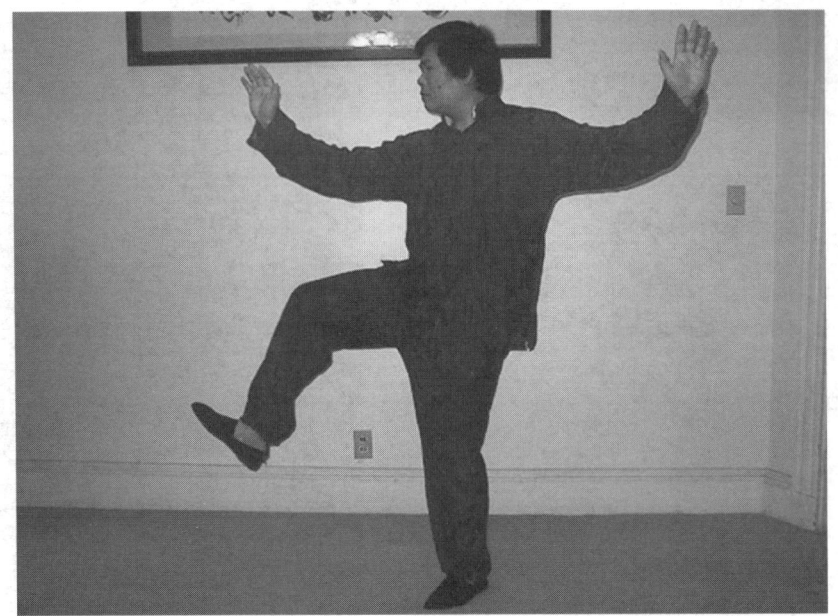

figure 203

29. Hitting Tiger

From the preceding movement, the right foot steps down, and the left hand moves across the chest with the palm face up as the right hand goes down to the hip *(fig 204)*. The left foot steps to the left *(fig 205)*. Shift the body weight onto the left foot as the right hand moves across the body with the arm straight and the left hand comes to the left hip *(fig 206)*.

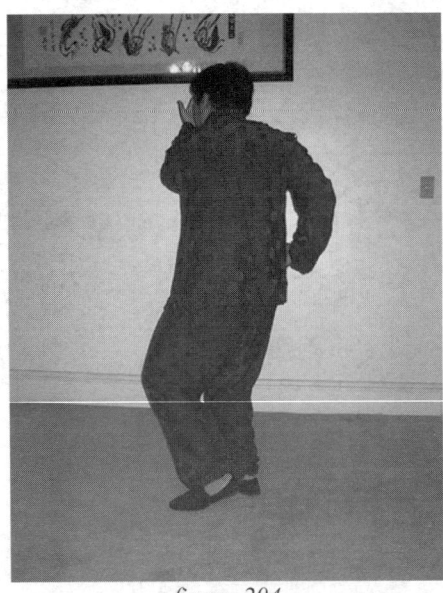

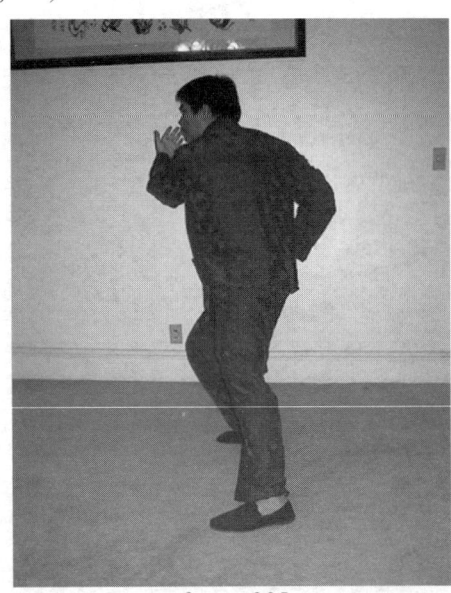

figure 204   *figure 205*

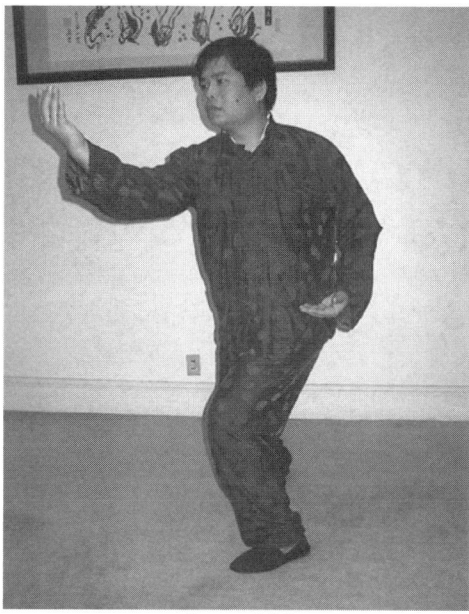

figure 206

Shift the body weight onto the right foot while the right hand comes to the right hip and the left hand crosses the body to the right *(fig 207)*. Close the hands into fists; then shift the body weight onto the left foot while moving the hands to the left, setting the left fist above the head and the right fist at the chest *(fig 208)*.

TAI CHI CHUAN – A COMPARATIVE STUDY

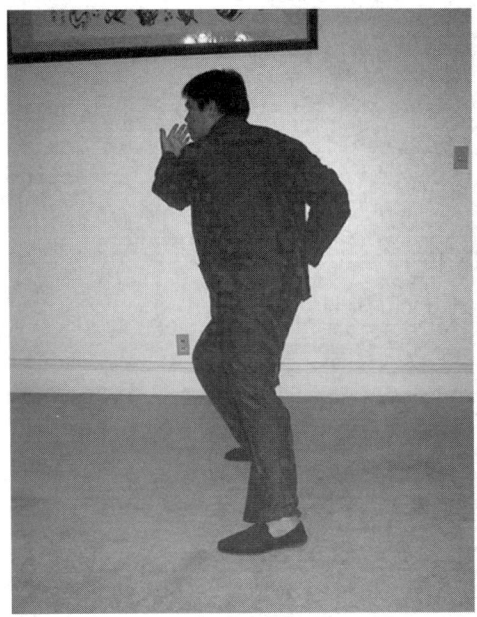

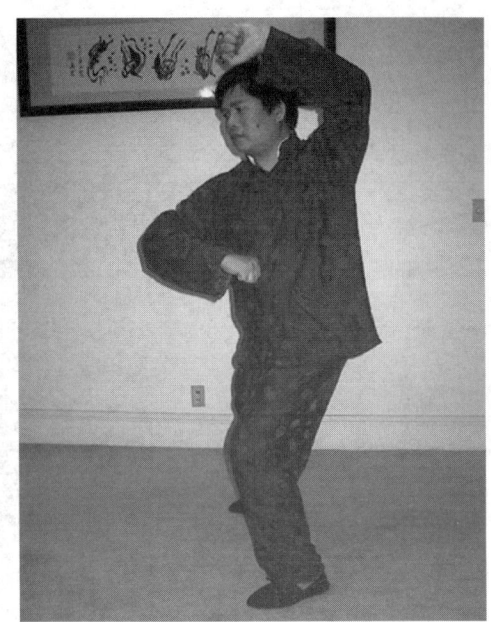

figure 207   *figure 208*

30. Hit the Ears with Two Fists

From the preceding movement, open the fists, and shift the body weight onto the right foot, pushing the hands forward to the corner *(fig 209)*. Turn the palms to face up; then pull the hands down, and shift the body weight back onto the left foot *(fig 210)*.

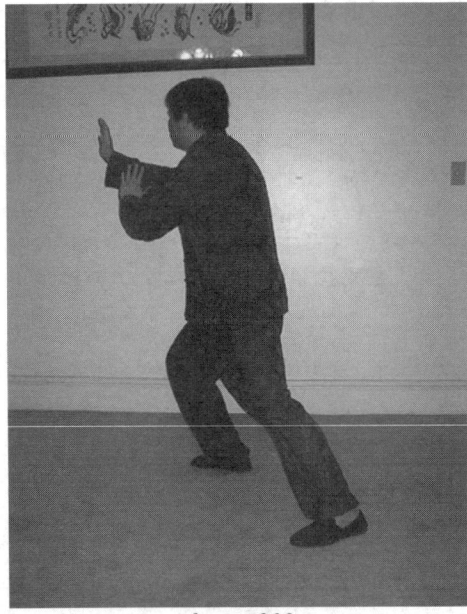

figure 209   *figure 210*

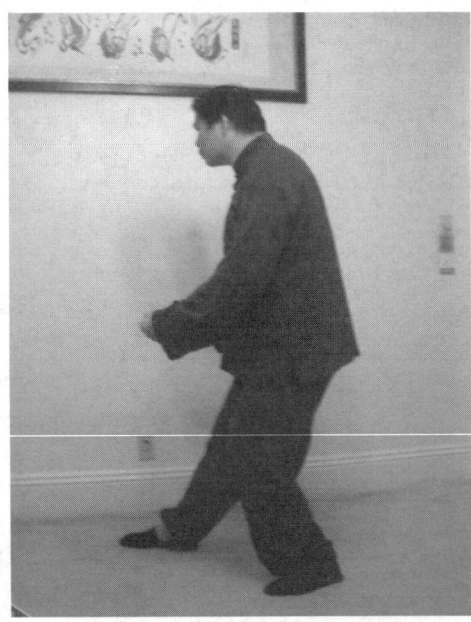

Raise the right knee up to the chest while pulling the hands down to each side of the right knee *(fig 211)*. The right foot steps forward to the right corner and the palms close into fists. Shift the body weight onto the right foot, bringing the fists up to ear level as the body weight arrives on the right foot *(figs 212 & 213)*.

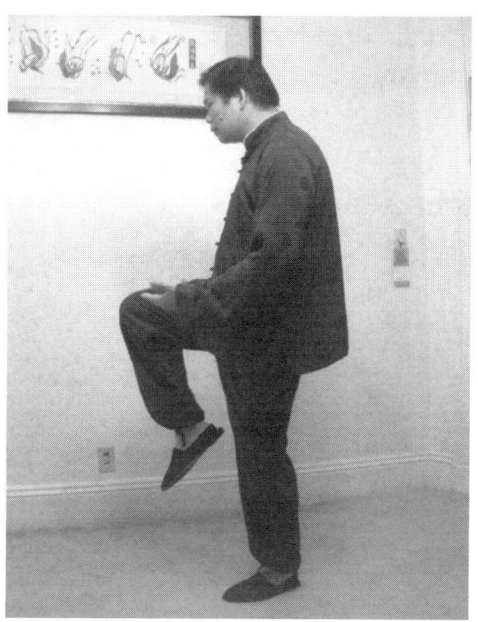

figure 211

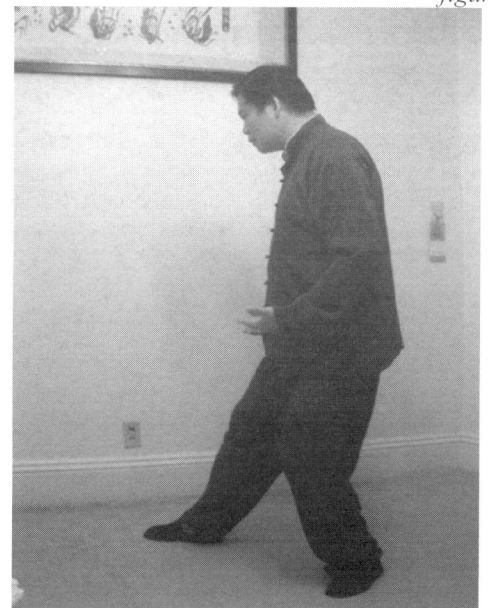

figure 212

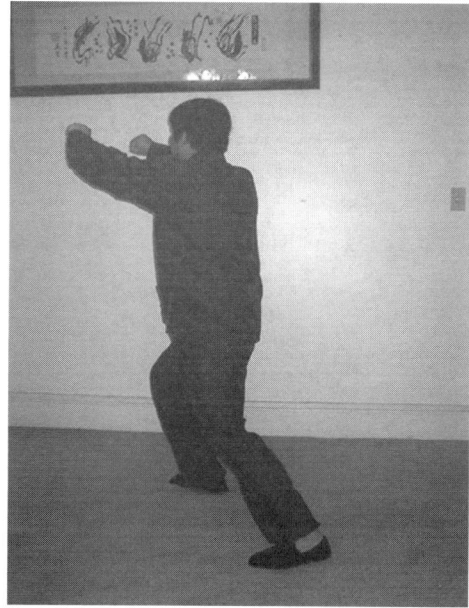

figure 213

31. Left Foot Kick

From the preceding movement, the left foot steps forward and lands on the toes; open the fists, and bring them down on top of the left knee, wrists crossing and palms facing in *(figs 214 & 215 show the same move from different angles)*. With the hands remaining crossed, bring them up in front of the face. The right hand is outside the left hand and the palms face in. Rotate the arms so the palms face out; then separate the hands with the left hand going to the front and the right hand going to the back *(fig 216)*. With the body weight still on the right foot, pick up the left foot and kick forward with the heel *(fig 217)*.

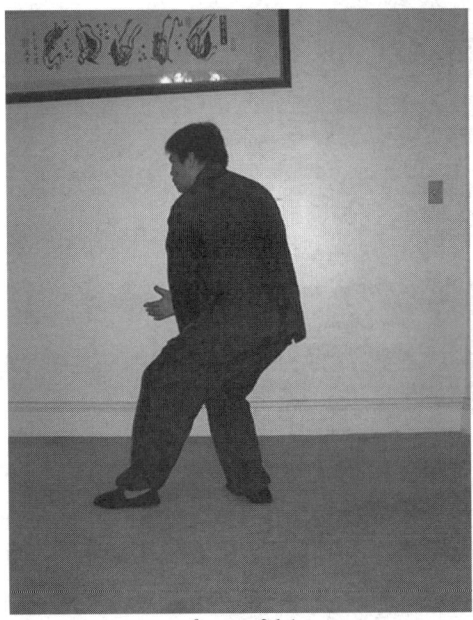

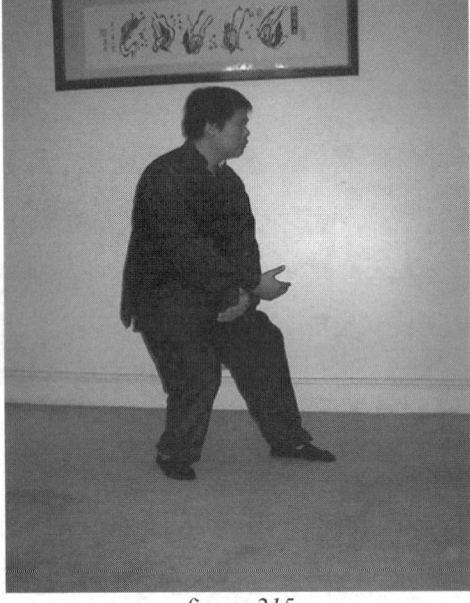

figure 214   *figure 215*

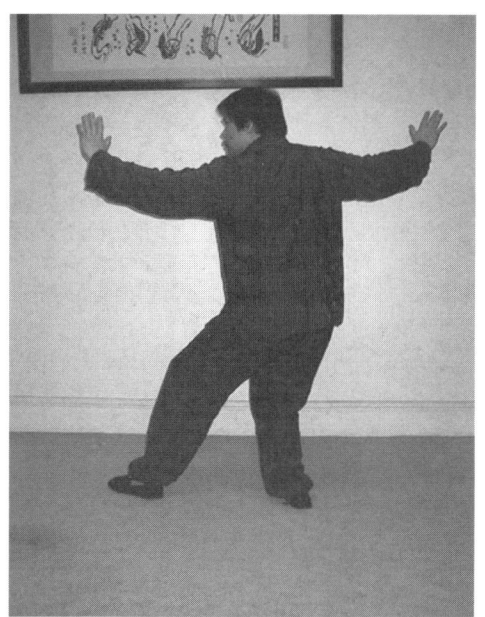

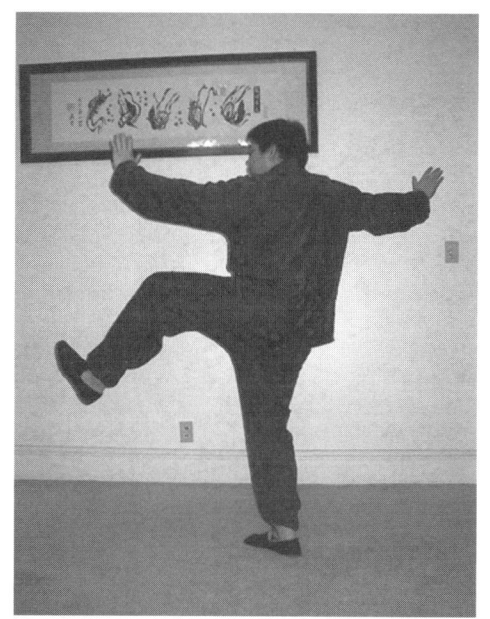

figure 216 *figure 217*

32. Brush Knee with Twist Step (2 times)
Part 1: Left Hand Brush Knee
From the preceding movement, the left foot steps down onto the toes, and the right hand moves across the chest. The left hand comes down to the hip, and the body turns to the left *(fig 218)*. Turn the body to the right with the body weight remaining on the right foot; the right hand moves down to the right hip, and the left hand comes up, moving across the chest with the palm facing in *(fig 219)*. The right hand then comes up next to the right ear, and the left hand arrives below it. Pick up the left foot, and step forward *(fig 220)*. As the left hand brushes down to outside the left knee and the right palm pushes forward to the center of the chest, shift the weight forward onto the left foot *(fig 221)*.

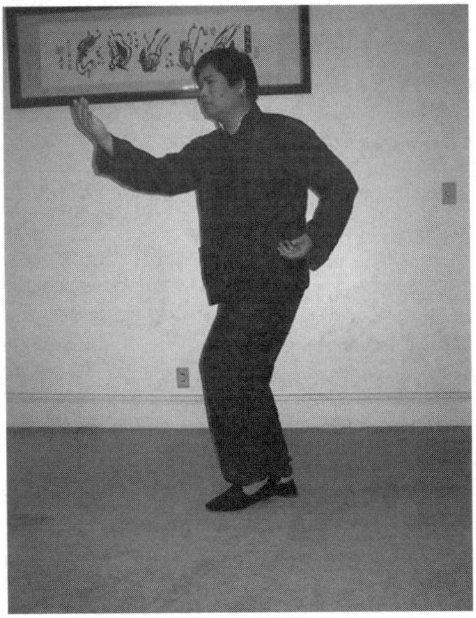

TAI CHI CHUAN – A COMPARATIVE STUDY

figure 218

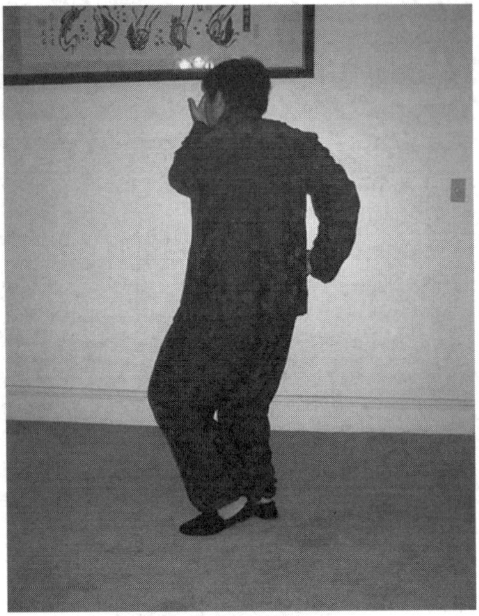

figure 219

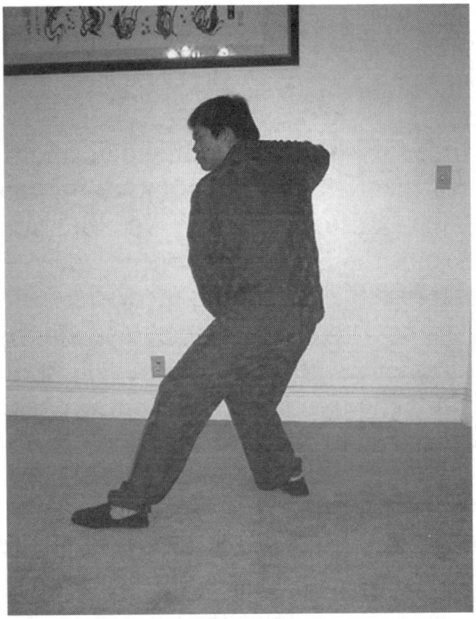

figure 220

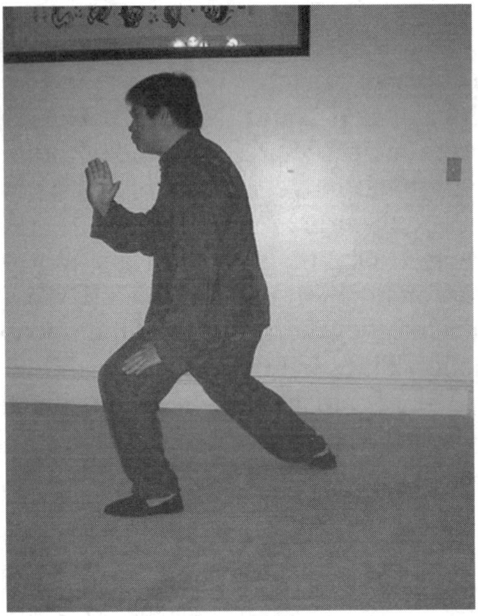

figure 221

Part 2: Right Hand Brush Knee
From the preceding movement, turn the left toes out; the left hand comes up next to the left ear, and the right hand comes up next to the left hand with the palm facing in *(fig 222)*. Pick up the right foot, and step forward *(fig 223)*. Shift

the weight forward as the right hand brushes down to outside the right knee, and the left palm pushes forward to the center of the chest *(fig 224)*.

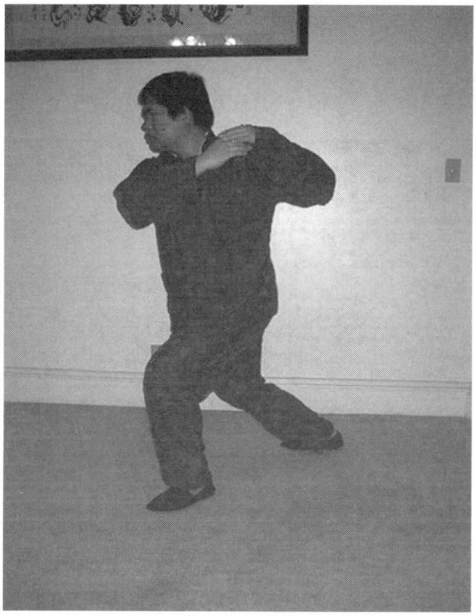

figure 222

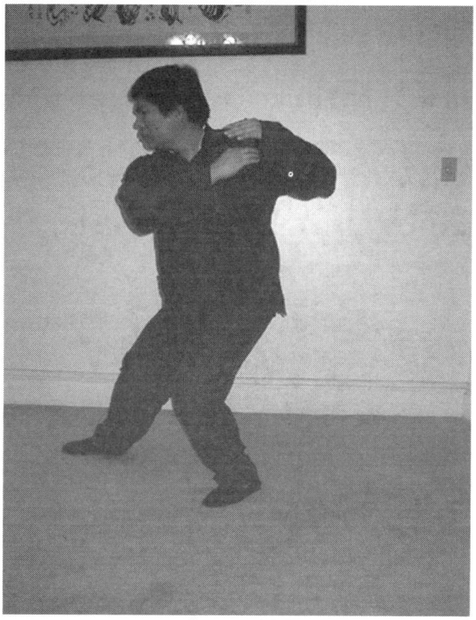

figure 223

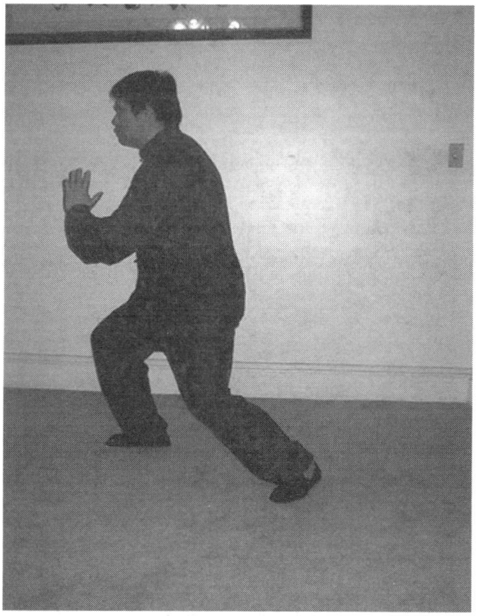

figure 224

33. Step Forward and Punch Down

From the preceding movement, turn the right toes out; the right hand comes up next to the right ear, and the left hand comes up under the right hand with the palm facing in *(fig 225)*. Pick up the left foot, and step forward *(fig 226)*. As the weight shifts forward, the left hand brushes down to outside the left knee, and the right hand closes into a fist and punches downward *(fig 227)*.

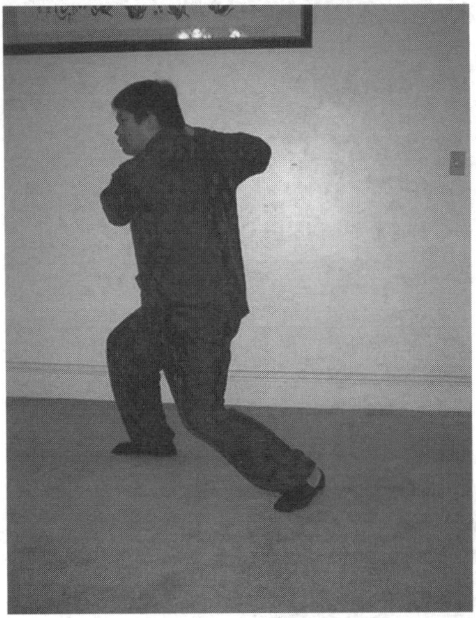

figure 225

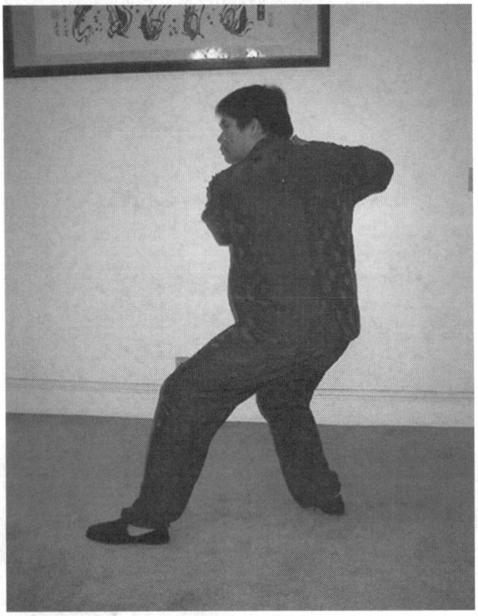

figure 226

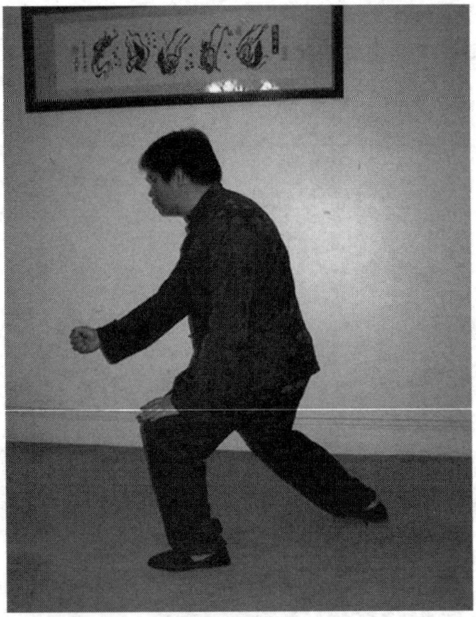

figure 227

34. Step Forward Grasp Sparrow's Tail
Part 1: Right Hand Warding Off

From the preceding movement, turn out the left toes, and open the right fist. With the body weight still on the left foot, the left hand comes up to the left ear, palm facing in. Pick up the right foot, and step forward *(fig 228)*. Shift the body weight onto the right foot, and bring both hands up to face level; the right palm faces in, and the left palm faces out *(fig 229)*.

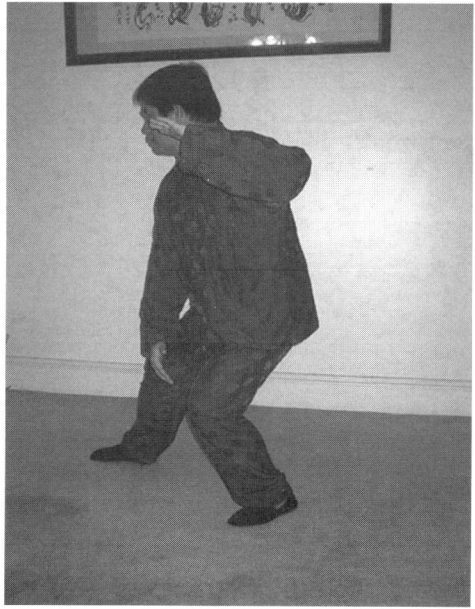

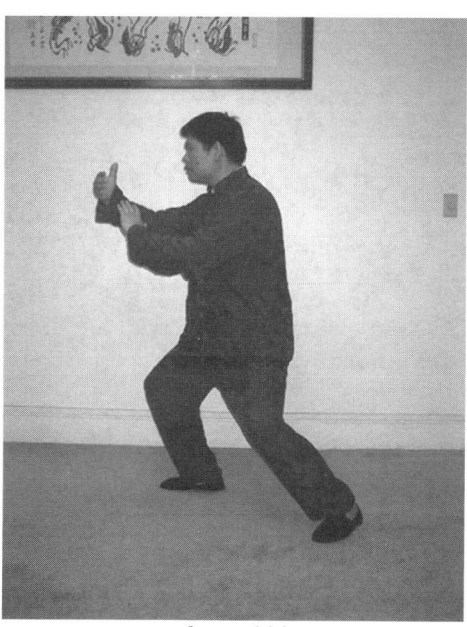

figure 228   *figure 229*

Part 2: Roll Back

From the preceding movement, turn both palms so that the left palm faces up and the right palm faces down *(fig 230)*. Bring the hands back to the left side of the hip, and at the same time, shift the body weight onto the left foot *(fig 231)*.

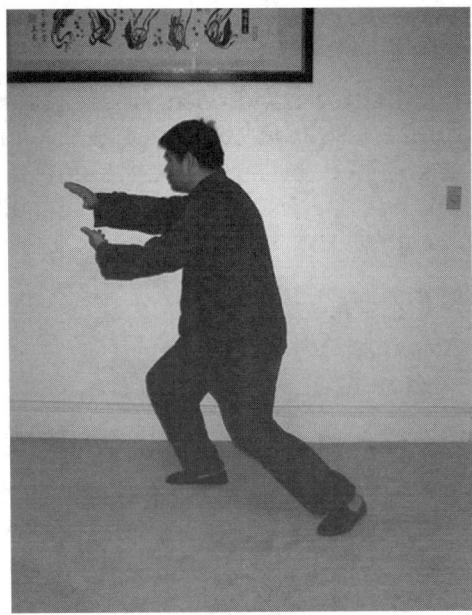

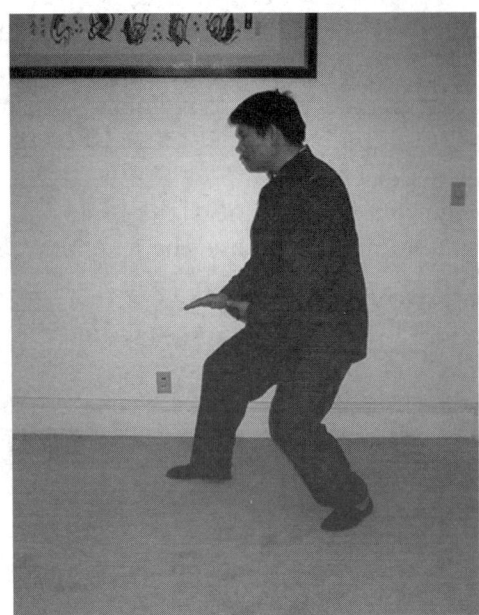

figure 230 *figure 231*

Part 3: Press
From the preceding movement, turn the left palm face down and the right palm face up, bringing the left above the right. The left hand sticks to the right wrist *(fig 232)*. Press the hands forward with the body weight shifting onto the right foot *(fig 233)*.

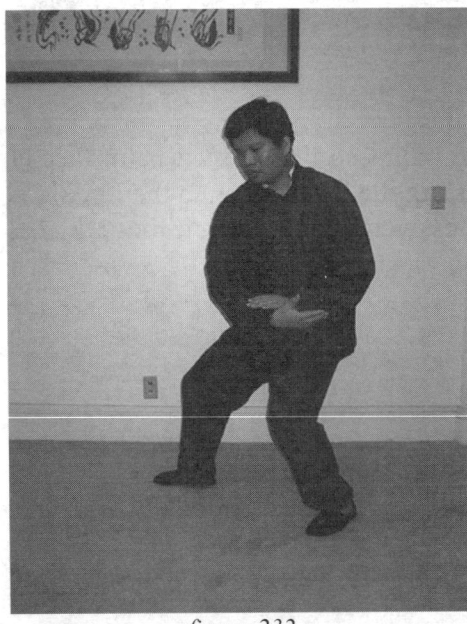

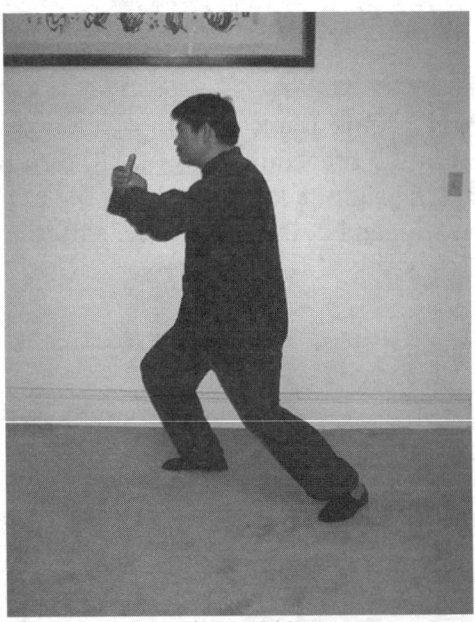

figure 232 *figure 233*

Part 4: Push

From the preceding movement, turn the palms face down, the left palm on top of the right, and bring them directly back to the chest with the palms facing down and the weight shifting onto the left foot *(figs 234 & 235)*. Separate the two hands at the chest with the wrists bent and the palms facing forward in front of the shoulders *(fig 236)*. Push the hands forward with the body weight shifting onto the right foot *(fig 237)*.

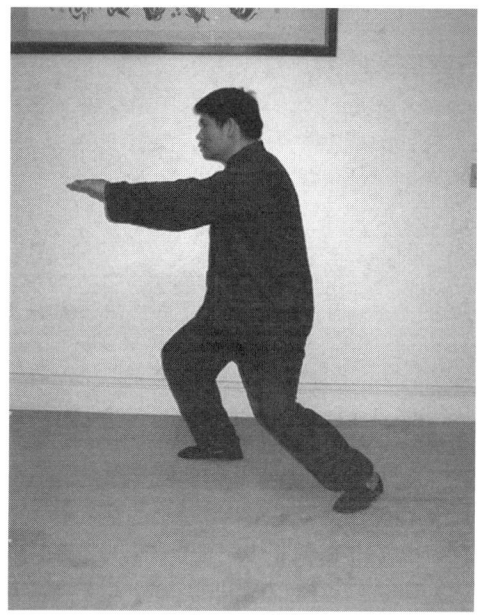

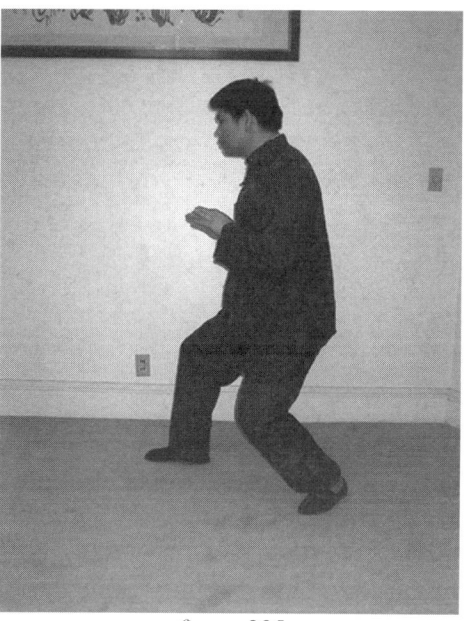

figure 234

figure 235

TAI CHI CHUAN – A COMPARATIVE STUDY

figure 236　　　　　　　　　　　*figure 237*

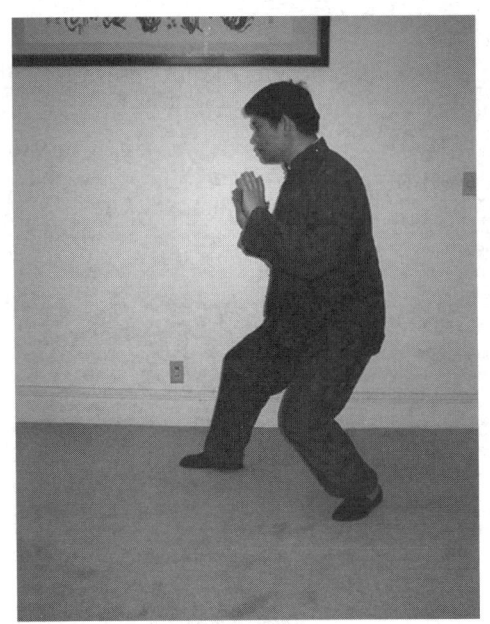

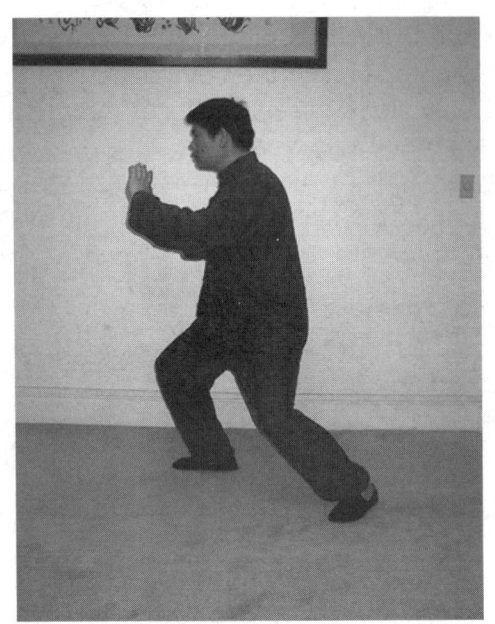

35. Single Whip

From the preceding movement, rotate the waist as the hands move in a complete counter clockwise circle over the head with the body weight shifting first onto the left foot *(figs 238 & 239)* then back onto the right foot *(fig 240)*. As the right fingers press together to form a beak, bend the wrist to form the hook. Extend the right arm, and set the left hand at the right hip with the palm facing in *(fig 241)*. Turn the head to the left, pick up the left foot, and step forward to the left *(fig 242)*. With the body weight shifting onto the left foot, move the left arm up and out to the left *(fig 243)*. Then with the body weight on the left foot, turn the left palm to face forward while the right hand hook remains the same *(fig 244)*.

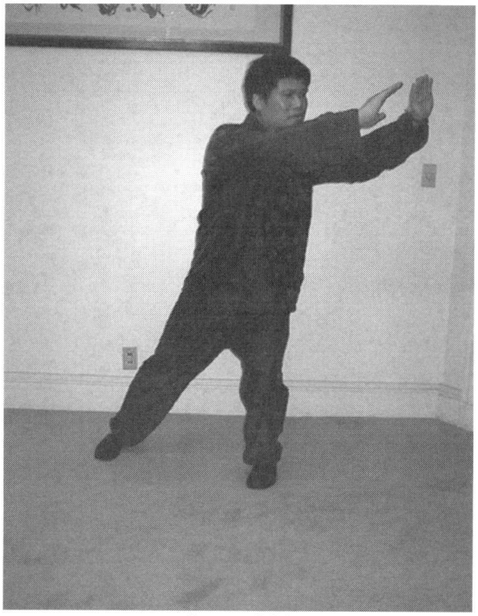

THE 43 MOVEMENT LARGE FRAME SOLO FORM

figure 238

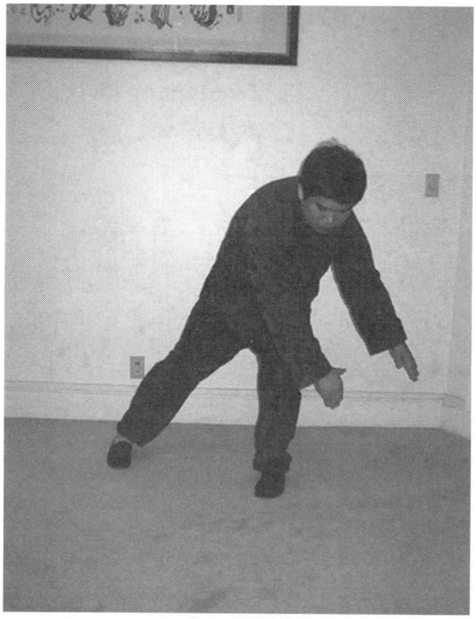

figure 239

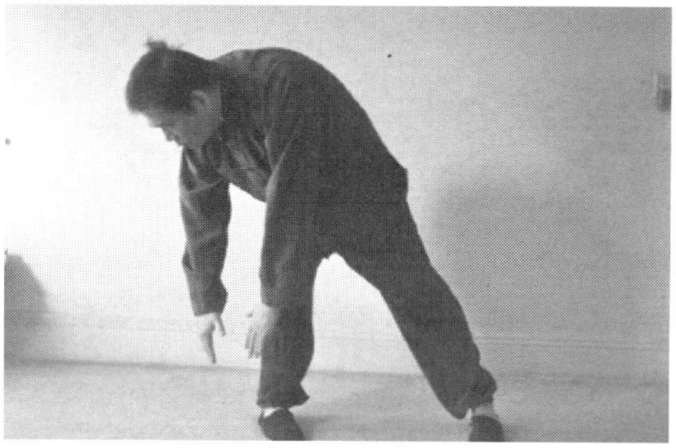

figure 240

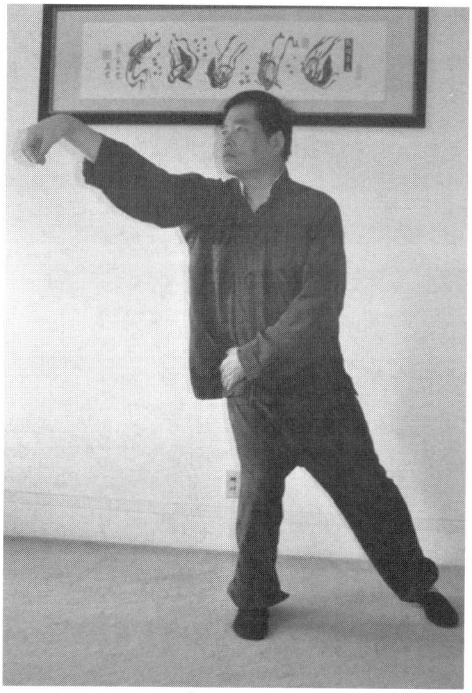

figure 241

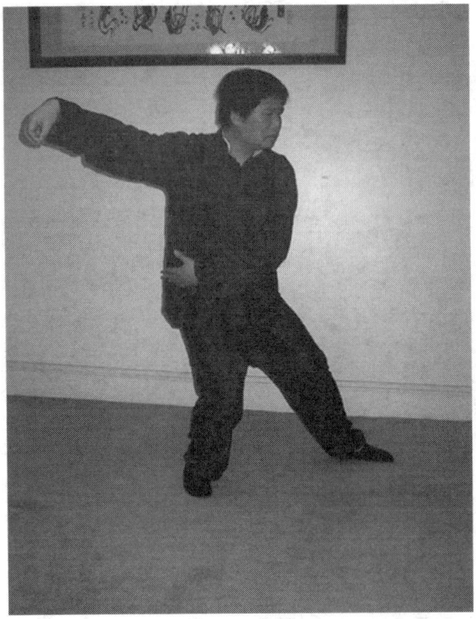

TAI CHI CHUAN – A COMPARATIVE STUDY

figure 242

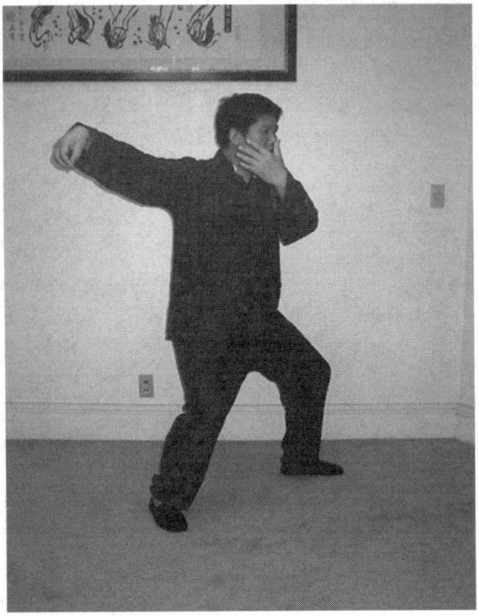

figure 243

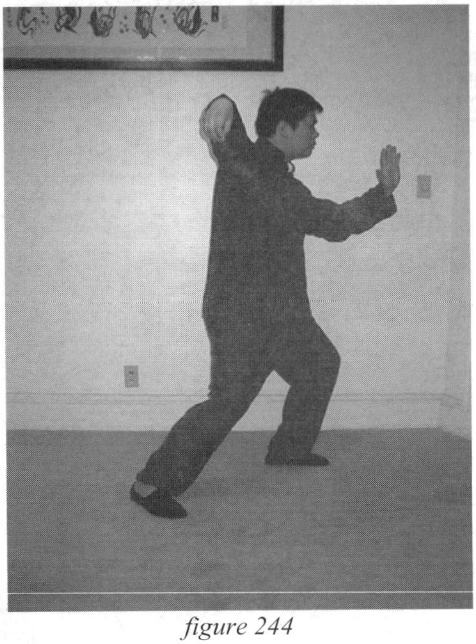

figure 244

36. Lower the Snake Body

From the preceding movement, turn the left palm to face up and the right toes out *(fig 245)*. Lower the body by lowering onto the right leg. Bring the left hand down to the left foot with the palm still facing up. The right hand remains the same *(fig 246)*.

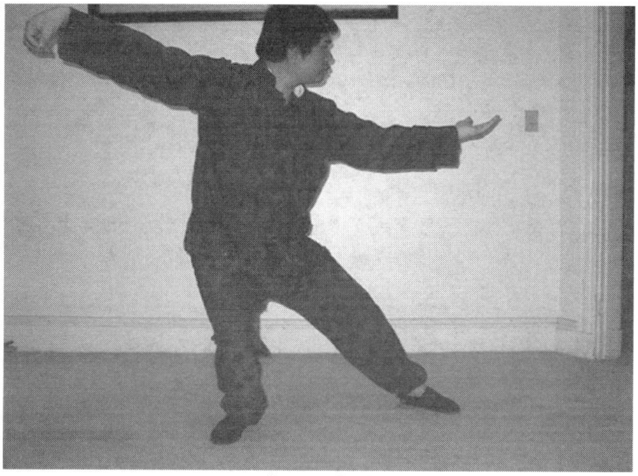

figure 245

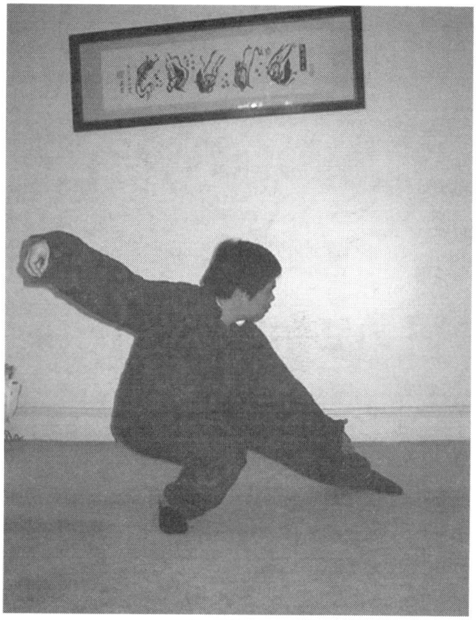

figure 246

37. Step Forward to become Seven Star

From the preceding movement, the body goes forward, shifting the weight onto the left foot. Open the right hand, and let it go forward to cross at the left wrist *(figs 247 & 248)*. Shift the body weight back onto the right foot, and pull the hands back to the hips. The left and right hands close to form fists *(fig 249)*. Turn the left toes out, shift the body weight onto the left foot again, pick up the right foot, and step forward, landing on the toes before the fists come together at chest level with the right fist below the left fist *(fig 250)*.

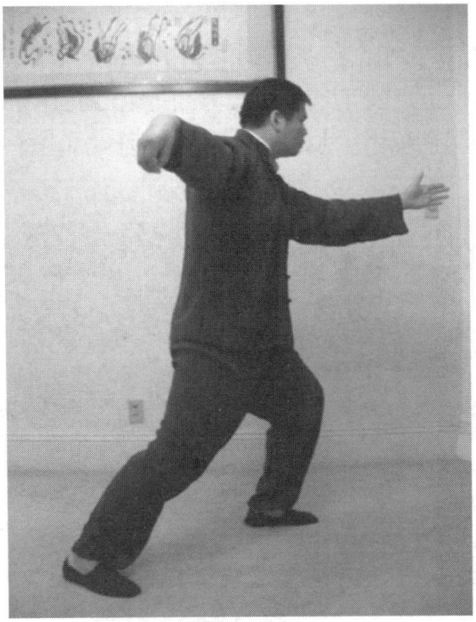

TAI CHI CHUAN – A COMPARATIVE STUDY

figure 247

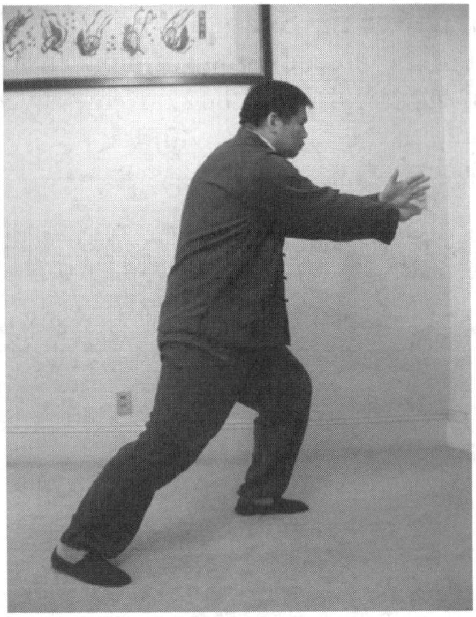

figure 248

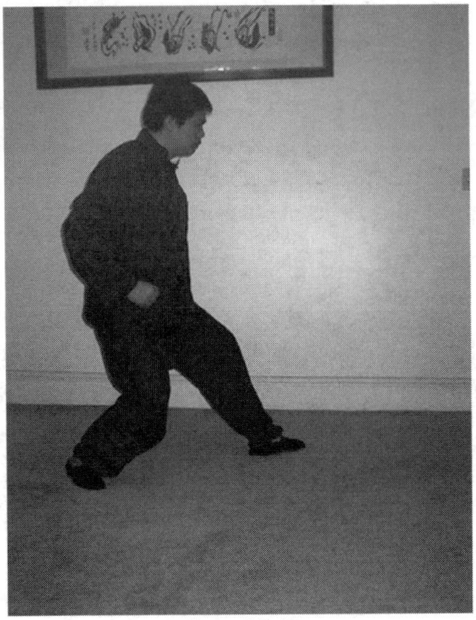

figure 249

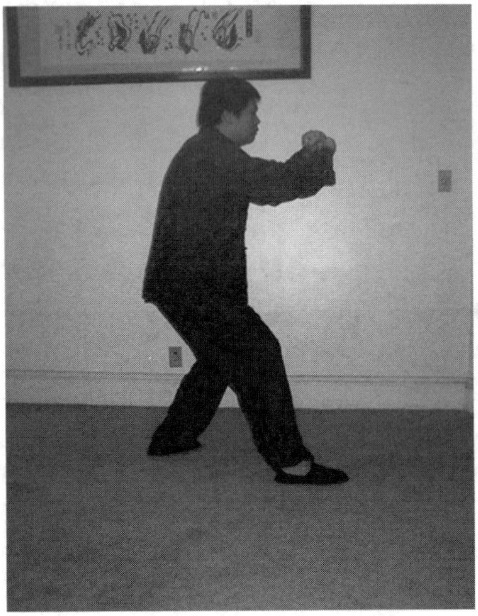

figure 250

38. Retreat to Ride the Tiger

From the preceding movement, open the fists with both palms facing out *(fig 251)*. With the body weight still on the left foot, pick up the right foot, and step backward. Shift the body weight onto the right foot, and at the same time, separate the hands, with the right hand going up to the right ear and the left hand going down to level with the left hip. With the body weight on the right foot, pick up the left foot, and land it on the toes a step closer to the right foot *(fig 252)*.

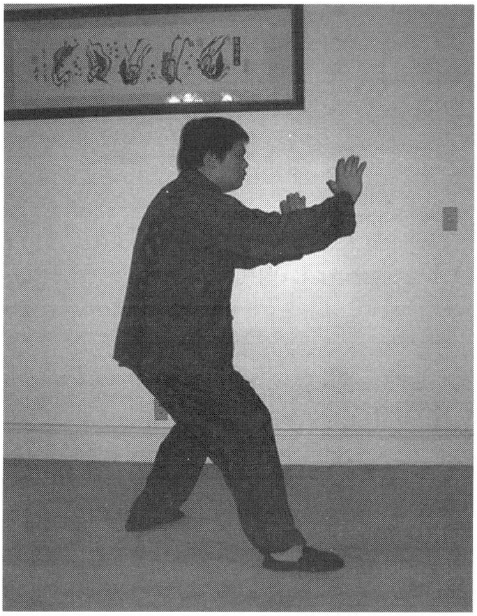

figure 251

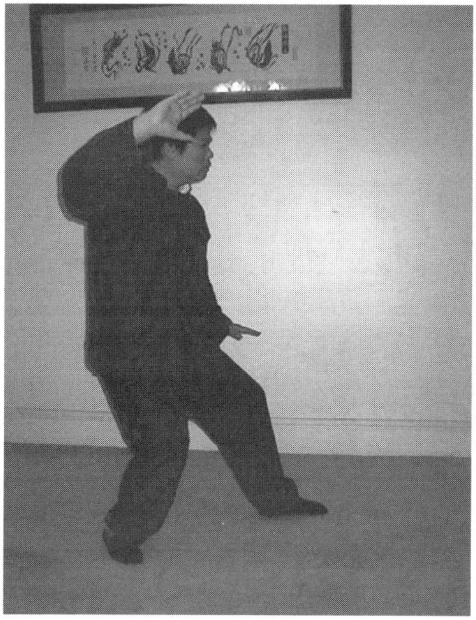

figure 252

39. Turn Around with Lotus Kick

From the preceding movement, bring the right hand to the chest with the palm facing down. Turn the right toes out before the left hand moves above the right hand and across the body, which turns right *(fig 253)*. With the body weight on the right foot, the left foot steps forward while the hands remain the same *(fig 254)*. With the body weight now on the left foot, turn the left toes inward, and move the hands to the right across the body, which turns right; the right foot positions to the right. The left palm now faces downward *(fig 255)*. With the body weight on the left foot, pick up the right foot and make a circle kick in front of the body from left to right as the hands move from right to left. The right palm ends facing downward *(fig 256)*.

figure 253

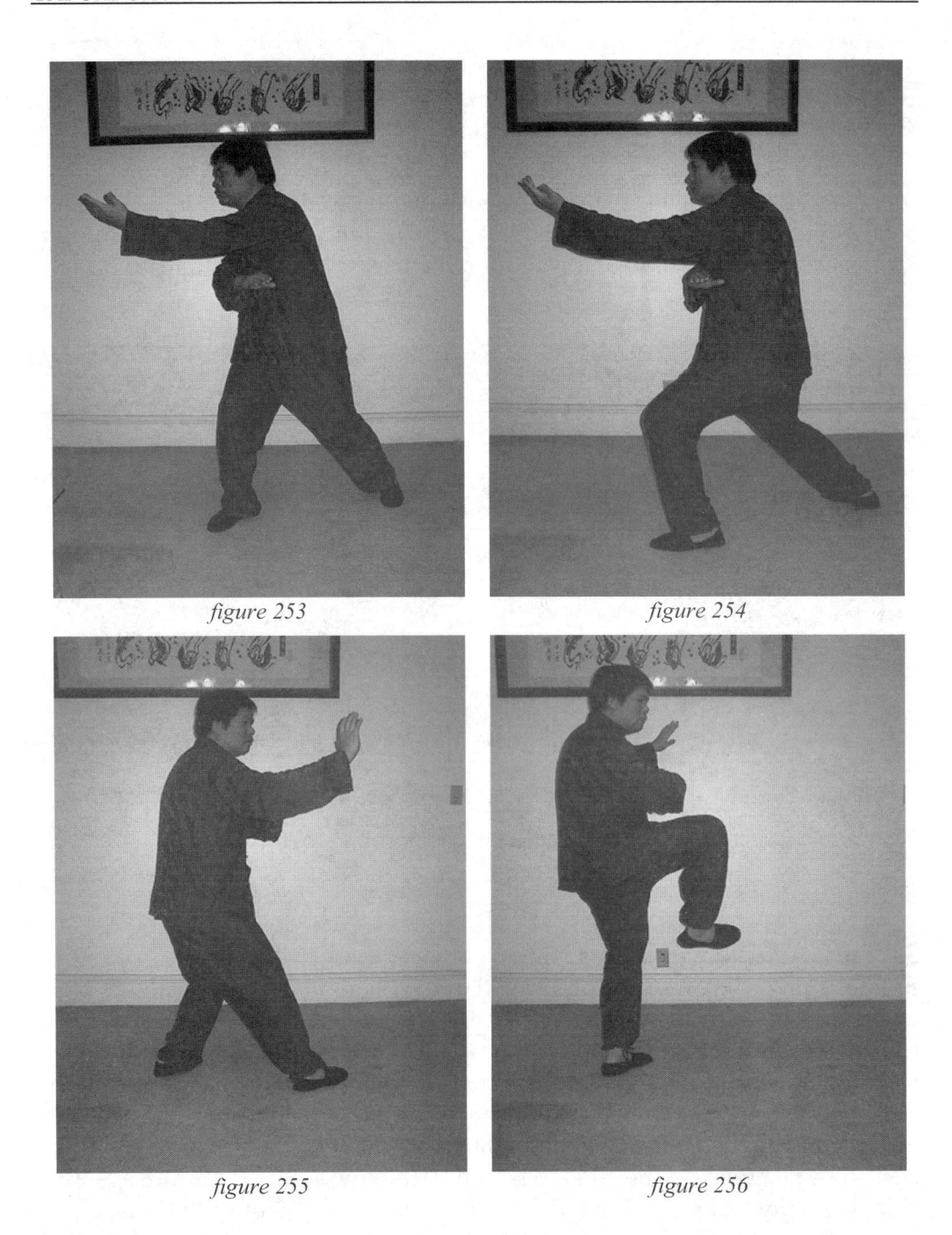

figure 254

figure 255

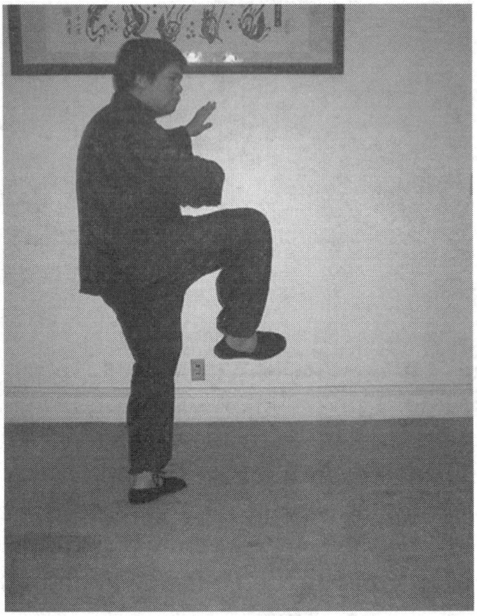

figure 256

40. Shooting Tiger
From the preceding movement, put the right foot down to the right corner, and bring the hands down to above the right knee *(fig 257)*. The body weight shifts onto the right foot; the two hands close into fists. Looking right, the right fist

comes up next to the right ear, and the left fist goes next to the right shoulder *(fig 258)*. Look forward before the left fist punches forward like a hammer at chest level *(fig 259)*.

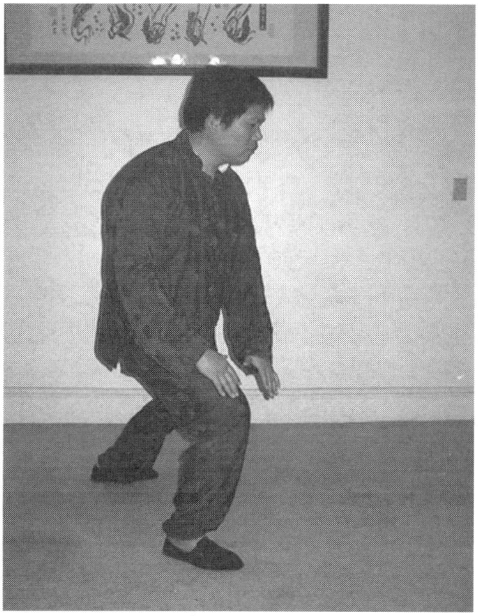

figure 257

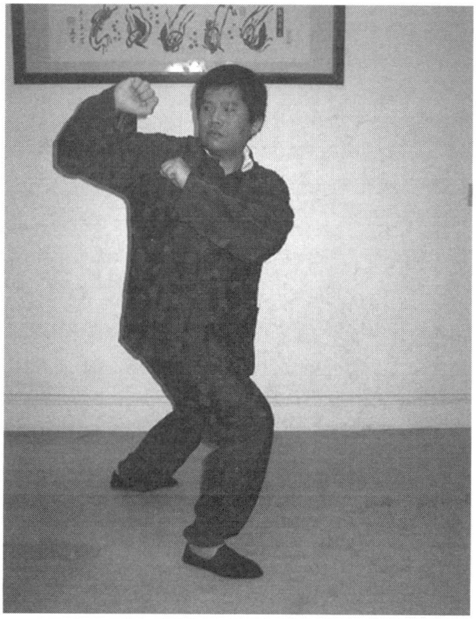

figure 258

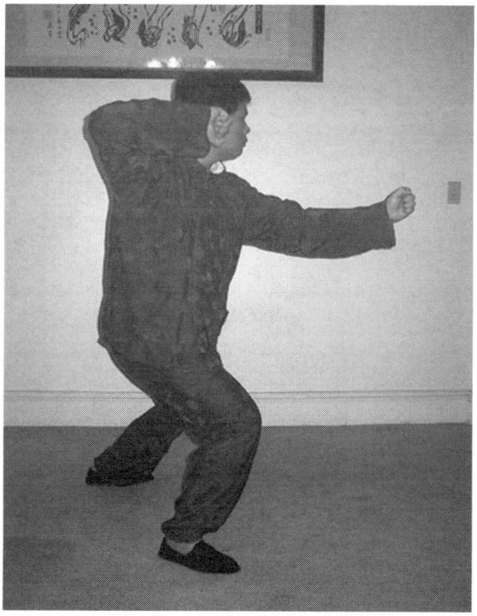

figure 259

41. Step Forward, Parry, Intercept and Punch

From the preceding movement, open the left fist with the palm facing up, and reach the right fist out over it *(fig 260)*. Bring the hands back to the left side of the hip, the left palm pressing against the right forearm. The right foot then steps forward with the toes pointing forward *(fig 261)*. Bring the hands up in front of the chest, and push forward as the body weight shifts forward *(fig 262)*.

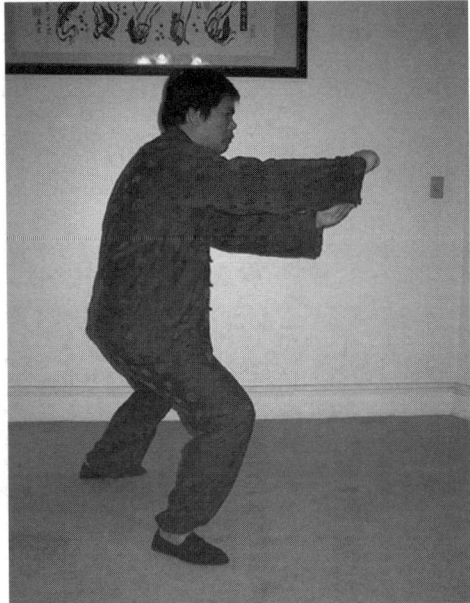

figure 260

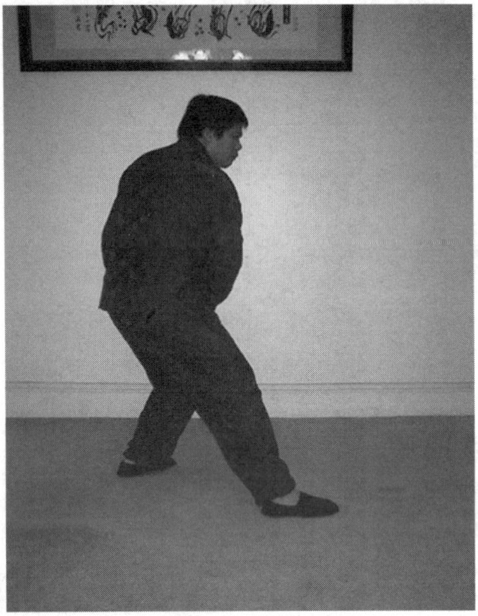

figure 261

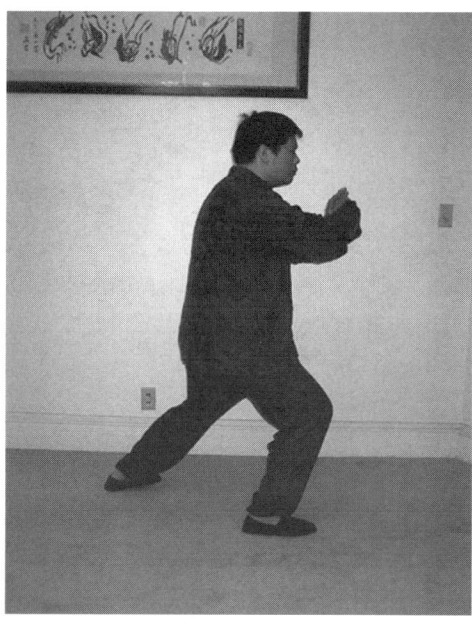

figure 262

With the body weight shifting onto the right foot, turn the right toes out; then separate the hands with the right fist coming back onto the right hip and the left hand pushing forward *(fig 263)*. Pick up the left foot; then make a clockwise sweep, and step forward. At the same time, the left hand makes a horizontal clockwise circle in front of the chest so that hand and foot mirror each other's motion *(fig 264)*. While the body weight is shifting onto the left foot, the right fist punches forward, and the left palm comes back next to the right elbow *(fig 265)*.

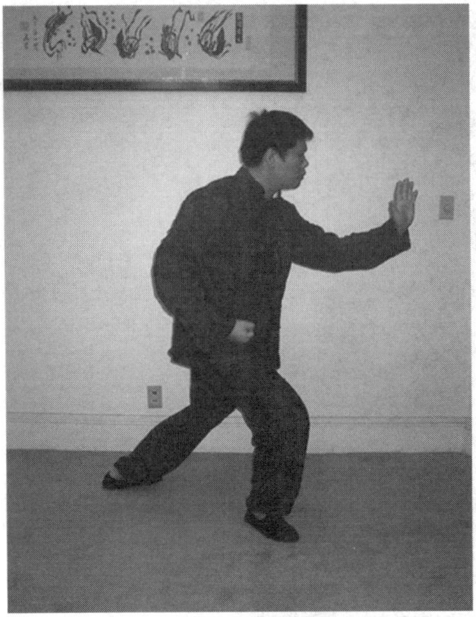

TAI CHI CHUAN – A COMPARATIVE STUDY

figure 263

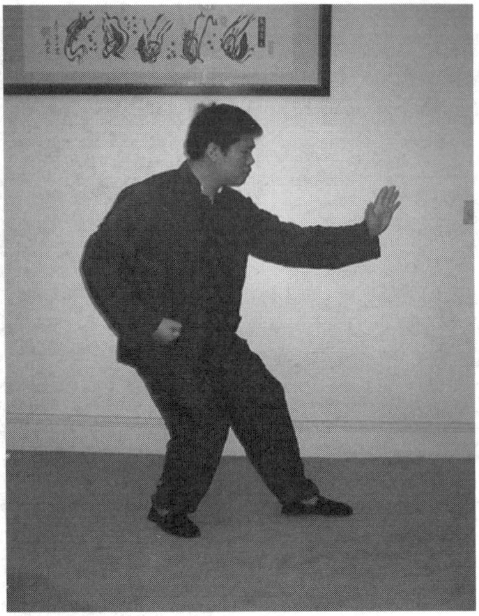

figure 264

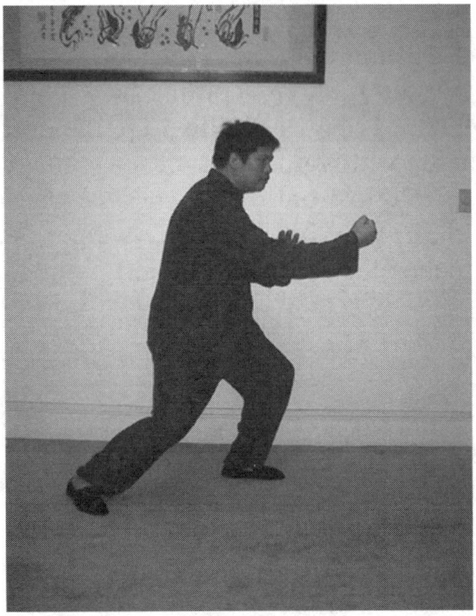

figure 265

42. Seal Tightly
From the preceding movement, put the left hand under the right elbow with the palm facing up *(fig 266)*. Open the right fist, and bring it back to the right side of the hip with the body weight shifting onto the right foot and the left

THE 43 MOVEMENT LARGE FRAME SOLO FORM

arm pushing forward with the palm facing in *(figs 267 & 268)*. Circle the hands in front of the chest so the palms face forward at the shoulders *(fig 269)*. Push the hands forward with the body weight shifting onto the left foot *(fig 270)*.

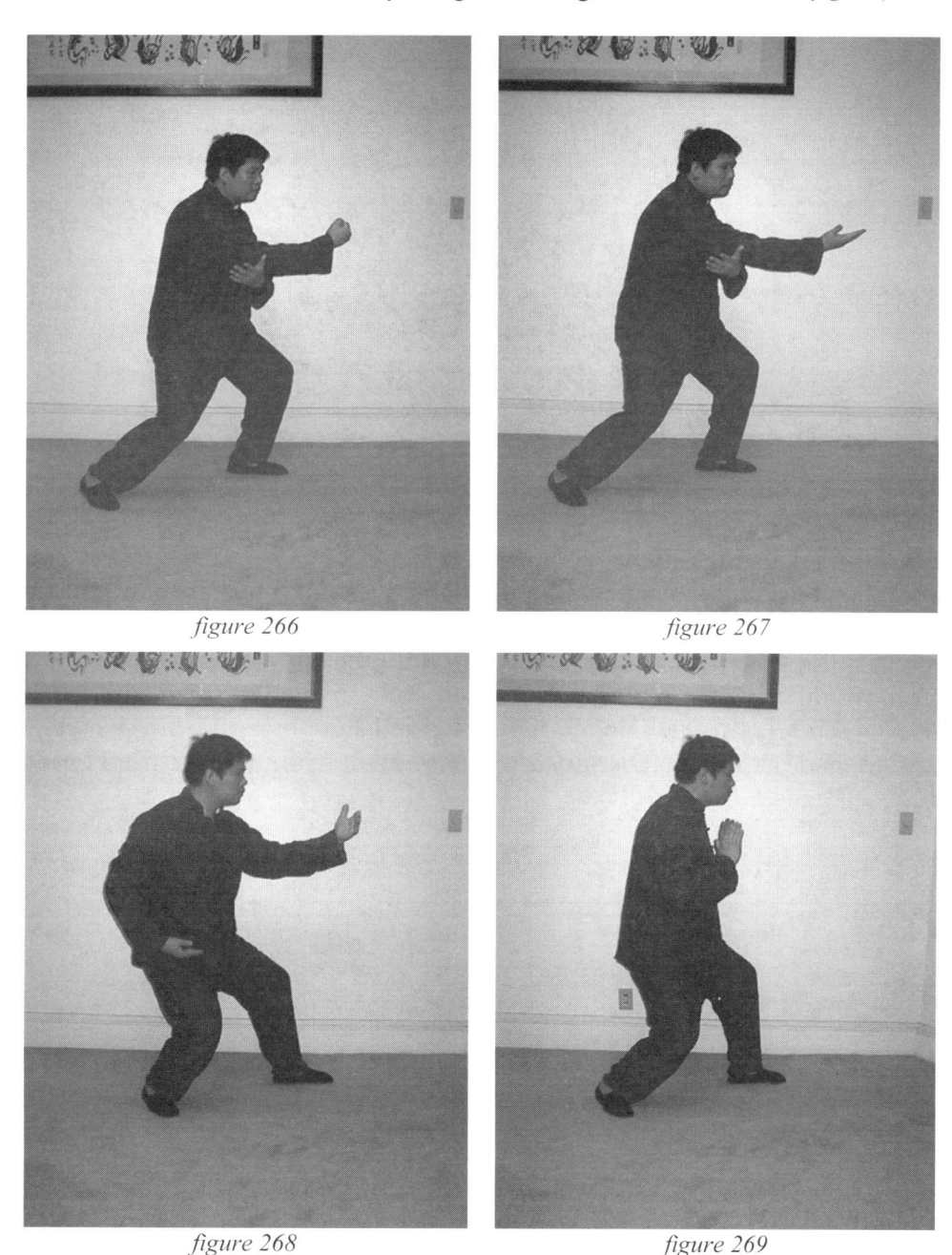

figure 266

figure 267

figure 268

figure 269

161

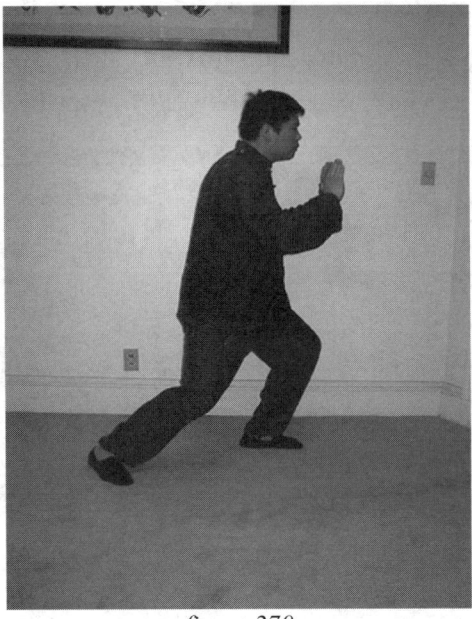

figure 270

43. Closing Tai Chi Chuan

From the preceding movement, the left hand does not move as the right hand moves to the right, and at the same time, the right toes turn out with the body weight shifting onto the right foot *(fig 271)*. Shift the body weight back onto the left foot, and bring the right hand back, crossing on the left wrist with the left wrist on top *(fig 272)*. Pick up the right foot, and step forward; shift the weight forward, and push the hands forward to face level with the right hand outside of the left hand *(figs 273 & 274)*.

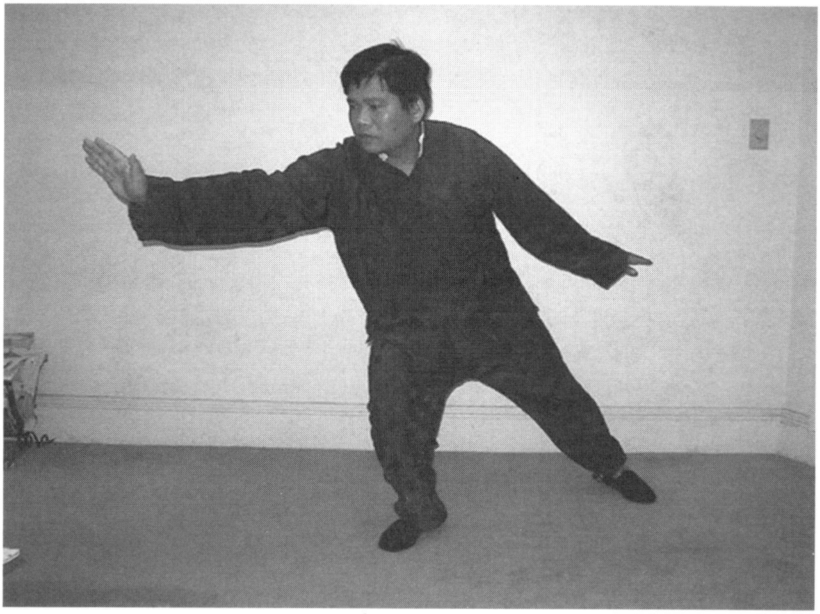

THE 43 MOVEMENT LARGE FRAME SOLO FORM

figure 271

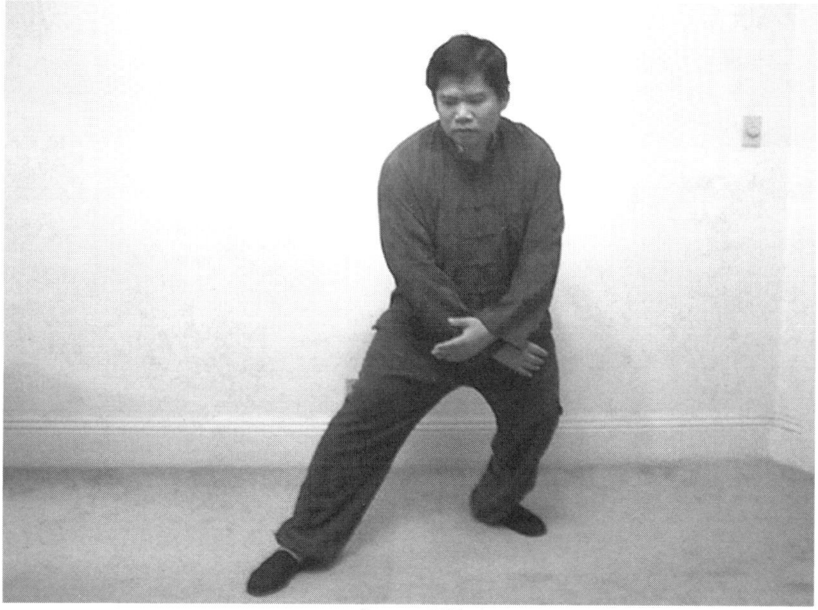

figure 272

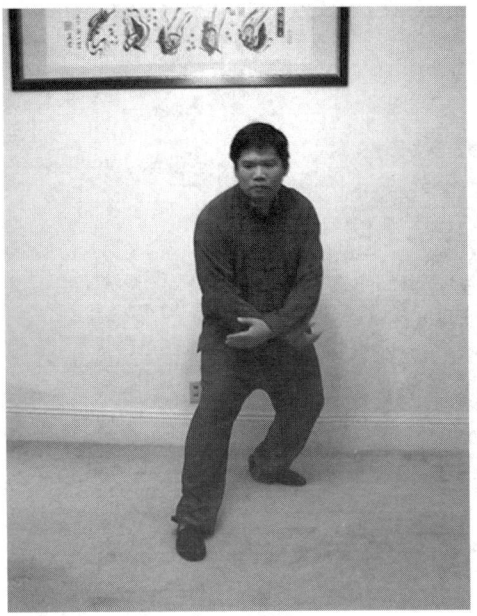

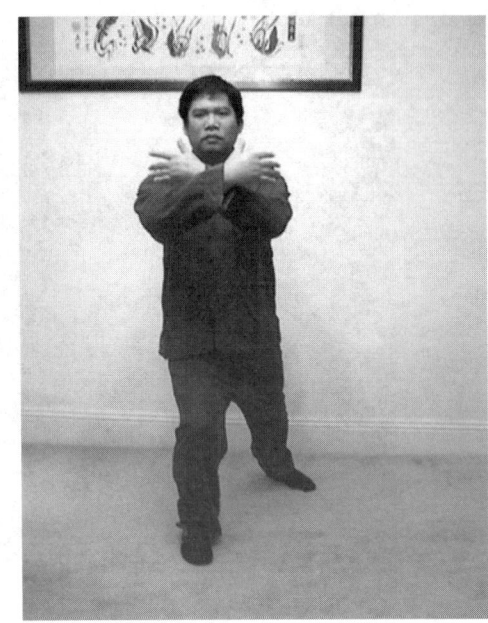

figure 273   *figure 274*

Pick up the left foot, and step up next to the right foot with the knees bent, the hands crossing on the wrists and the elbows pointing down *(fig 275)*. Turn the palms to face out. Separate the hands, and bring them down to the legs with the palms facing down; at the same time, straighten the knees to stand up *(figs 276 & 277)*.

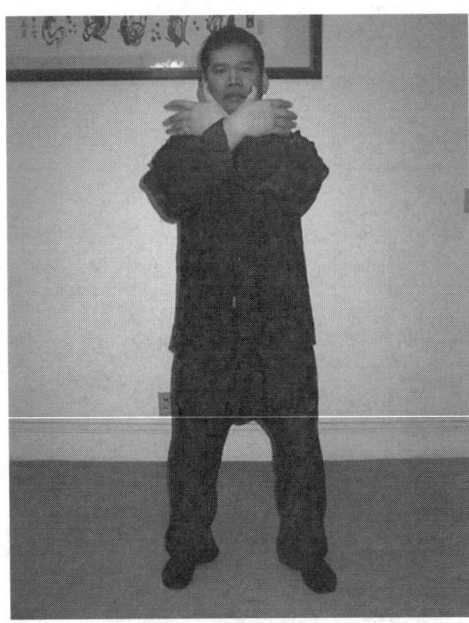

figure 275   *figure 276*

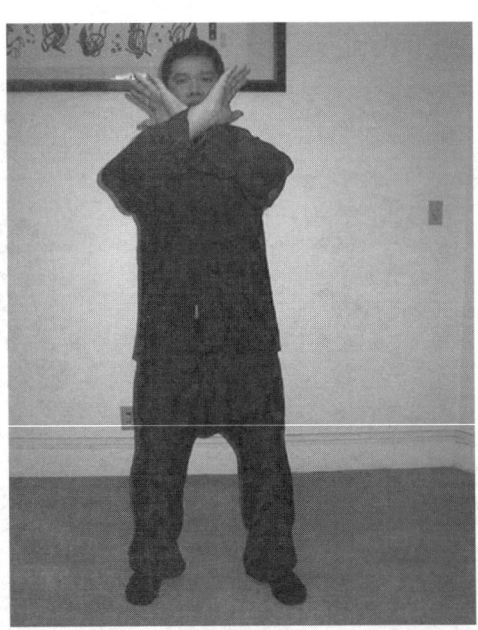

THE 43 MOVEMENT LARGE FRAME SOLO FORM

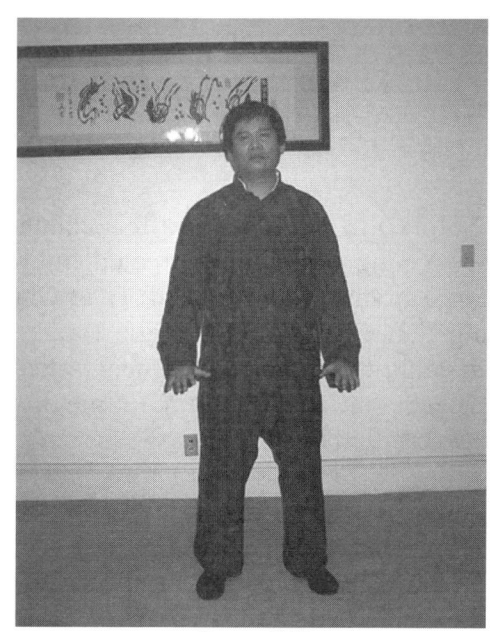

figure 277

Chapter 6
The 42 Movement Medium Frame Solo Form

A. Introduction

The Medium Frame Solo Form introduced in this chapter is based on Yeung Sau Chung's teaching. Yeung Sau Chung created this Medium Frame Solo Form based on the Large Frame Solo Form of Yang Cheng Fu, his father. In his own words, Yeung Sau Chung said that the Large Frame Solo Form is "too loose." It is difficult to focus and concentrate to discharge power. Therefore, he emphasized that the Medium Frame Form facilitates power mobilization.

Since this Medium Frame Solo Form is based on the Large Frame Form, it shares many characteristics with the Large Frame Form of Yang Cheng Fu. Today, many people mistake this Medium Frame Form for the Large Frame Form of Yang Cheng Fu. When compared to the Large Frame Form, the obvious distinctive characteristic lies in the execution of the movement. The Medium Frame Form has more square components than the Large Frame Form, which has more round components. It is often said among experienced Tai Chi Chuan practitioners that round components are for *chi* circulation and square components are for power delivery.

The second characteristic is excellent postural alignment. The body's weight is well-supported in every position. The posture is well-balanced, comfortable and powerful, and clearly distinguishes empty and full.

The third characteristic is the degree of waist rotation, which in the Large Frame sometimes compromises the execution of a movement. The rotation is not large as in the Large Frame Form which stretches the tendons and ligaments, and it is not compact as in the Small Frame Form which stretches the muscle groups.

My father Gin Soon Chu summarized the characteristic of the Medium Frame Solo Form as follows:

> The philosophy of the Medium Frame Solo Form is similar to borrowing money from a bank. Although a shorter term loan has a lower interest rate, the bank does not earn much money from it.

> Although a longer term loan earns more money for the bank, it is in risk of losing the principle. The middle term loan is better. It is flexible so it can follow the market trend easily.

The Medium Frame Solo Form can be easily mobilized for martial combat. It functions as both a health maintenance exercise and a training art for martial skill as well.

Practicing the Medium Frame Solo Form is meant to train the body to prepare for and to understand the martial application of Tai Chi Chuan. Executing each movement mobilizes the body for offensive and defensive maneuvers. From this, one can see that the Medium Frame Solo Form is an application training form. It trains the body to mobilize the power quickly and efficiently.

B. The Principles and Concepts of the Medium Frame Form

Tai Chi Chuan has many functions. It is a Chinese martial art system, a health maintenance exercise, and a discipline to improve temperament. More specifically, it can increase blood circulation, restore all the vital organs and glands, nourish the skin and hair, revitalize the eyes, stabilize the body temperature, and greatly increase a person's energy level. It also improves body balance and alertness, and stimulates the central nervous system. It is a unique physical art guided by intangible principles. Following are some of the principles and concepts for bettering oneself in Tai Chi Chuan training.

1. **The body should be upright**
   In practice, the body has to be upright. Upright refers to the body being straight, not leaning to the left, right, front, or back. The back and the coccyx are in a straight line. It does not matter how one maneuvers the body, the back should always remain straight. This is what the *Tai Chi Chuan Classics* refer to as the coccyx being straight. When the coccyx is straight, the center of gravity is lower, and the body has better balance and stability. If the center is not balanced, it is easy for the opponent to take advantage. In order for the body to be upright, internally, the spirit should be awakened and calm; externally, the head suspended from above, the back raised, the *chi* sunk to the *dan tien* (an area three inches below the navel), and the waist and hips lowered.

2. **The body should be comfortable, relaxed, and tranquil**
   Tai Chi Chuan is an exercise to work on the physical body, *chi*, and spirit. When one practices the solo form, all the movements should be natural so that the practitioner is comfortable, relaxed, and tranquil. Relaxation has to happen throughout the whole body, inside as well as outside. The head, shoulders, waist, hips, knees, hands, elbows, wrists, feet, and all the joints must be completely relaxed so that there is no stiffness. The whole body is so relaxed that it does not appear to have any bone. Tranquility requires all distractions be removed so that the practitioner is able to concentrate fully on the Tai Chi Chuan Solo Form and bring out the intent's creativity.

3. **The body should be nimble, and the head suspended from above**
   In practice, the body should be nimble and the head suspended so that the spirit reaches to the top of the head. To have a nimble body and suspend the head from above means to have the head in an upright position, similar to having a glass of water on top of the head when any small movement of the head will cause the glass to fall and the water to spill. To be able to support the glass of water on top of the head, the jaw should not tilt in any direction. Relax the neck, and keep its muscles flexible. The intent is to imagine that the head is supporting the sky, and one is standing firmly on the ground. When one is able to maintain this condition throughout practice, the spirit is awakened, and the *chi* and blood circulate.

4. **Sink the *chi* to the *dan tien***
   Practicing Tai Chi Chuan requires the practitioner to be able to suspend the head from above and sink the *chi* down to *dan tien*, an area three inches below the navel. During practice, the intent guides the breathing and directs the *chi* to the *dan tien*. Tai Chi Chuan is based on natural breathing, or the process of inhalation when the abdomen expands, and exhalation when the abdomen contracts. If one finds this difficult to do, one should not force it to happen. As long as one relaxes the body, keeping it calm and tranquil by first relaxing the nervous system and second the physical body, complete body relaxation will result, and the *chi* will automatically sink down to the *dan tien*.

5. **Relax the shoulders and lower the elbows**
   Relax the shoulders means to have the shoulders sink downward. Many beginners raise the shoulders when they move the hands. If the

shoulders do not sink, the body has no rooting, the center of gravity is high, there is no balance or stability, and the *chi* and blood circulations are poor. To lower the elbows means to have the elbows pointing downward. To lower the elbows does not mean to have locked and straight arms, but flexible and stretching arms. With time, one will feel that the arms are heavy and have a lot of power. To be sure the shoulders are sinking and the elbows are pointing downward, check that the hand is always higher than the elbow.

6. **Hollow the chest and raise the back**
   Sink the chest and raise the back are two components that always go together. Many practitioners incorrectly assume that they are two separate entities. When one is able to sink the chest, one is able to raise the back. To sink the chest is to have the chest go inward naturally so that the body and *chi* will sink down. The chest should not be thrust outward, for this can cause the *chi* to come up to the chest; the breathing will not be smooth, and the top of the body will become heavier than the bottom. Neither should one force the chest inward as this will narrow the chest's cavity and the diaphragm will not sink. This inhibits breathing and blood circulation. To raise the back is to spread the back so that the *chi* will be circulated better in this area. Generally, when one has a relaxed and natural posture, the chest sinks and the back is raised.

7. **Inside and outside harmony**
   Inside refers to the internal components such as power, *chi*, mind and spirit. Outside refers to the physical components such as head, hands, hips, elbows, knees, fists, and feet. All movements and strikes must have elements from these two components to be powerful.

8. **Top and bottom coordinate**
   In practice, all movements must be coordinated and unified. When one part of the body moves, all other parts move. When one part does not move, no part moves. All movement is centered on the waist so that when the waist moves, all parts follow.

9. **Apply intent, not physical power**
   One can practice Tai Chi Chuan at three levels. At the beginning, the student works on the physical components of the body. Next, the student works on the *chi* circulation, or the energy level. Finally, the student works on the intent creativity, or the invisible components

level. The definition of intent practices is infinite; it can be practicing a concept such as soft, or it can be practicing a martial technique. This highlights the importance of the insubstantial aspects over the substantial aspects in Tai Chi Chuan. This is the same in our physical world: the insubstantial aspect is more important than the substantial aspect.

10. **Walk like a cat**
All the stepping in Tai Chi Chuan is stable, light, and nimble. It is so light that one does not make any sound in stepping forward or backward. Generally, stepping forward begins with the body's weight on one foot. Then lightly pick up the empty foot, and step forward; gently place the foot down without any sound, and slowly shift the body's weight onto the forward foot. The body remains upright without bobbing up and down. When one practices this regularly, the legs will be stronger, and one is able to walk like a cat.

11. **All the movements are slow and even like pulling silk from a cocoon**
Practicing Tai Chi Chuan correctly requires a certain standard. Therefore, practice of the Tai Chi Chuan Solo Form should develop stability, rooting, and nimbleness. The practitioner must be fully aware of all the motions, so maximum concentration is required. This is like the work of pulling silk from a cocoon: one should be able to pull the silk from the cocoon without breaking it. In order to execute this in practice, one must relax the body and apply the intent to direct all the physical movements.

12. **All the movements should be continuous**
Another name for Tai Chi Chuan is Chung Chuan. This means Infinite or Long Fist. This is to symbolize the infinite progression of the Tai Chi Chuan Solo Form movements. It is often compared to ocean waves: one wave comes after another in an infinite process. In order to practice Tai Chi Chuan as an infinite process, apply the intent to guide the *chi* to circulate throughout the body. It is often said by many experienced practitioners that when the physical movement is broken, the *chi* is not; when the *chi* broken, the intent is not; when the intent is broken, the spirit is not. Here, "not" means not correct or not present. It does not matter whether a movement is advance or retreat, forward or backward; apply the technique of "folding" to connect it so that all the movements will be continuous.

13. **All the motions have lightness**
A correct method to practice Tai Chi Chuan is to apply intent over the physical power, suspend the head from above and sink the *chi* down to *dan tien*, walk like a cat, assume an upright body position, relax and move in a circular motion. When one can do that, obviously all the movements will be light and nimble and clearly distinguish empty and full, unweighted and weighted.

14. **All the motions should be slow and even**
The primary object in Tai Chi Chuan practice is to have a nimble body, full of spirit and intent. To achieve this objective, one must bring the characteristics of spirit, intent, and a flexible body to each practice experience. Slow and even motions, natural breathing, and calmness are but some of the characteristics required.

15. **Breathe Naturally**
Tai Chi Chuan requires deep, even, and natural breathing. It is not necessary to practice synchronized breathing with movements as advocated by some of the contemporary practitioners. Breathing naturally will sink the *chi* down to the *dan tien*, and with time, the breathing will complement the movement. In inhalation, the body performs closing motions; in exhalation, the body performs opening motions. On occasion, multiple breaths may occur in one movement. This is done by not deliberately incorporating breathing with all physical movements.

C. The Fundamentals

The obvious characteristic of the Tai Chi Chuan Medium Fame Solo Form is its forward leaning posture to focus the power in one direction. This action follows the principle of engaging the enemy. When we are engaging an enemy, we apply everything we have so the strike is very powerful and devastating.

Tai Chi Chuan fundamentals consist of movements of the hands, eyes, body position, and stance and step. It is often said that when one executes a hand technique without moving the feet, one is looking for trouble. If the head is looking down like a dog and the body is stretching like a cat, one's skill is very poor. Therefore, one must spend time practicing the fundamentals.

1. Basic Hand Techniques and Positions

Tai Chi Chuan involves many hand techniques. It is necessary to get them right so that a movement will be performed properly and executed correctly in martial application. The hand techniques are divided into the fist *(fig 1)*, the palm *(fig 2)*, and the hook *(fig 3)*. The common Tai Chi Chuan techniques are ward off, roll back, press, push, pull down, split, elbow strike, shoulder strike, palm strike, punching, kicking, and hooking. When closing the fingers into a fist, the fingers should not be too tight. When forming a palm strike, bend the wrist so that the power goes directly into the center of the palm.

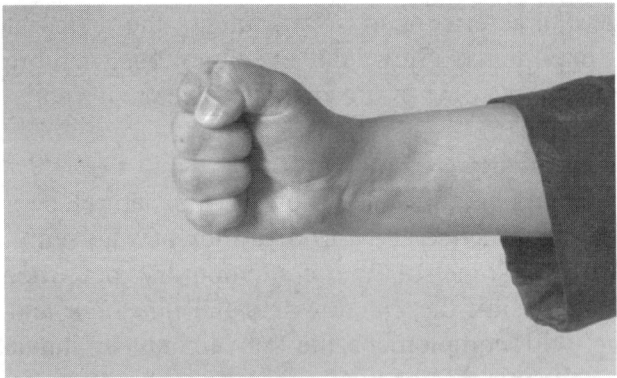

figure 1

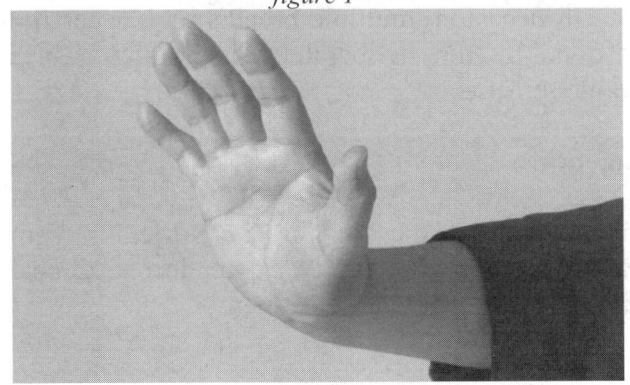

figure 2

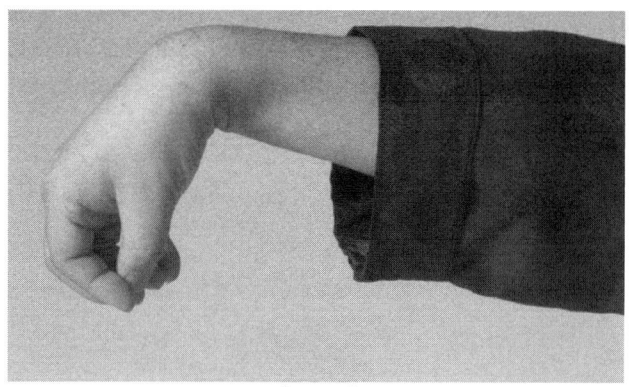

figure 3

a. The Fists

The fist is a most important weapon in bare hand combat. There are several techniques involving the fist in Tai Chi Chuan. Here is the list.

i. Hidden Fist: The fist rests by the waist. It is face up.

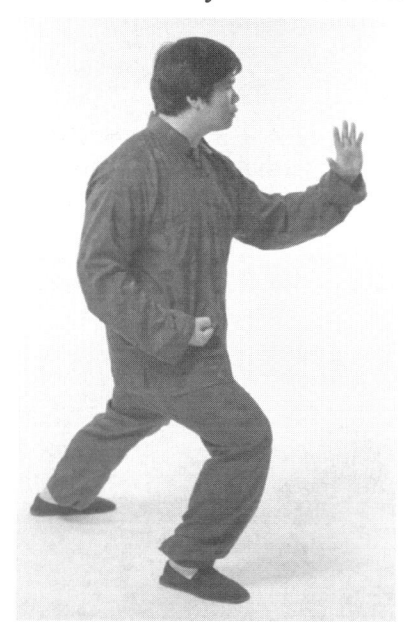

ii. Thrusting Fist: The fist is resting by the waist then goes forward. Its position is not higher than the shoulder and not lower than the chest.

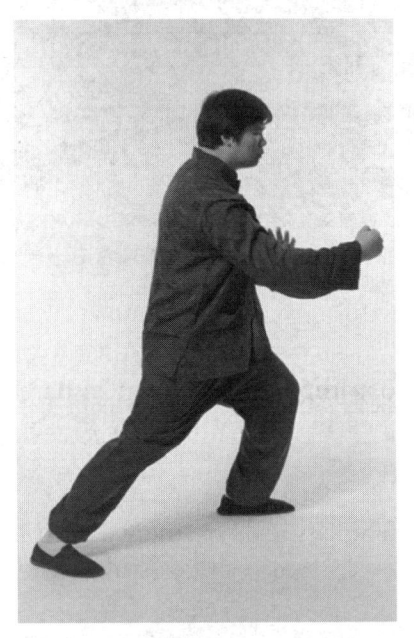

iii. Downward Fist: The fist is resting by the waist then goes downward. It faces either to the left or right. It arrives level to the front knee.

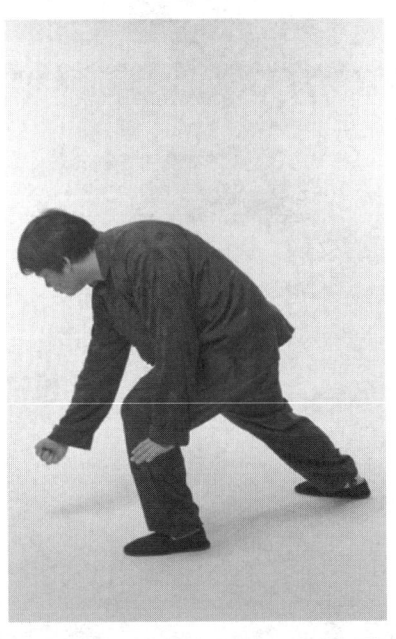

iv. Parry Fist: The fist comes up in an arc. It begins with the fist facing down and ends with the fist facing up to the front or side.

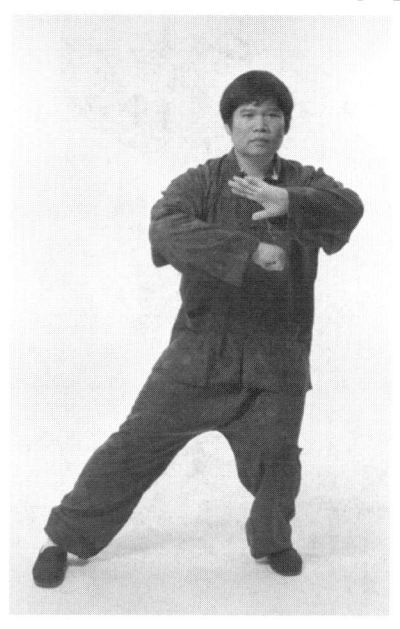

v. Back Fist: The fist moves upward then downward in an arc. It begins with the fist facing down and ends with the palm of the fist facing up.

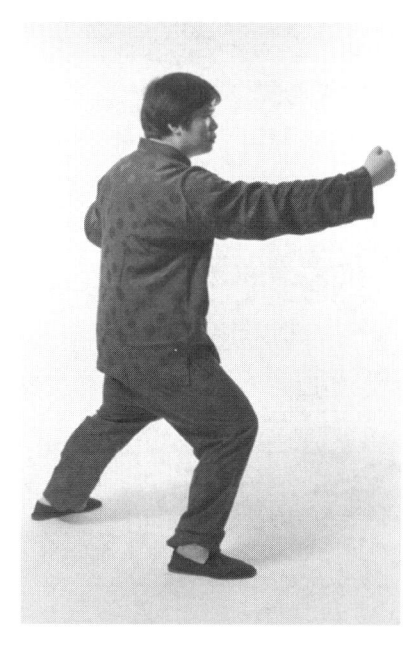

vi. Double Fist: The two fists go upward to ear level.

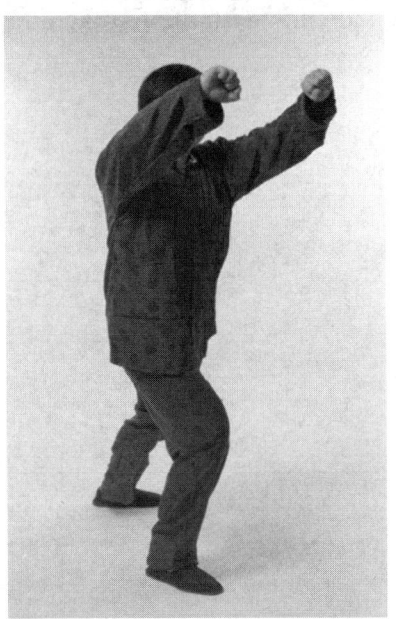

vii. Horizontal Fist. The fists move horizontally to the left or right.

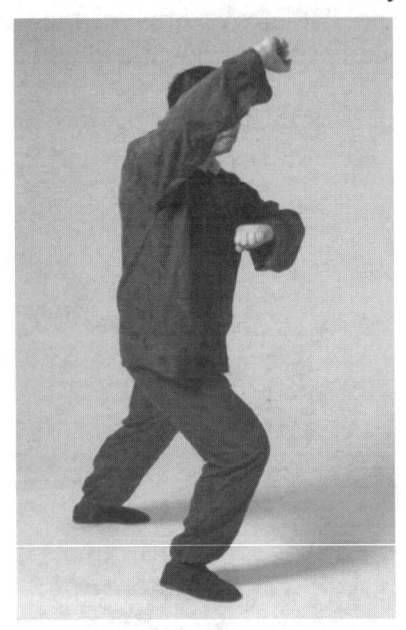

b. The Palms

Although the name implies that Tai Chi Chuan uses the fist, most of the hand techniques in Tai Chi Chuan prefer the palm. Internal martial art practitioners recognize that a palm can easily be transformed into more options than a fist. Here is the list of common techniques involving the palm.

i. Single Palm Push: Bend the elbow and wrist with the fingers pointing up. The palm pushes forward on level with the shoulder.

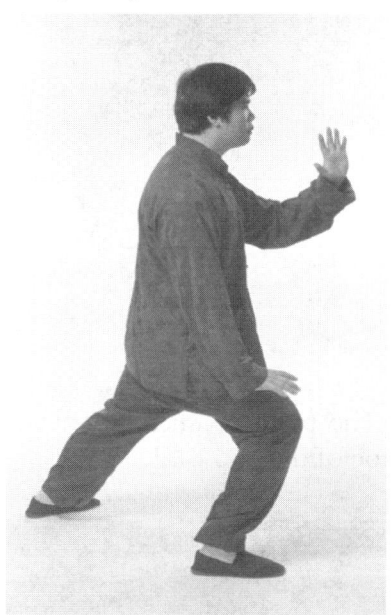

ii. Double Palm Push: The two palms push forward from the shoulders with the fingers pointing up.

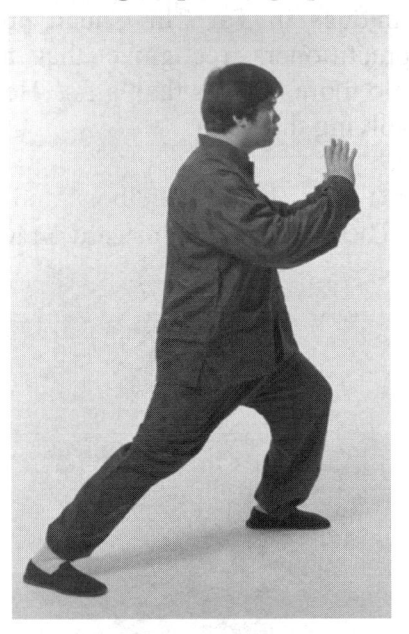

iii. Brush Palm: The palm brushes downward from the center of the body to the side of the body.

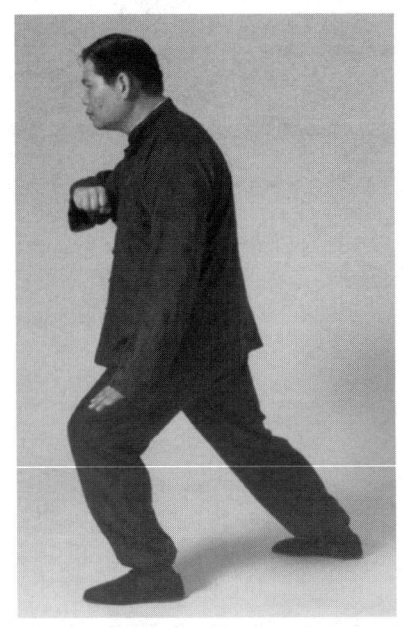

iv. Intercepting Palm: The palm comes from the side of the body to the chest with the palm facing down and forward. The fingers are pointing to the side.

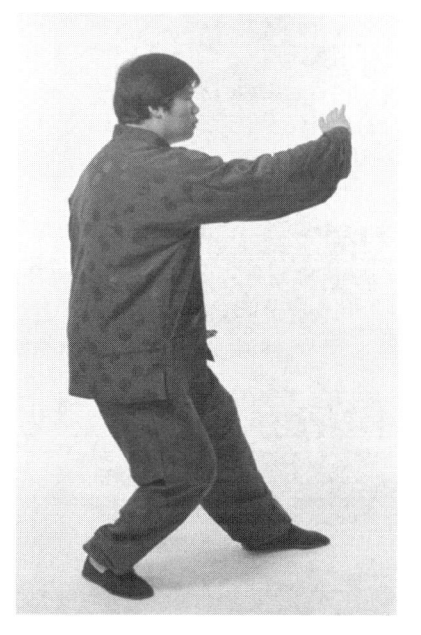

v. Separating Palm: The two palms begin from the center of the body, separating into two sides with the palms facing away from the body and the fingers pointing up.

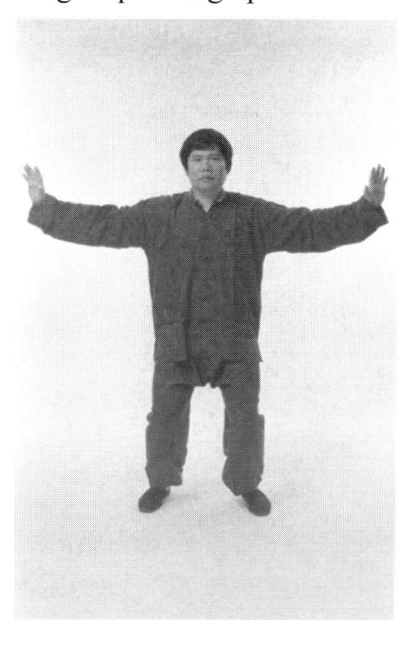

vi. Diagonal Separating Palm: The two palms begin from the center of the body, separating into top and bottom.

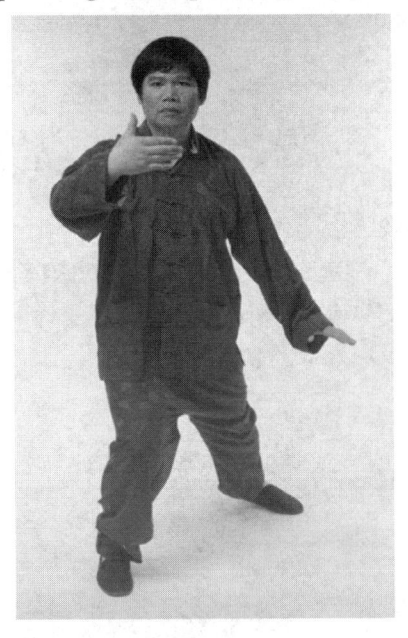

vii. Vertical Cloud Palm: The palms go up and down. The upper palm faces out.

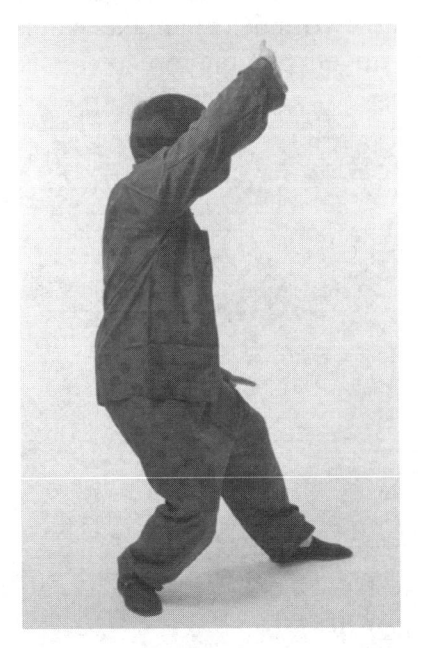

viii. Horizontal Cloud Palm: The palms move horizontally to the left or right. The palms face out and down.

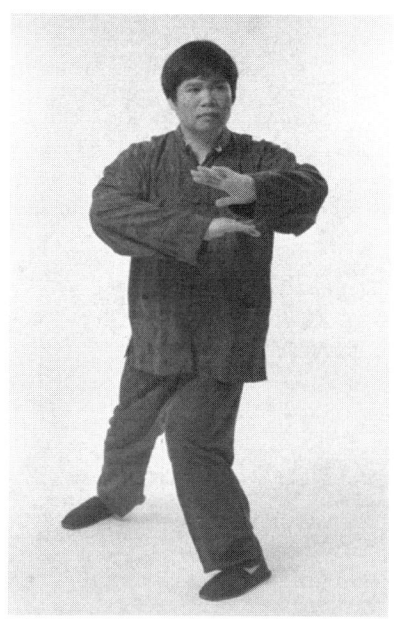

ix. Thrusting Palm: The palm thrusts forward with the fingers pointing upward.

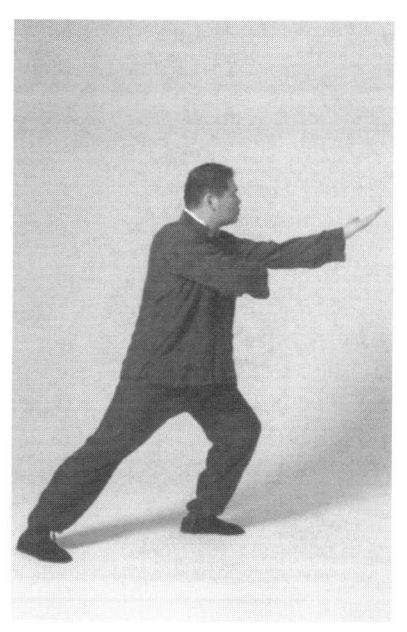

x. Blocking Palm: The palm goes upward above the head, facing out.

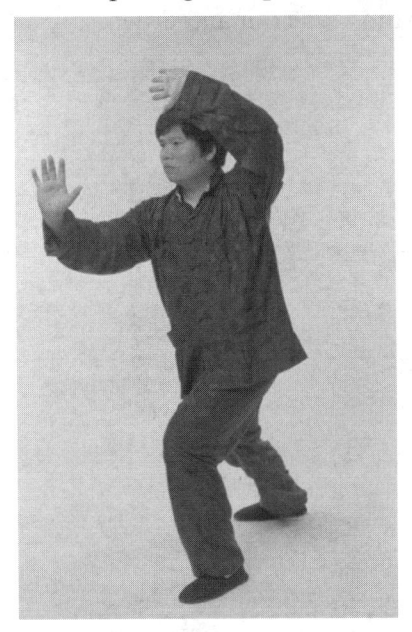

xi. Embracing Palm: The palm faces inward with the fingers pointing to the side.

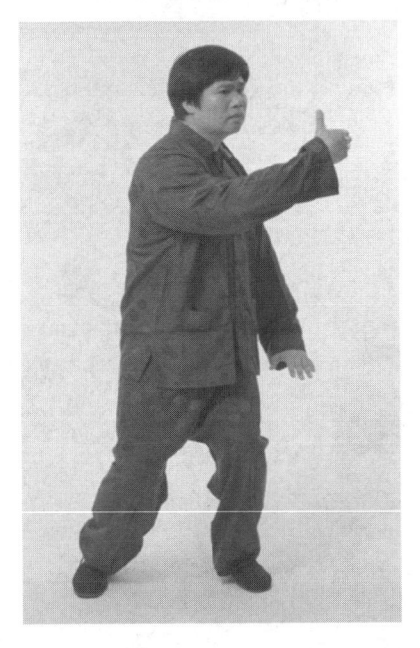

xii. Downward Palm: The palm goes down with the fingers pointing to the left.

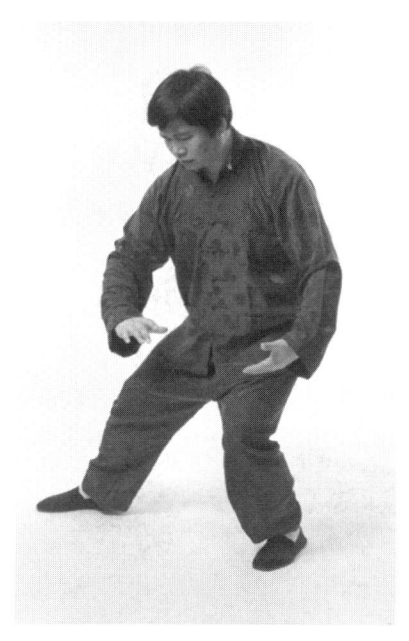

xiii. Lift Palm: The palm goes upward with the fingers pointing up.

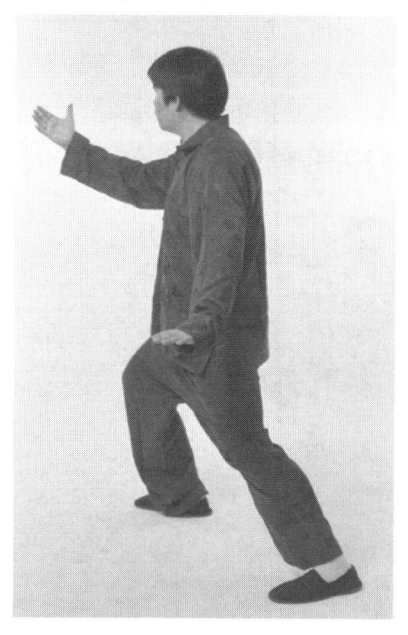

xiv. Yin Yang Palm: One palm faces up, and the other palm faces down.

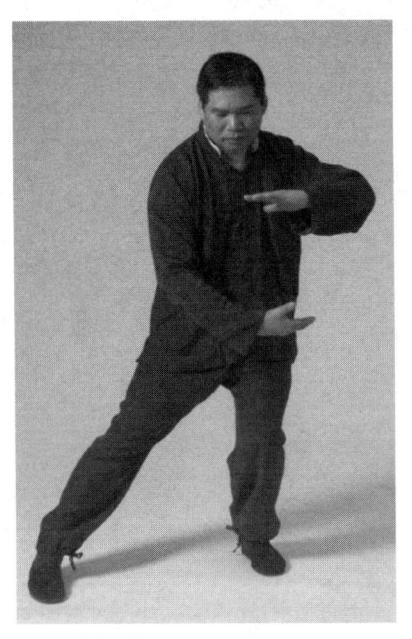

xv. Press Palm: The right palm faces in, joined at the wrist by the left palm facing out (press).

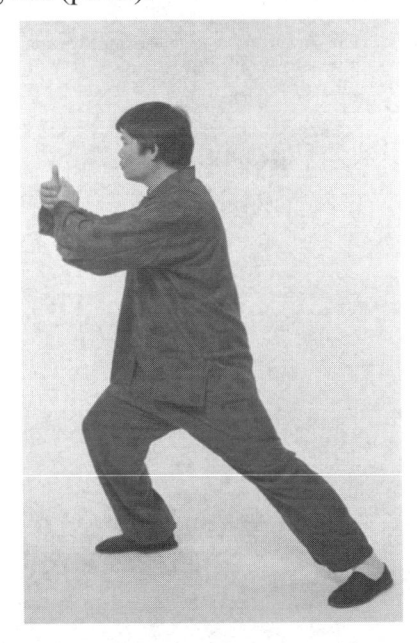

c. **The Arms**

In Tai Chi Chuan, the arm movements are often incorporated to execute the techniques of split, shoulder strike, and elbow strike. Here are some of the common arm movements.

i. Embracing: The palms face inward.

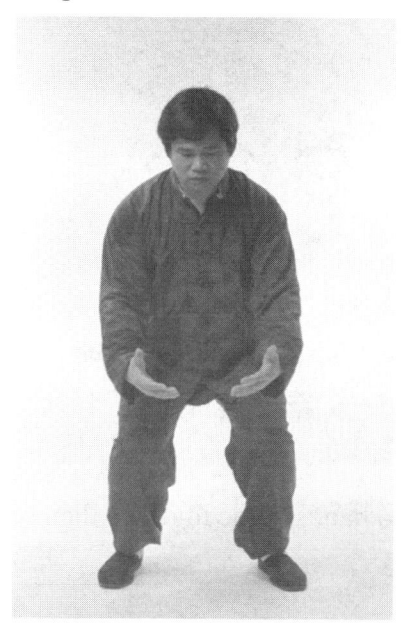

ii. Push: The two arms come together in front of the chest.

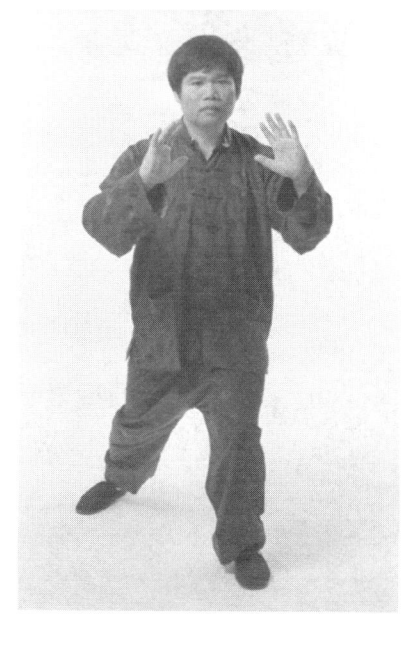

iii. Separation: The two hands separate into front and back.

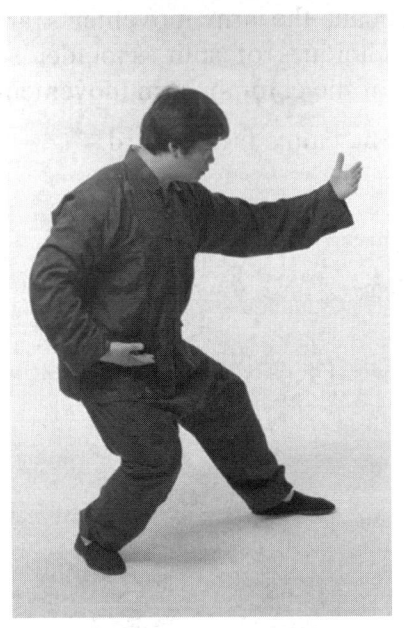

iv. Split: The two hands come together then separate to the sides.

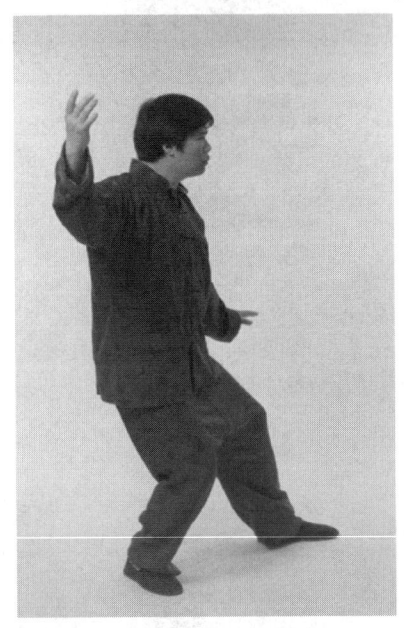

2. Eye and Body Techniques and Positions

a. Eye Position
As in all Chinese martial art systems, the eyes are very important in Tai Chi Chuan. They are related to the expression of *chi* and spirit in power delivery. In practice, it is necessary to concentrate the spirit and mind. Each movement coordinates with the intent and is natural so that the hands, feet, and body are all in unison.

b. Body Position
  i. The head always remains upright with the eyes looking forward and far off so the spirit can reach to the top of the head. This means the head remains upright following the intent. When the top of the head is slightly lifted upward, the jaw tilts inward, and the tongue touches the hard palate. The trunk is leaning forward so the whole body is aimed forward.
 ii. The neck is relaxed and straight. There is no tension on the neck muscles so that it is easy to rotate the neck to either side without stiffness.
iii. The shoulders are relaxed and sunk. If the shoulders do not sink, this inhibits the blood flow, and the *chi* will rise. This will inhibit the whole body from sinking downward to a better rooting.
 iv. The elbows should sink and point downward. Otherwise, they cause the same problem as the shoulders.
  v. The chest should be relaxed and natural so that the *chi* can sink to the *dan tien*, an area three inches below the navel. Make sure the chest does not go outward or sink inward.
 vi. The back should be spread evenly so that the *chi* will be able to penetrate into the bones. It is said that as long as one has the chest relaxed, the back is automatically raised.
vii. The waist should be relaxed so that it is flexible. All Tai Chi Chuan Solo Form movements are initially based on the rotation of the waist. Therefore, the more flexible and loose the waist, the better and more efficiently one will be able to execute the solo form movements.
viii. The hip and buttocks must tuck under so that all the postures are connected. Otherwise, if the posture is not properly connected, issuing power is difficult. Therefore, the hip should relax and sink to get a better balance and the buttocks should not be protruding. Overall, the body should be relaxed and natural, and the coccyx in

a straight and upright position so that all the movements are nimble and start from the waist.

3. **Step and Stance**

   Step and stance cover some important areas of Tai Chi Chuan training. Stance training refers to the stationary postures in the solo form, and step training refers to the movements involved with body weight transition in the solo form. Stance is the lower-body posture, and step is the movement of the lower-body posture. In Tai Chi Chuan training, when a beginner is unable to master the stance and step training, it is difficult to maintain body balance, correctly execute the movement, and progress in training. Therefore, stance and step skills are the basic requirements for body balance and mobility. They are so vital that all martial art systems require beginning students to spend many years on stance and step skill training before being allowed to learn any routine. In the high standard of Tai Chi Chuan practices, principles such as walk like a cat and pulling silk from a cocoon require a lot of control and coordination. If the stance and step skills are not strong and correct, one cannot practice the principles properly.

   a. **Stance Position**

      In the Tai Chi Chuan Medium Frame Solo Form, the front knee is aligned with the toes, the back leg is straight, and the trunk leans forward. There are several different types of stances. A list of the common stances follows:

      i. Forward Bow Stance:
         Bend the front leg with the foot flat on the floor and the knee aligned to the toes. The back leg is straight. Generally, 60% of the body's weight is on the front leg, and 40% of the body's weight is on the back leg.

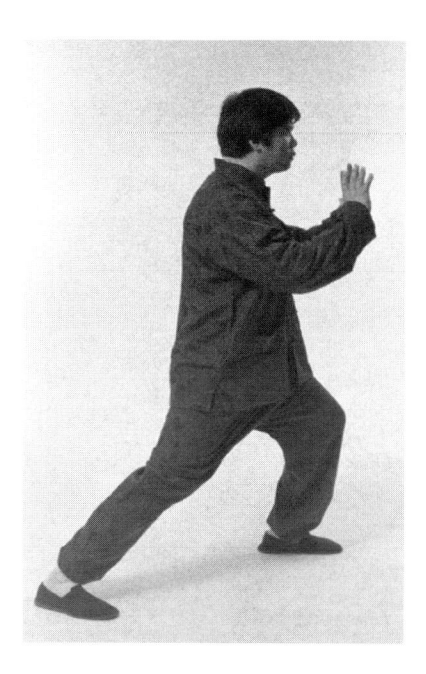

ii. Backward Bow Stance:
   Bend the back leg with the foot flat on the floor and the knee pointing to the same direction as the toes. The front leg is straightened but without the knee being locked. Generally, 60% of the body's weight is on the back foot, and 40% of the body's weight is on the front foot.

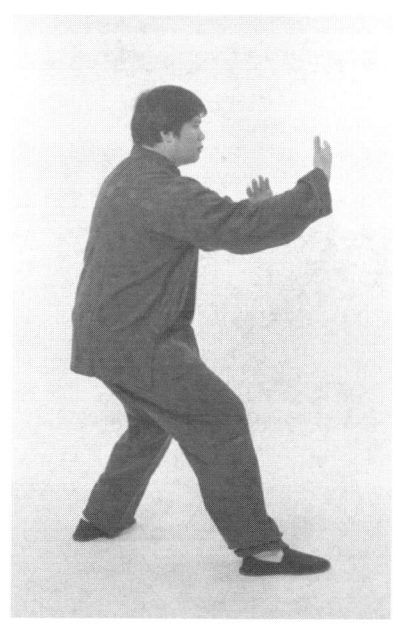

iii. Horse Stance:
Separate the feet as wide as the shoulders. Bend the legs, and line the knees up with the toes.

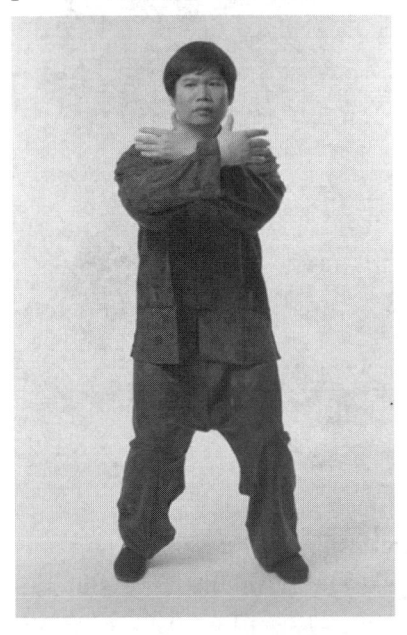

iv. Stand Up on One Leg:
As the name implies, the body's weight is supported on one leg with the other leg suspended. The weighted foot is turned out 45 degrees.

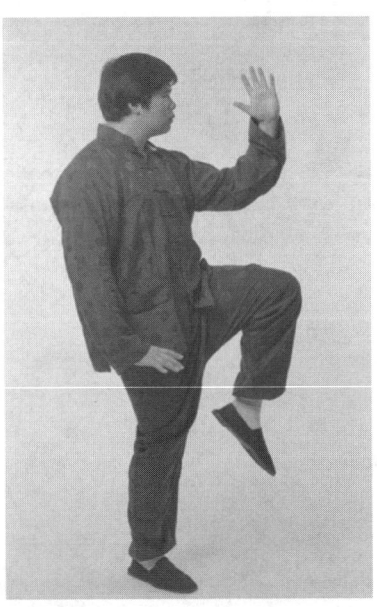

v. Low Stance:
One leg supports the body's weight lower to the ground. The other leg is extended straight forward.

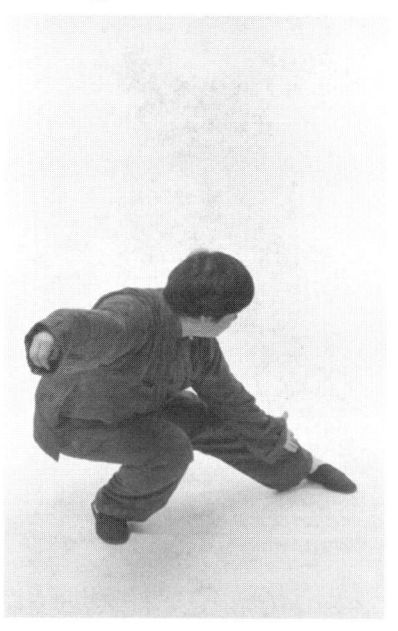

vi. Seven Star Stance:
The back leg supports the body's weight; the front leg rests on its heel, its toes are off the ground. The fist is under the elbow.

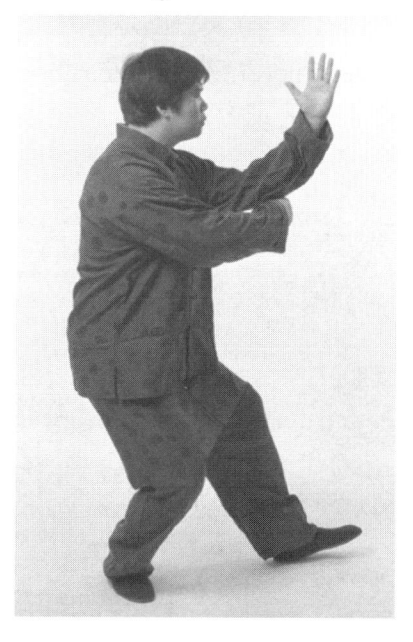

vii. Cat Stance:
The back leg supports the body's weight. For the front leg, only the toes touch the ground.

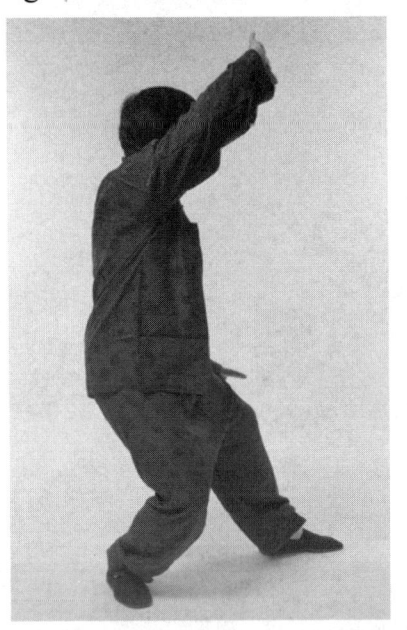

b. Step Techniques

Mobility is very important in all Chinese martial art systems. It is the ability for one to get close to or away from an opponent. It is often said that if one is launching a strike without moving the feet, one is looking for trouble. Therefore, moving the feet is very important. It is the soul of martial art.

i. Forward Step:
   The rear leg steps forward.

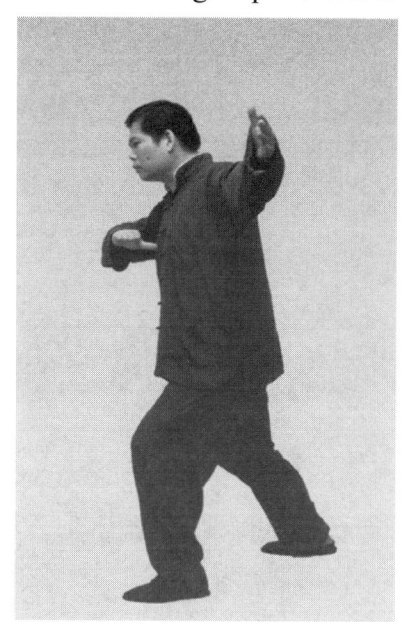

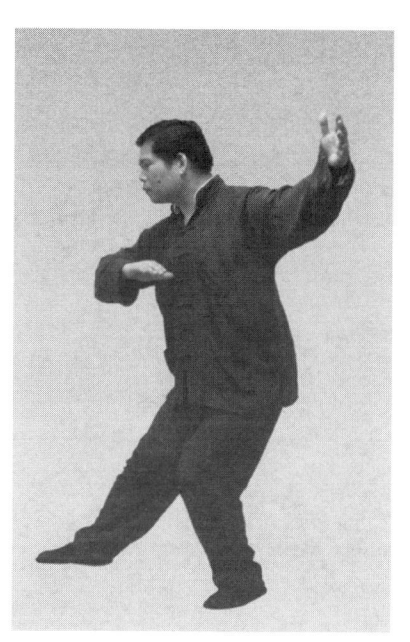

ii. Backward Step:
    The front leg steps backward.

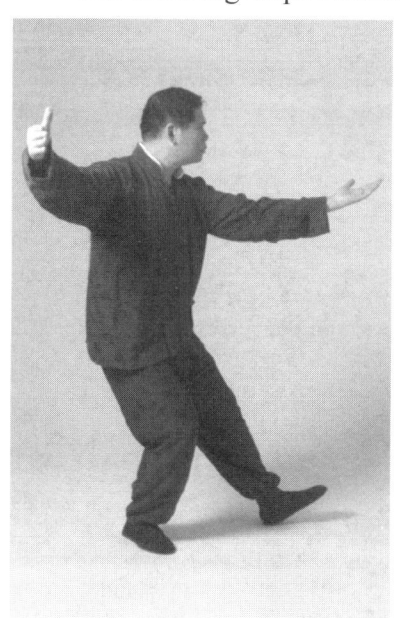

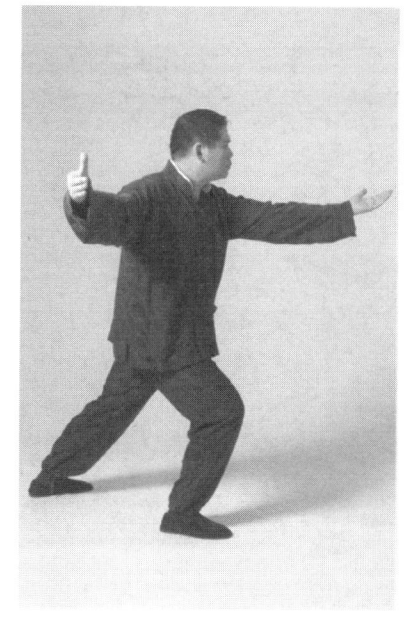

iii. Retreating Step:
   The front or back leg takes a half step back.

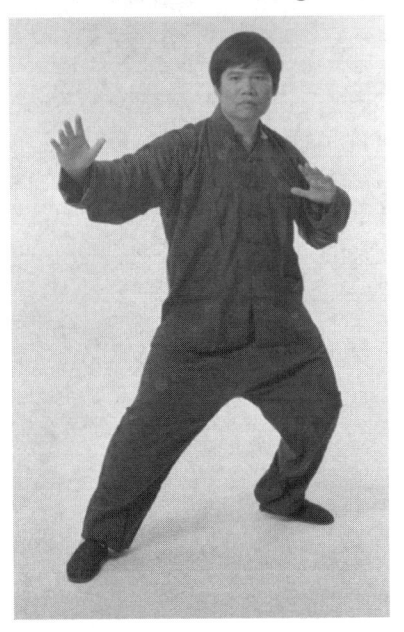

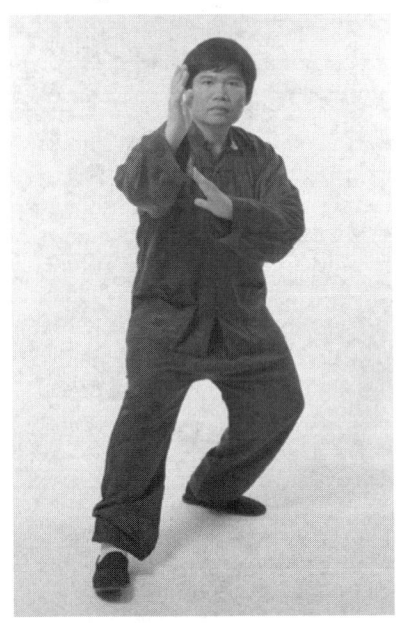

iv. Following Step:
   The back leg takes a half step forward.

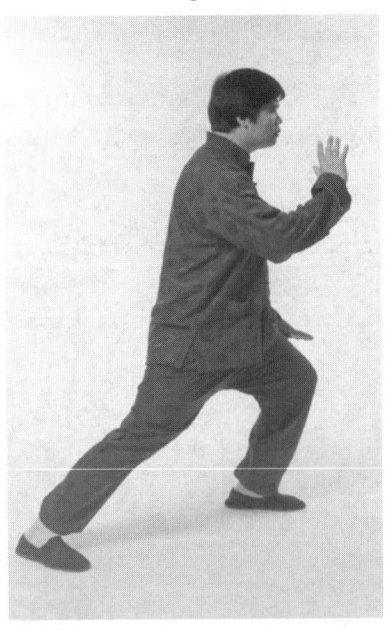

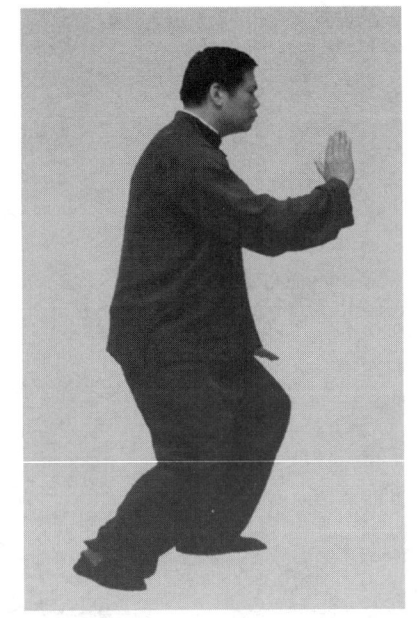

v. Side Step:
   Either foot steps to the side.

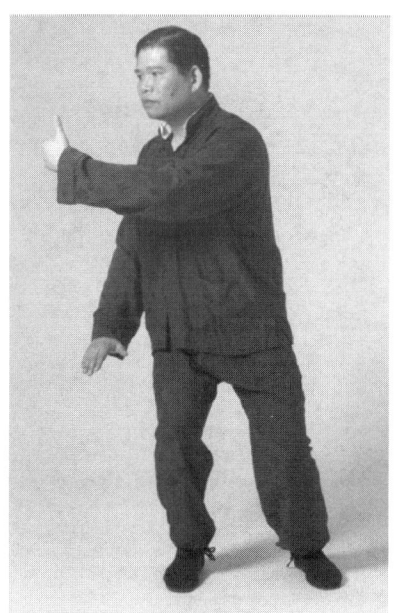

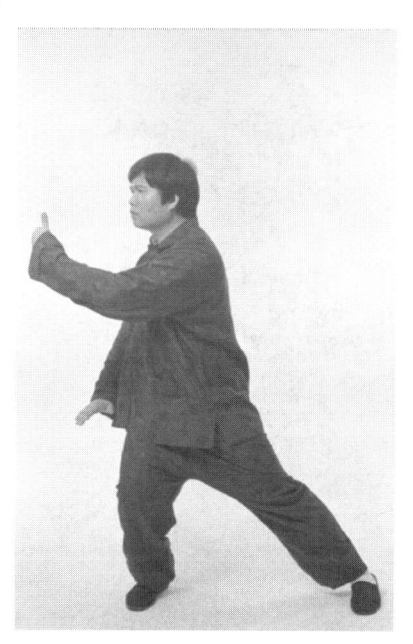

These are the common steps in Tai Chi Chuan. They must be executed slowly and evenly, distinguishing empty and full. When stepping forward, the front heel touches the ground first. When stepping backward, the back toes touch the ground first. When shifting the body weight from one foot to another, do it slowly and maintain balance. The distance between the two feet generally corresponds to the width of the shoulders. If the distance is too wide, it affects mobility. If it is too narrow, it will not develop any skill. The rotations on the heels and the toes have to be done correctly.

c. Kicking

In Tai Chi Chuan practices, the body is often supported by one leg. Therefore, there are many hidden low kicks in the Tai Chi Chuan Solo Form. The common kicks that one can see in the solo form follow:

i. Separation Kick:
   Kick with the side of the foot. Target the foe's rib cage.

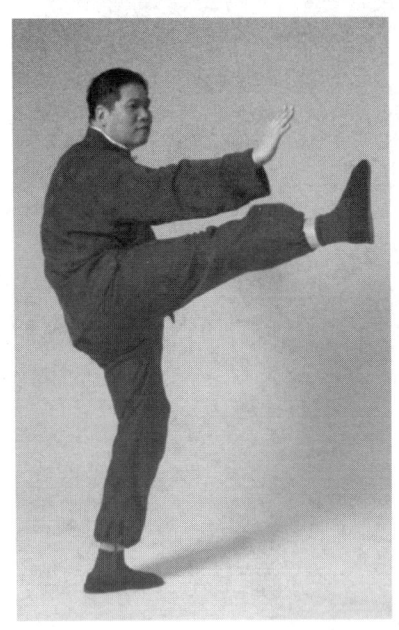

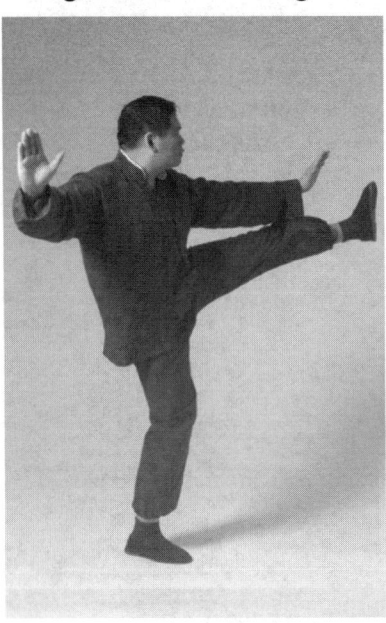

ii. Heel Kick:
   As its name indicates, kick with the heel. One should try to pull the toes inward to expose the heel for kicking.

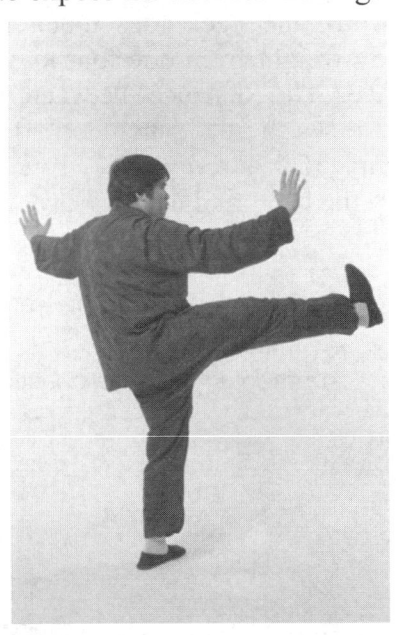

iii. Round Kick:
   This is a kick in a half circle motion by the right leg and foot. The leg and foot sweep upward and across from left to right at chest level or higher. The hands sweep across from right to left, striking the top of the right foot when they meet at the body's centerline.

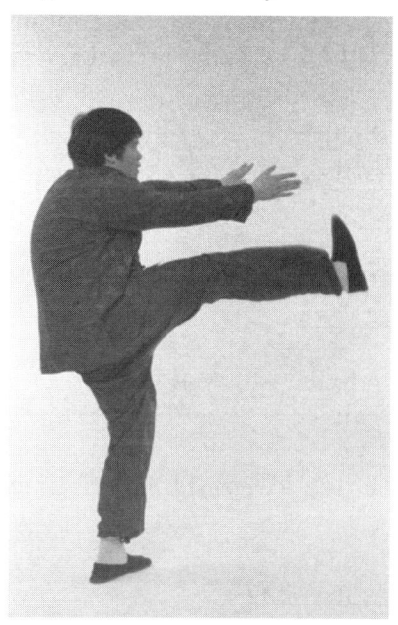

TAI CHI CHUAN - A COMPARATIVE STUDY

The 42 Movement Tai Chi Chuan Medium Frame Solo Form

This condensed Medium Frame Solo Form was developed in 1988 for intermediate level students at the Brookline Adult and Community Education Program. In that program, students begin with the 22 Movement Medium Frame Solo Form, and for those wishing to continue after the introductory level, I teach this condensed 42 Movement Medium Frame Solo Form:

1. Beginning Tai Chi Chuan
2. Grasp the Sparrow's Tail
3. Single Whip
4. High Pat Horse
5. Step Forward, Parry, Intercept, and Punch
6. Seal Tightly
7. Cross Hands
8. Embrace Tiger Return to the Mountain
9. Grasp the Sparrow's Tail
10. Fist under Elbow
11. Step Backward and Drive Away Monkey (3 times)
12. Diagonal Flying
13. Lift Hands
14. White Crane Spreads Its Wing
15. Brush Knee, Twist Step, and Push Right Hand Forward
16. Pick up Needle in Sea Bottom
17. Fan Back
18. Turn Around and Chop
19. Right Part the Wild Horse's Mane
20. Left Warding Off
21. Waving Hands Like Clouds (7 times)
22. Single Whip
23. High Pat Horse
24. Side Kicks
25. Fair Lady Works on Shuttles (2 times)
26. Left Warding Off
27. Right Foot Kick
28. Left Hitting Tiger
29. Hit the Ears with Two Fists
30. Left Foot Kick
31. Brush Knee with Twist Step (2 times)
32. Step Forward and Punch Down
33. Step Forward and Grasp the Sparrow's Tail

34. Single Whip
35. Lower the Snake Body
36. Step Forward to Become Seven Stars
37. Retreat to Ride the Tiger
38. Turn Around with Lotus Kick
39. Shooting Tiger
40. Step Forward, Parry, Intercept, and Punch
41. Seal Tightly
42. Closing Tai Chi Chuan

1. Beginning Tai Chi Chuan

Begin with the feet standing parallel to the shoulders and the body facing forward *(fig 1)*. Slowly raise the hands up to level with the shoulders *(fig 2)*. Turn the palms face down, and drop the hands down to the sides of the hip with the palms face down *(figs 3 & 4)*.

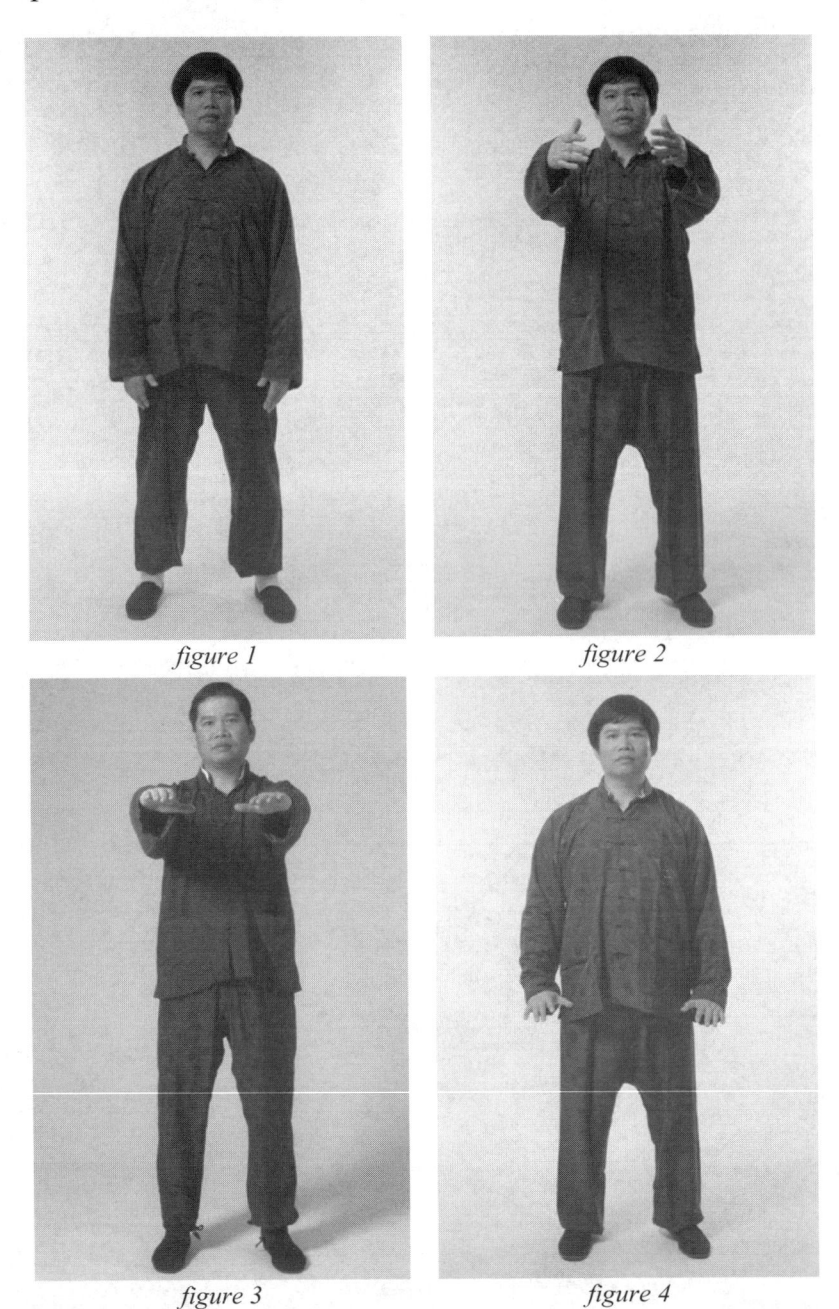

figure 1

figure 2

figure 3

figure 4

Bring the left hand up to the left of the body with the fingers pointing up and level with the left shoulder. Simultaneously, the right hand comes up to the chest with the palm facing down *(fig 5)*. Turn the right foot out 45 degrees, bend the knees, and bring the left hand under the right hand so the palms face each other *(fig 6)*.

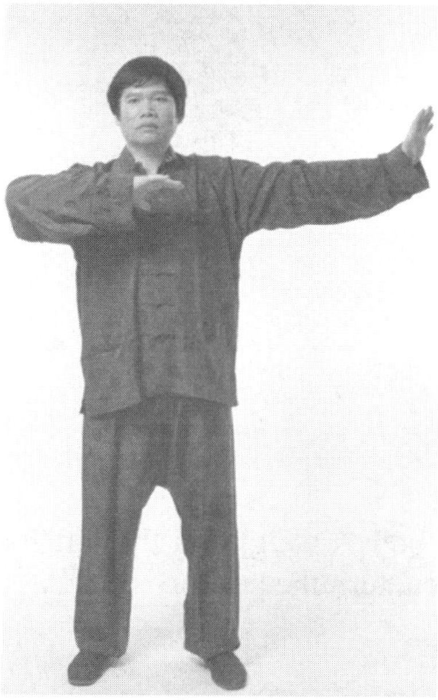

figure 5

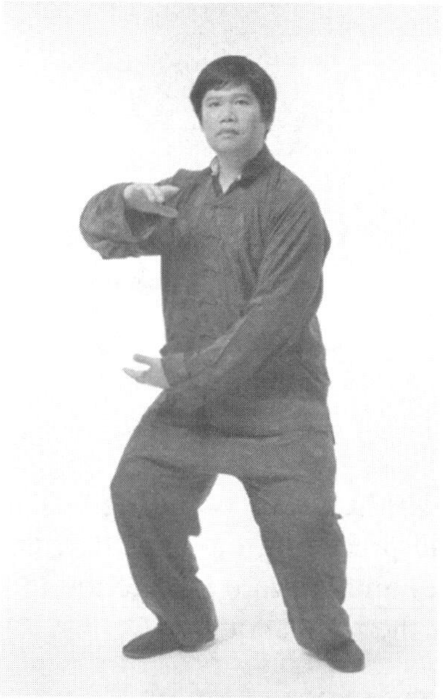

figure 6

2. Grasp the Sparrow's Tail
Part 1: Left Hand Warding Off

From the preceding movement, with the body's weight on the right foot, pick up the left foot, and step forward *(fig 7)*. As the body's weight shifts onto the left foot, separate the hands with the left hand coming up while the right hand goes down to the right side of the hip *(fig 8)*.

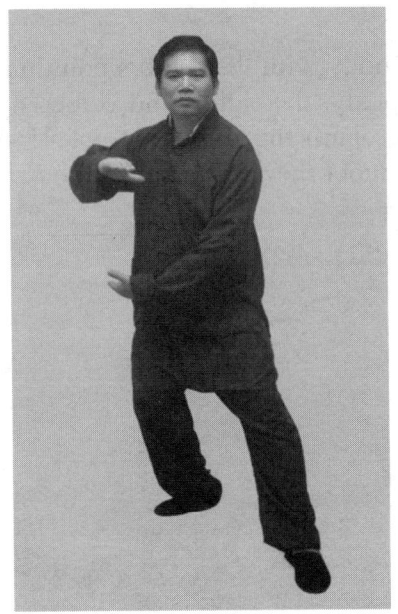

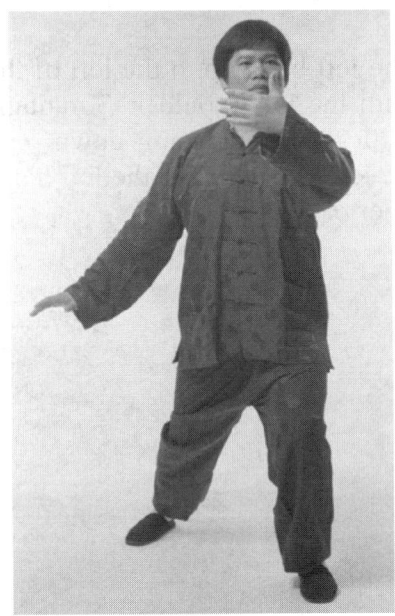

figure 7 *figure 8*

Part 2: Right Hand Warding Off
From the preceding movement with the body's weight on the left foot, bring the right hand forward next to the left knee, turn the head to the right, and look out over the right shoulder *(figs 9 & 10)*.

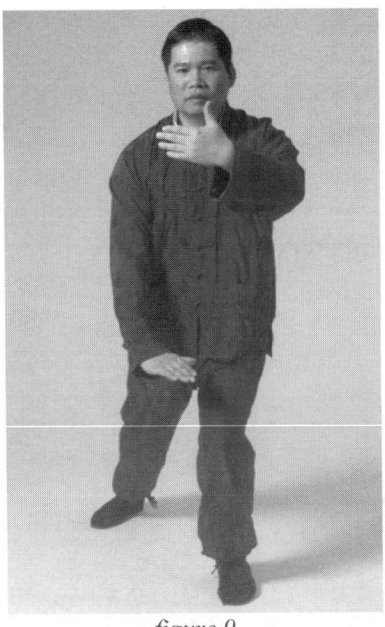

figure 9 *figure 10*

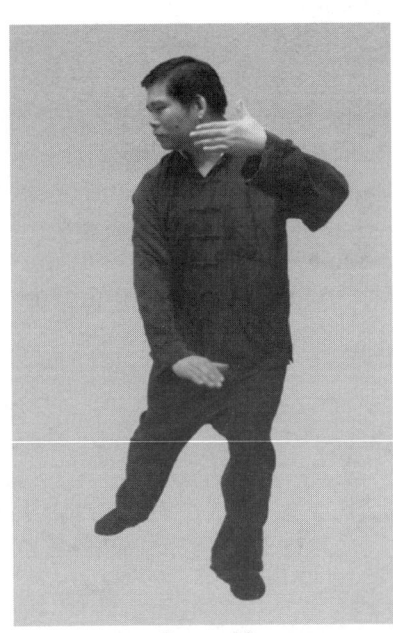

The right foot steps forward *(fig 11)*. While the body's weight is shifting onto the right foot, bring both hands up to face level. The right palm faces in, and the left palm faces out *(fig 12)*.

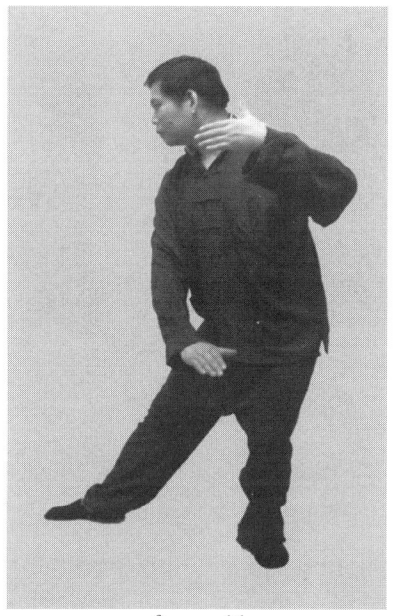

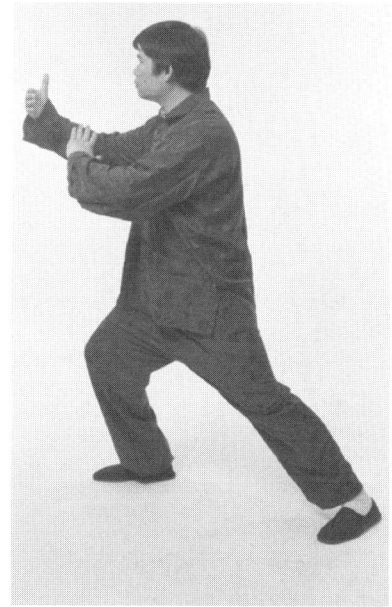

figure 11   figure 12

Part 3: Roll Back

From the preceding movement, turn both palms so the left palm faces up and the right palm faces down *(fig 13)*. Bring the hands back to the left side of the hip while shifting the body's weight onto the left foot *(figs 14 & 15)*.

TAI CHI CHUAN - A COMPARATIVE STUDY

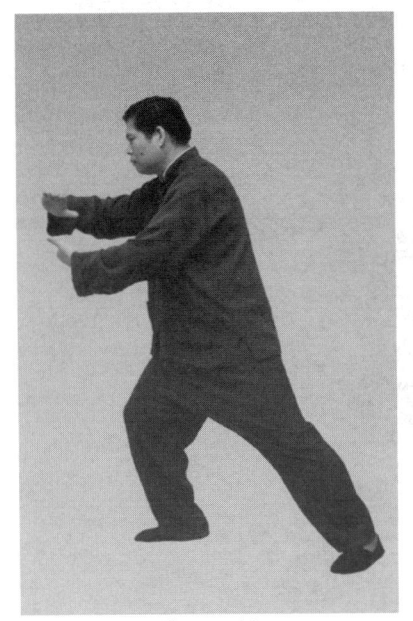

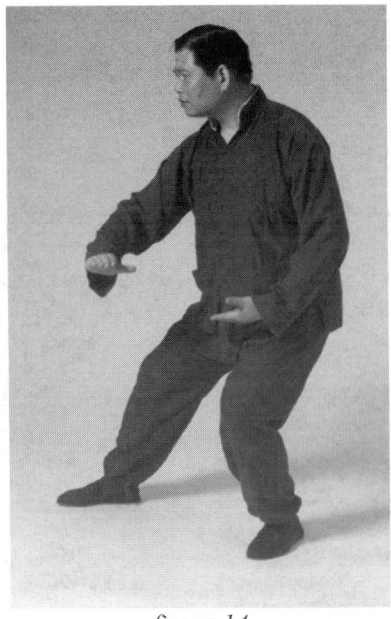

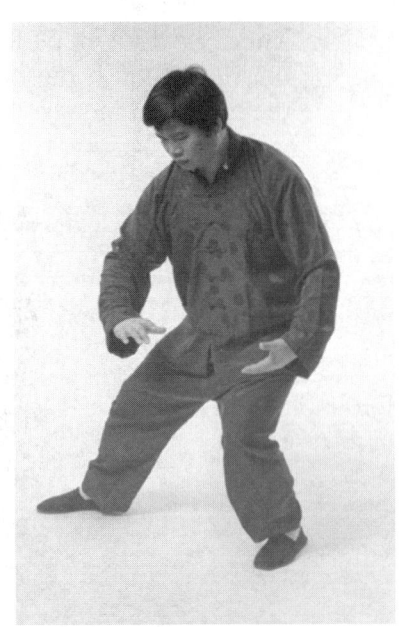

figure 13   *figure 14*   *figure 15*

Part 4: Press

From the preceding movement, turn the right palm face up, and the left palm face down, bringing the left above the right. The left hand then sticks to the right hand *(fig 16)*. Press the hands forward with the body's weight shifting onto the right foot *(fig 17)*.

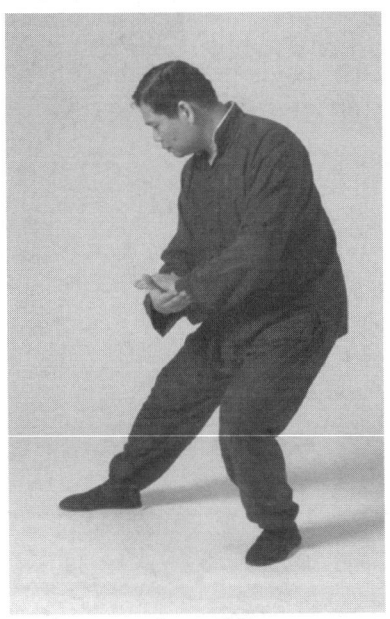

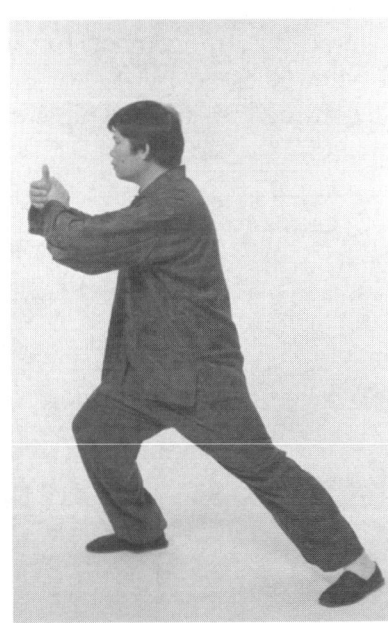

figure 16   *figure 17*

Part 5: Push

From the preceding movement, separate the two hands *(fig 18)*. Bring the hands back to the chest with the body's weight shifting onto the left foot. Bend the wrists so the palms face forward *(fig 19)*. Push the hands forward with the body's weight onto the right foot *(fig 20)*.

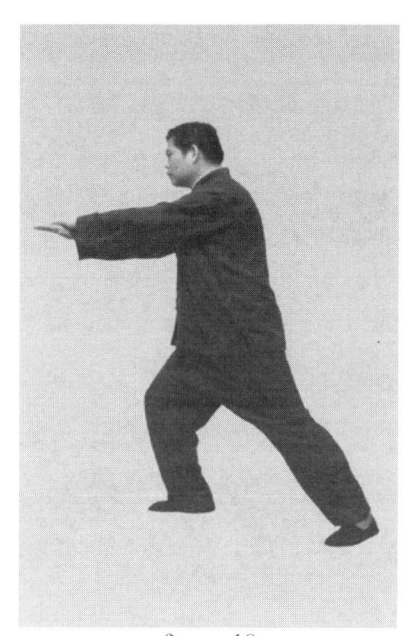

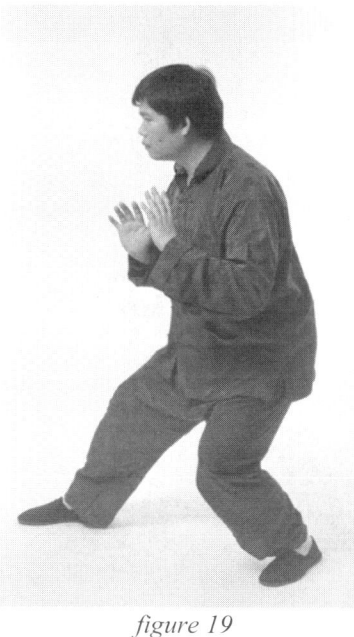

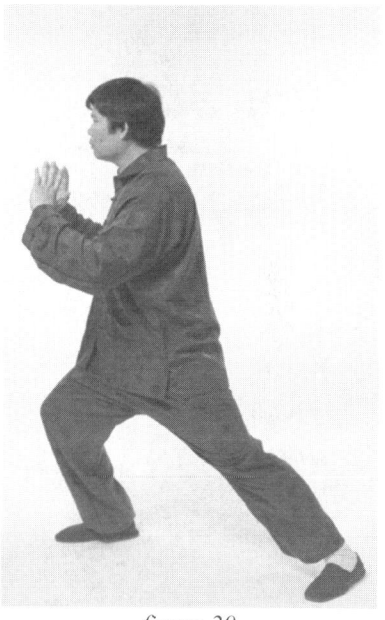

figure 18 *figure 19* *figure 20*

3. Single Whip

From the preceding movement, bring the left hand back next to the right elbow while shifting the body's weight onto the left foot *(fig 21)*. Rotate the waist to the left along with the hands while turning the right toes in *(fig 22)*. Rotate the waist back to the right with the body's weight shifting onto the right foot *(fig 23)*.

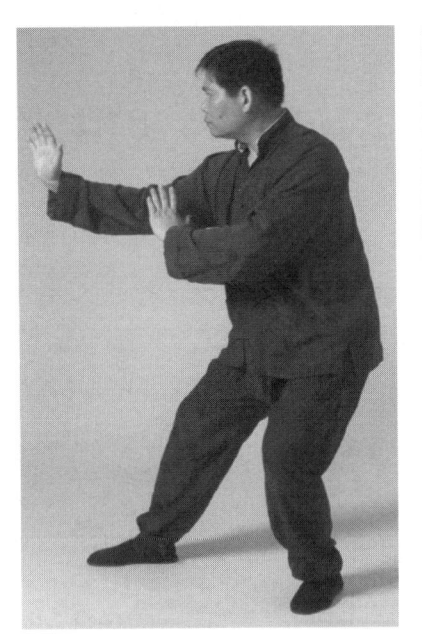

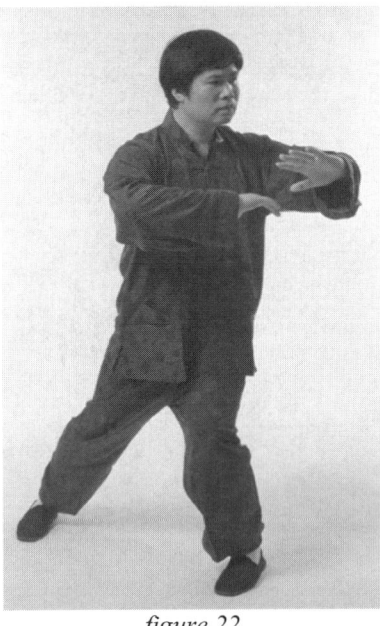

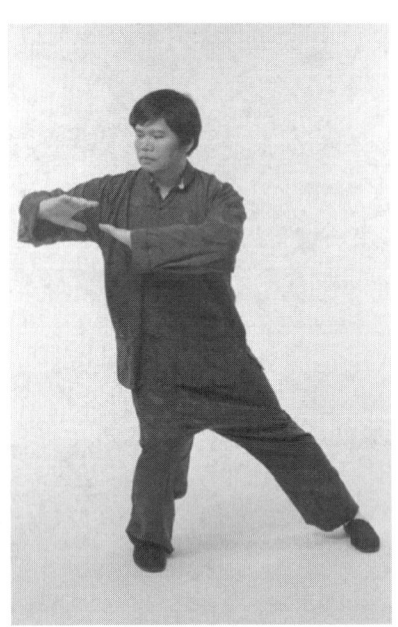

figure 21   *figure 22*   *figure 23*

Bring the right hand's fingers together to form a beak, and bend the wrist to form a hook, extending the right arm *(fig 24)*. Set the left hand in front of the face with the palm face in. Turn the head to the left; then pick up the left foot and step to the left *(fig 25)*. When the body's weight has shifted forward onto the left foot, turn the left palm to face forward. The right hand's hook remains the same *(fig 26)*.

THE 42 MOVEMENT MEDIUM FRAME SOLO FORM

figure 24　　　*figure 25*　　　*figure 26*

4. High Pat Horse

From the preceding movement, with the body's weight on the left foot, turn the left palm to face up, and shift the body's weight back onto the right foot *(fig 27)*. With the body's weight shifted onto the right foot, open the right hand, and bring it on top of the left shoulder with the palm face down. Set the left foot on its toes; then push the right hand forward with the palm face out, while bringing the left hand back to the left side of the waist *(fig 28)*.

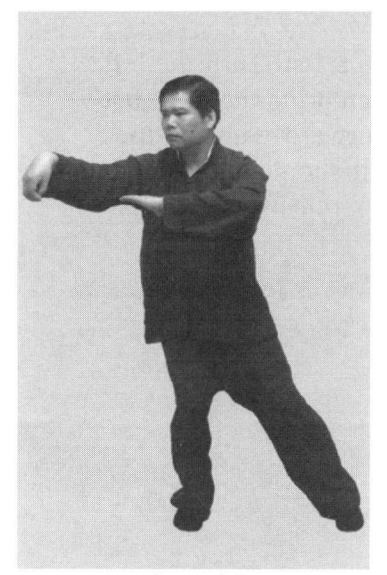

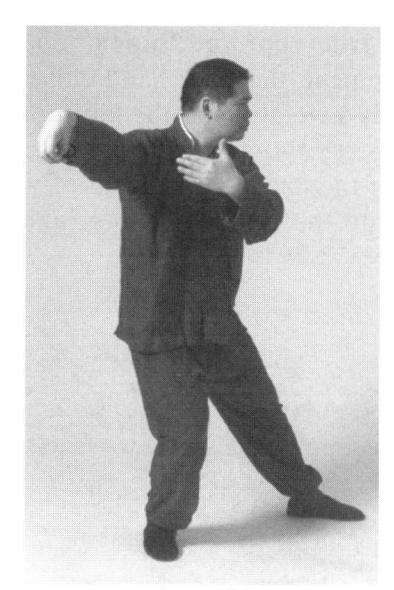

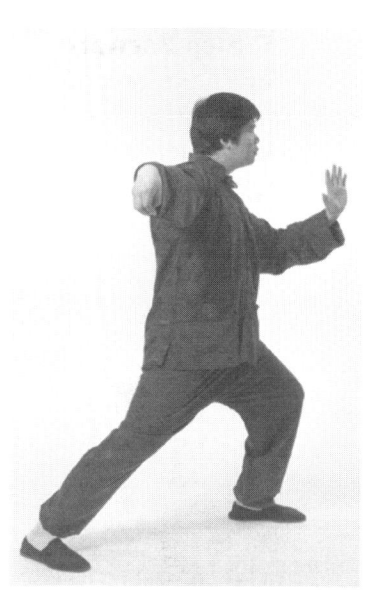

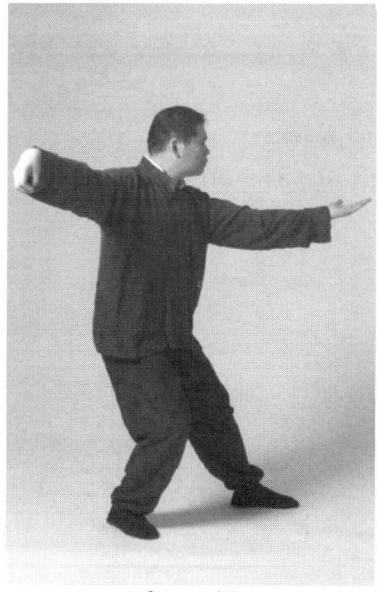

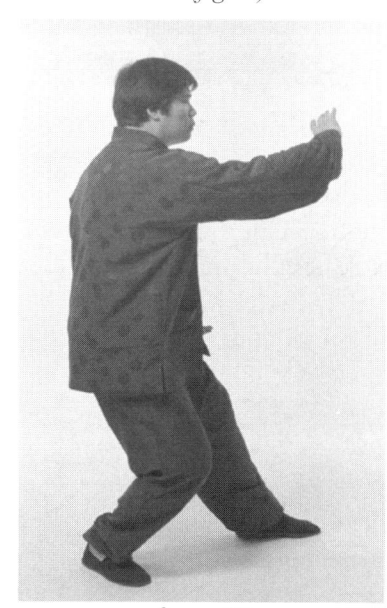

figure 27　　　*figure 28*

5. Step Forward, Parry, Intercept and Punch

From the preceding movement, the right hand closes into a fist. Turn the left toes out, and shift the body's weight onto the left foot. Then bring the right fist to the left side of the hip *(fig 29)*. The right foot steps forward with the toes pointing out *(fig 30)*; bring the hands up in front of the left shoulder. With the body's weight shifting onto the right foot, the right fist circles forward then down *(fig 31)*.

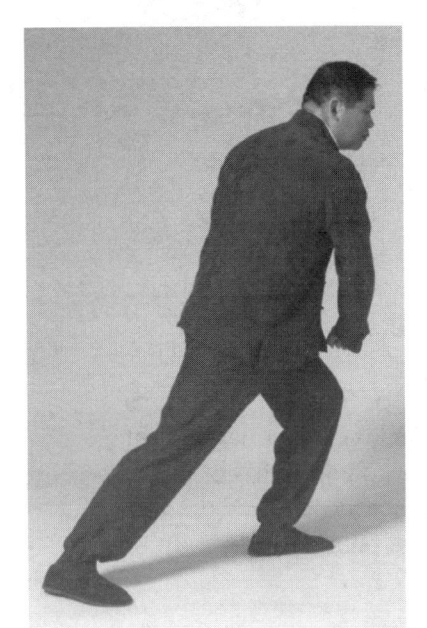

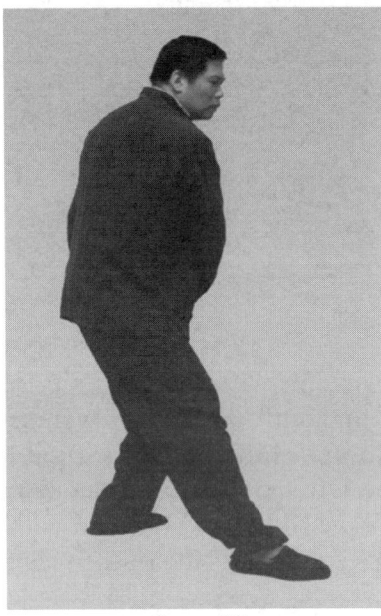

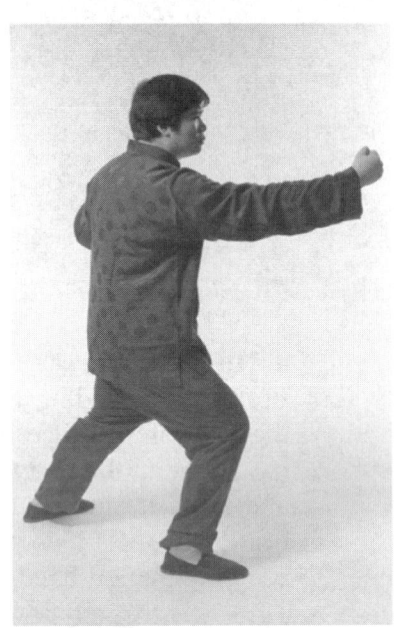

figure 29 *figure 30* *figure 31*

Bring the right fist back onto the right side of the hip and push the left hand forward from the left shoulder *(fig 32)*. With the body's weight on the right foot, pick up the left foot, and step forward *(fig 33)*. While the body's weight is shifting onto the left foot, the right fist punches forward, and the left palm comes back next to the right elbow *(fig 34)*.

THE 42 MOVEMENT MEDIUM FRAME SOLO FORM

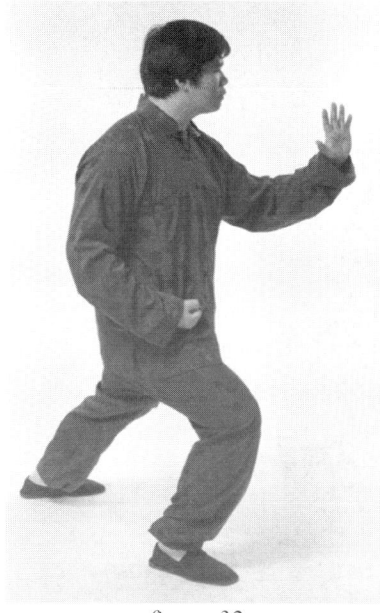

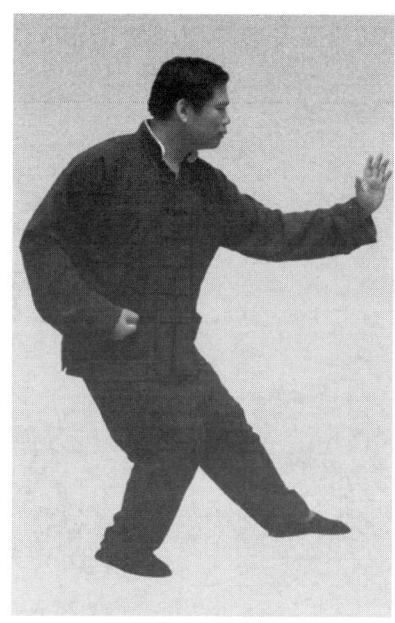

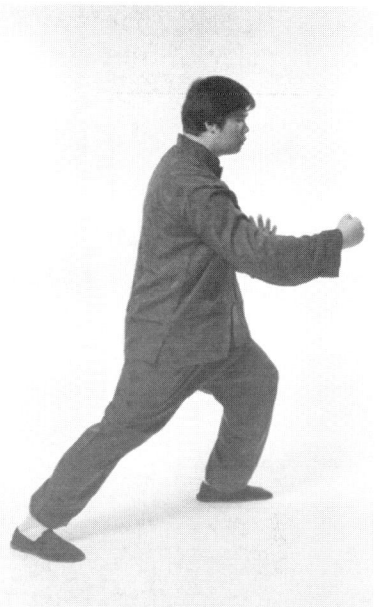

figure 32 *figure 33* *figure 34*

6. Seal Tightly

From the preceding movement, put the left hand under the right elbow with the palm face up *(fig 35)*. Open the right fist, and bring it back to the right side of the hip with the body's weight shifting onto the right foot and the left arm pushing forward with the palm face in *(figs 36 & 37)*.

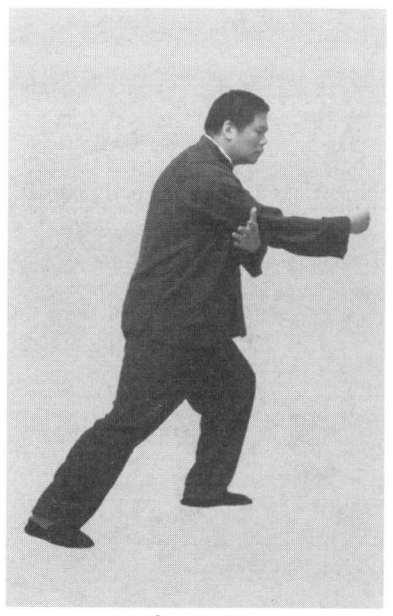

figure 35 *figure 36* *figure 37*

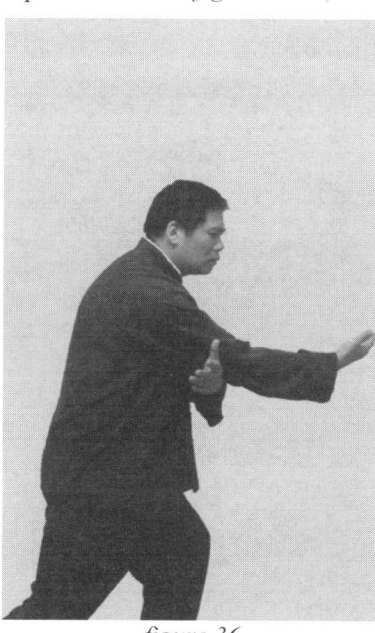

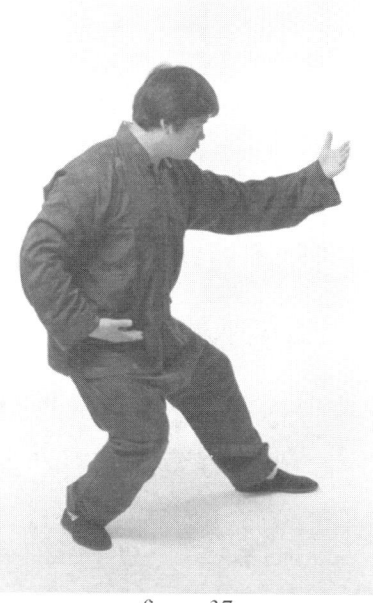

Bring the hands in front of the chest with the palms face forward *(fig 38)*. Push the hands forward with the body's weight shifting onto the left foot *(fig 39)*.

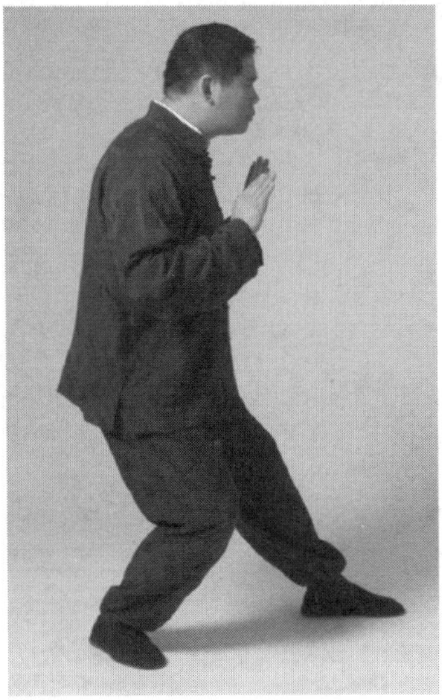

figure 38

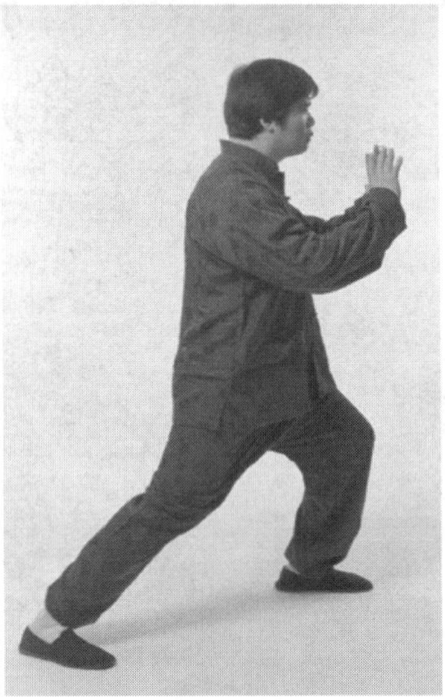

figure 39

7. Cross Hands

From the preceding movement, bring the hands back to the chest with the palms still facing forward as the weight shifts back onto the right leg *(fig 40)*. Rotate the waist to the right, turning the left toes in and pushing the right hand out *(fig 41)*. Shift the body's weight onto the left foot, and push the left hand out; the right hand remains the same *(fig 42)*.

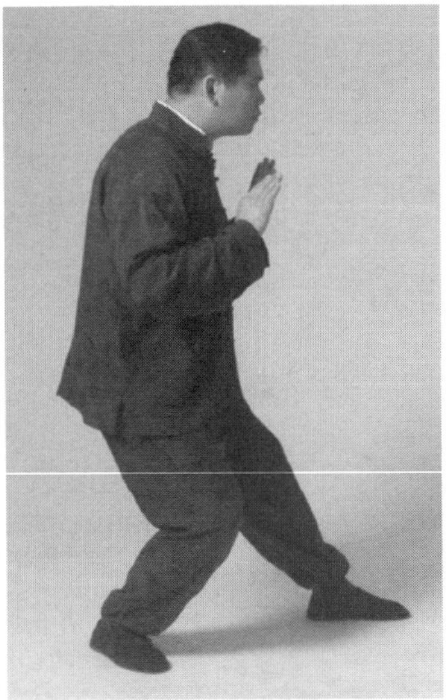

figure 40

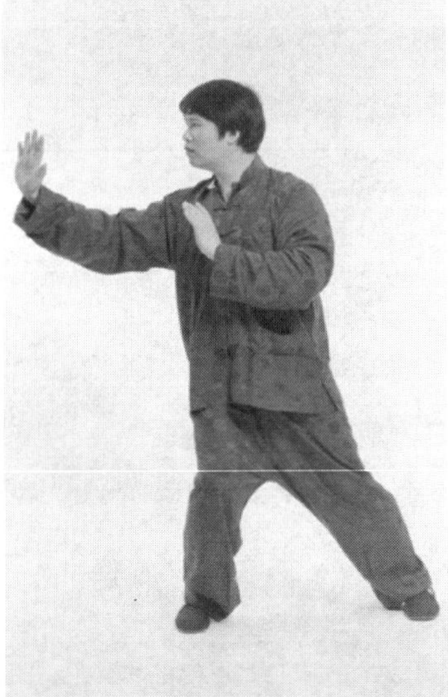

figure 41

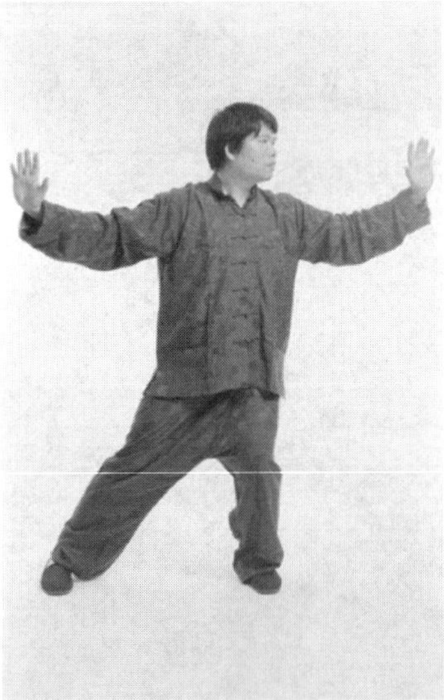

figure 42

With the eyes and body facing forward, pick up the right foot, and step next to the left foot at a width parallel to the shoulders *(fig 43)*. The two hands come down to the abdomen. Cross the hands together at the wrists, the left wrist on top of the right wrist *(fig 44)*. Turn the wrists to bring the hands up to face level with the palms facing in *(fig 45)*.

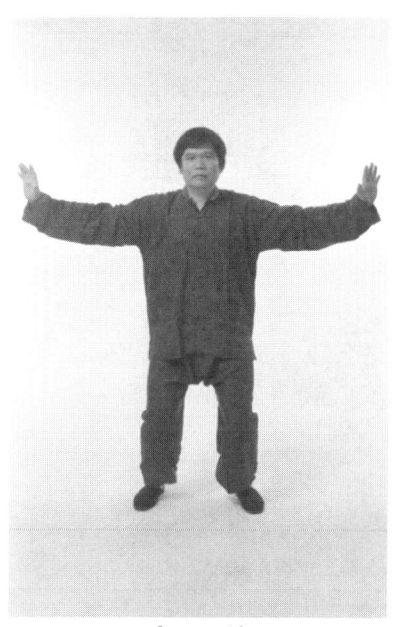

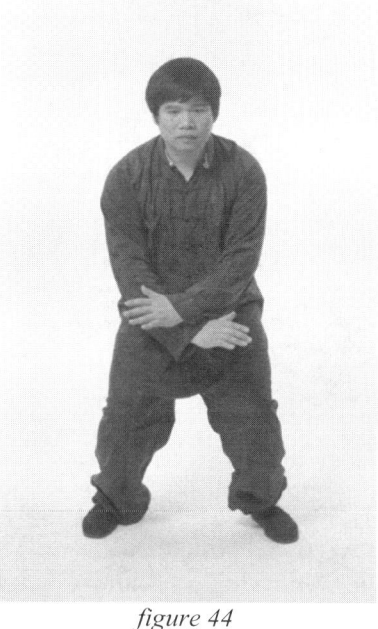

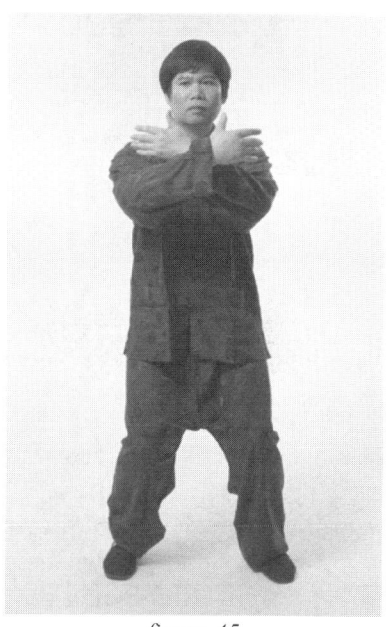

figure 43 *figure 44* *figure 45*

8. Embrace Tiger Return to the Mountain

From the preceding movement, turn the left foot in, and bring the left hand outside the right hand, turning the right palm down *(fig 46)*. Turn the head to the right corner, and with the body's weight on the left foot, pick up the right foot, and step forward *(fig 47)*. While shifting the body's weight onto the right foot, the right hand goes down to the right side of the right knee, and the left hand pushes forward from the left shoulder *(fig 48)*.

TAI CHI CHUAN - A COMPARATIVE STUDY

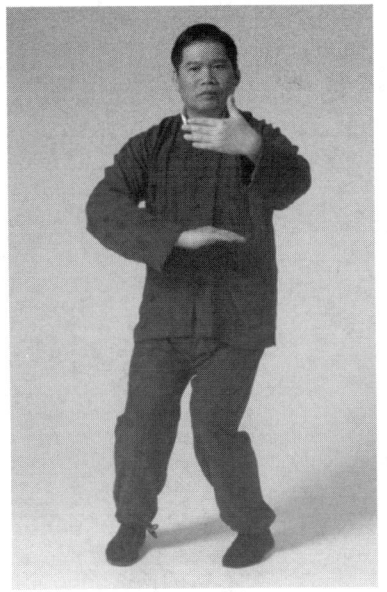

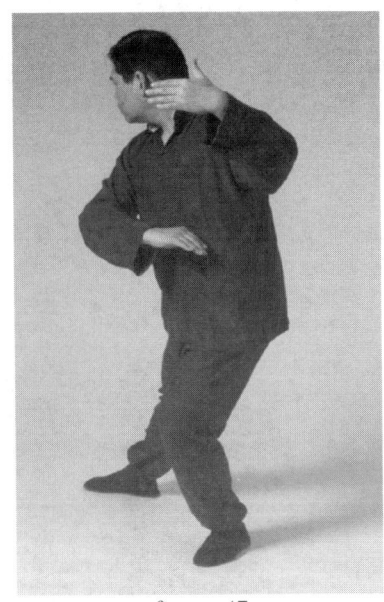

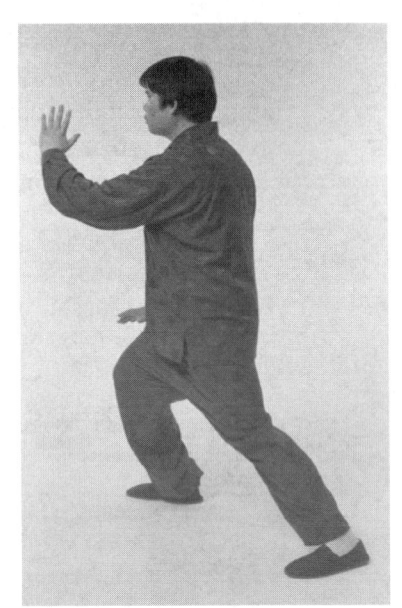

figure 46   *figure 47*   *figure 48*

9. Grasp Sparrow's Tail
Part 1: Roll Back

From the preceding movement, bring the right hand in a hook up above the left hand *(fig 49)*. Open the right hand; turn the left palm to face up with the right palm facing down *(fig 50)*. Bring the hands back to the left side of the hip, and at the same time, shift the body's weight onto the left foot *(fig 51)*.

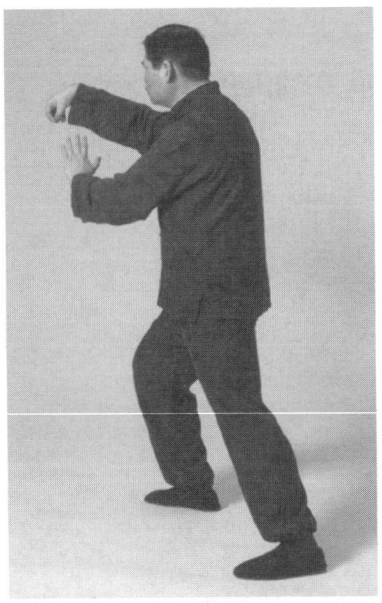

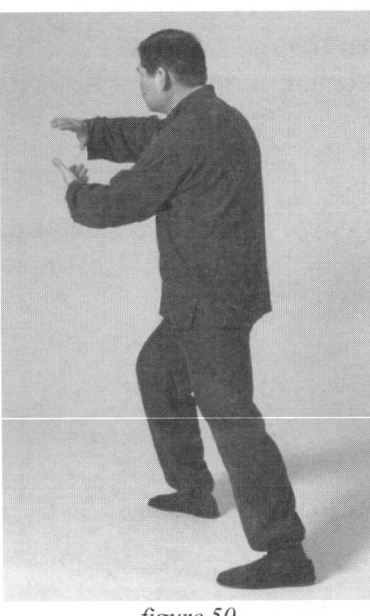

figure 49   *figure 50*   *figure 51*

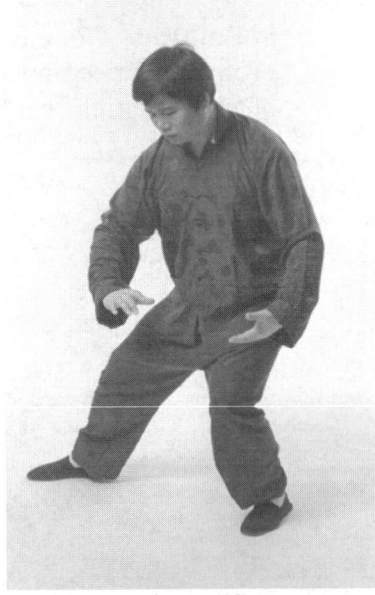

212

THE 42 MOVEMENT MEDIUM FRAME SOLO FORM

Part 2: Press

From the preceding movement, turn the right palm face up and the left palm face down. The left hand then sticks to the right hand *(fig 52)*. Press the hands forward with the body's weight shifting onto the right foot *(fig 53)*.

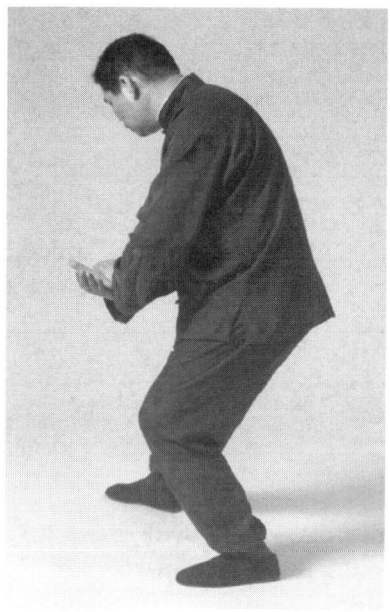

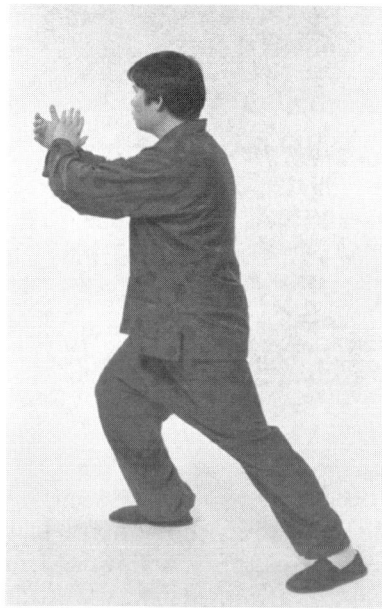

figure 52   *figure 53*

Part 3: Push

From the preceding movement, separate the two hands *(fig 54)*. Bring the hands back to the chest with the body's weight shifting onto the left foot. Bend the wrists so the palms face forward *(fig 55)*. Push the hands forward with the body's weight shifting onto the right foot *(fig 56)*.

TAI CHI CHUAN - A COMPARATIVE STUDY

figure 54 *figure 55* *figure 56*

Part 4: Push

From the preceding movement, bring the left hand back next to the right elbow with the body's weight shifting onto the left foot *(fig 57)*. Rotate the waist to the left with the hands following along and right toes turning in *(fig 58)*.

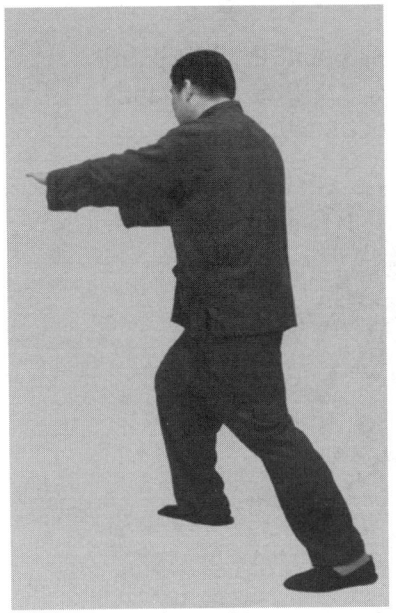

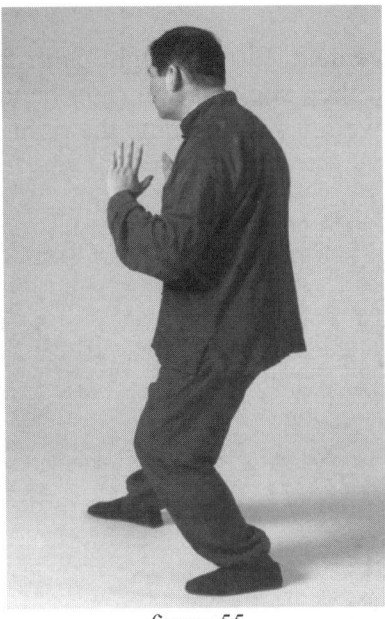

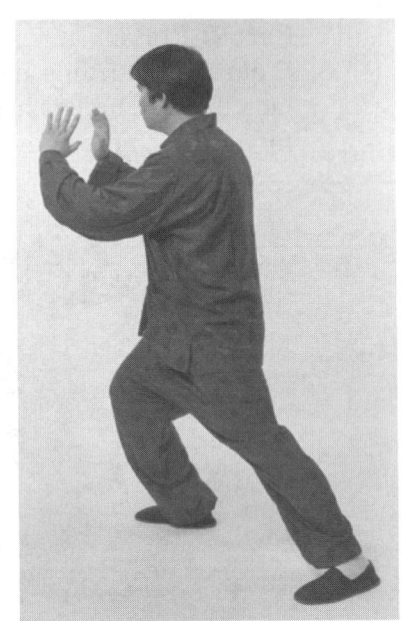

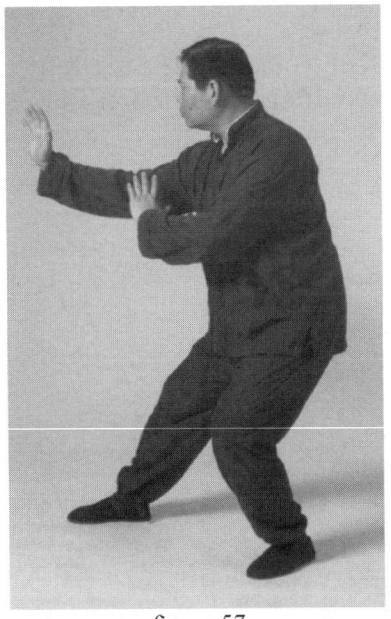

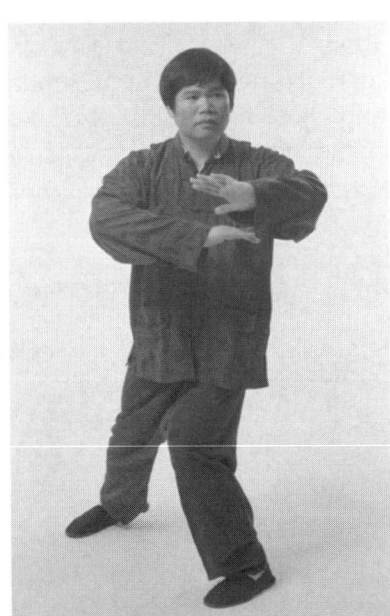

figure 57 *figure 58*

THE 42 MOVEMENT MEDIUM FRAME SOLO FORM

Rotate the waist back to the right with the body's weight shifting onto the right foot *(fig 59)*. Turn the head to look to the left, pick up the left foot, and step forward. The body's weight then shifts onto the left foot, and the hands push forward *(fig 60)*.

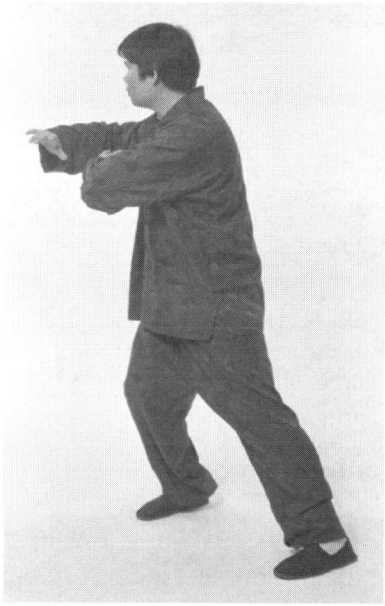

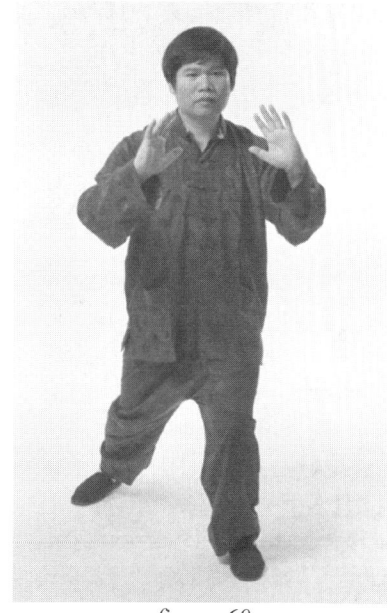

figure 59   *figure 60*

10. Fist under Elbow

From the preceding movement, pick up the right foot, and step in front of the left foot *(fig 61)*. Close the right hand into a fist, and shift the body's weight onto the right foot. Look out from the left shoulder *(fig 62)*; pick up the left foot, and land it on the heel with the body's weight remaining on the right foot; bring the right fist under the left elbow *(fig 63)*.

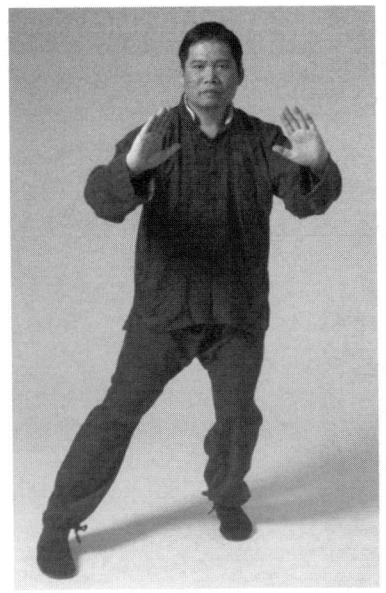

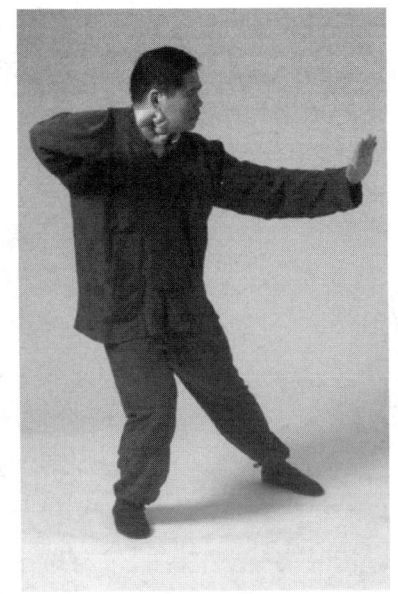

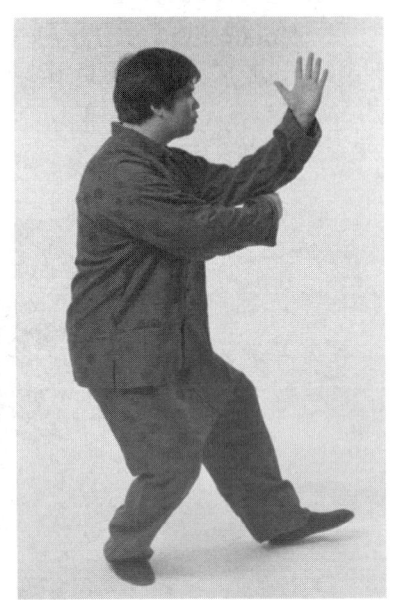

figure 61　　　　　*figure 62*　　　　　*figure 63*

11. Step Backward and Drive Away Monkey (three times)
Part 1: Left Step Backward
From the preceding movement, open the right fist, swing it out to the right, and make it level with the right shoulder; extend the left hand forward, facing the palm up *(figs 64 & 65)*. With the body's weight on the right foot, pick up the left foot, and step backward *(fig 66)*.

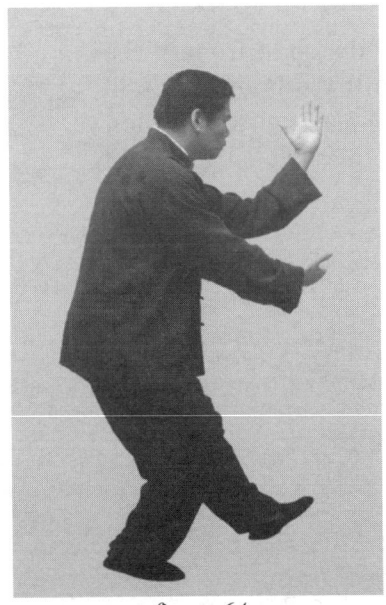

figure 64　　　　　*figure 65*　　　　　*figure 66*

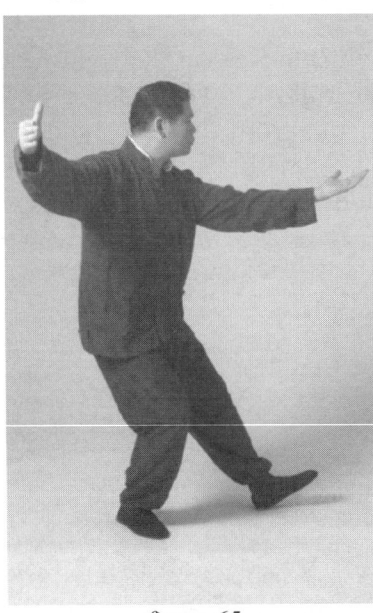

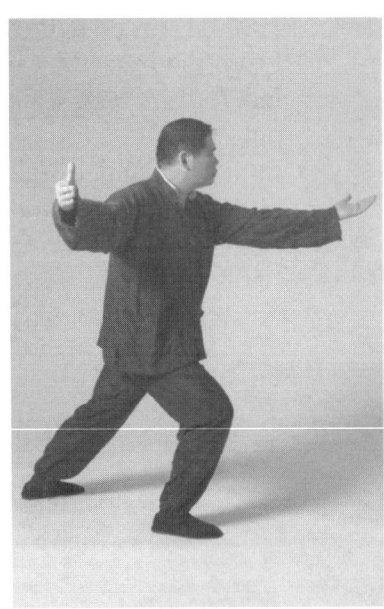

Bring the right hand in front of the right shoulder *(fig 67)*, and shift the body's weight onto the left foot. Push the right hand forward with the palm face forward, and at the same time, bring the left hand back to the left side of the hip with the palm face up *(fig 68)*.

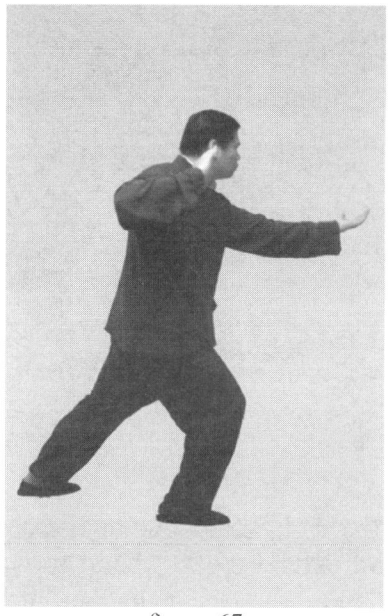

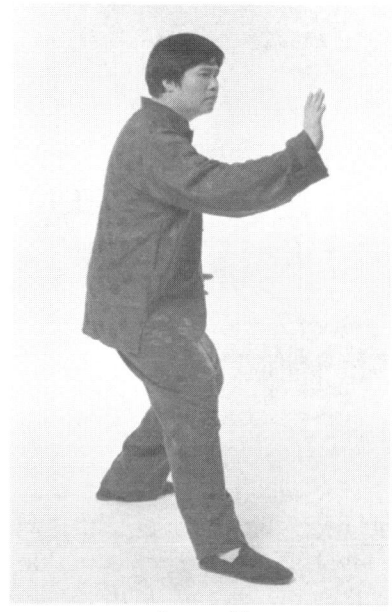

figure 67   *figure 68*

Part 2: Right Step Backward

From the preceding movement, swing the left hand out to the left, make it level with the left shoulder, and extend the right hand straight forward with the palm face up *(fig 69)*. With the body's weight on the left foot, pick up the right foot, and step backwards *(fig 70)*. Shift the body's weight onto the right foot, and bring the left hand in front of the left shoulder. Push the left hand forward with the palm face forward, and at the same time, bring the right hand back to the right side of the hip with the palm face up *(fig 71)*.

TAI CHI CHUAN - A COMPARATIVE STUDY

figure 69   *figure 70*   *figure 71*

Part 3: Left Step Backward
From the preceding movement, swing the right hand out to the right side, make it level with the right shoulder, and extend the left hand forward with the palm face up *(fig 72)*. With the body's weight on the right foot, pick up the left foot, and step backwards *(fig 73)*.

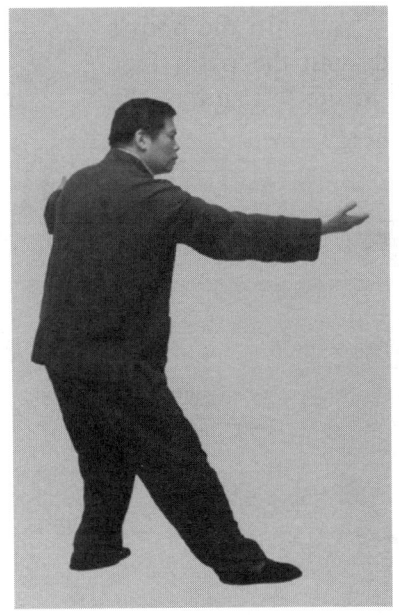

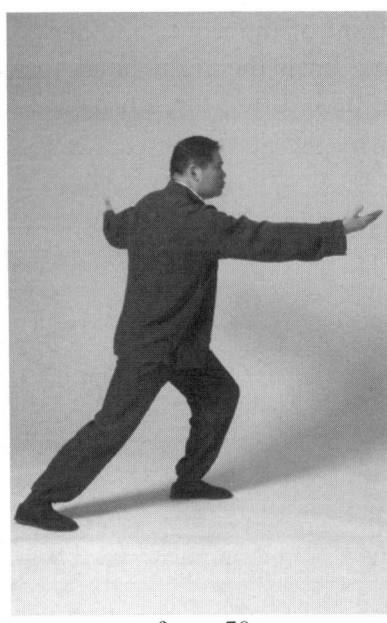

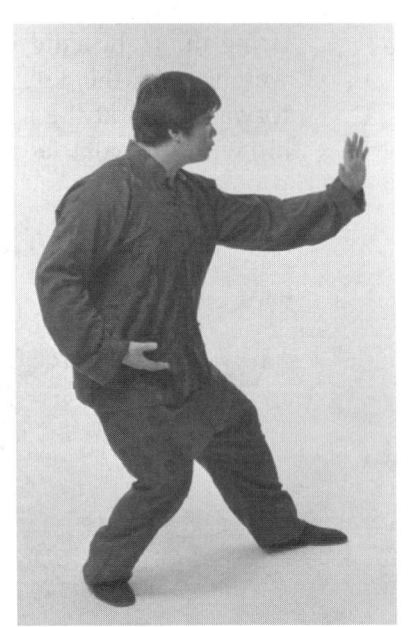

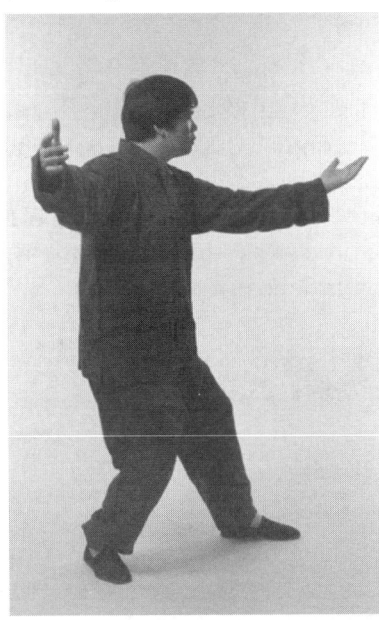

figure 72   *figure 73*

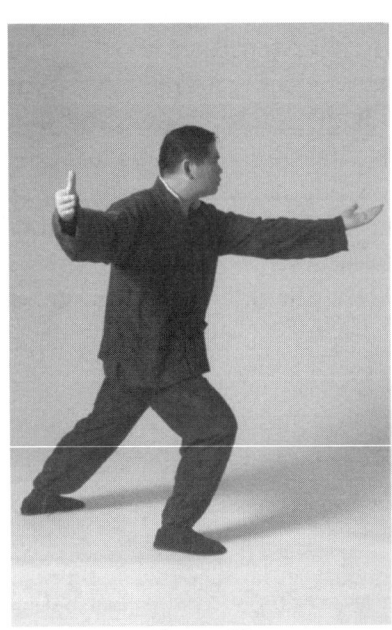

218

Bring the right hand in front of the right shoulder *(fig 74)*, and shift the body's weight onto the left foot. Push the right hand forward with the palm face forward, and at the same time, pull the left hand back to the left side of the hip with the palm face up *(fig 75)*.

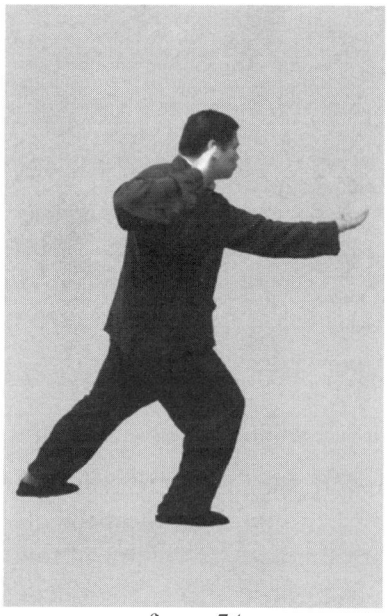

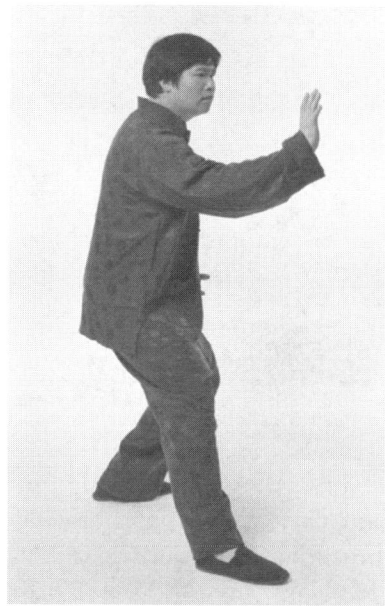

figure 74   *figure 75*

12. Diagonal Flying

From the preceding movement, bring the right hand under the left hand with the palms facing each other *(fig 76)*. Turn the head, and look out from the right shoulder with the body's weight on the left foot; pick up the right foot, and step to the right corner *(fig 77)*. Shift the body's weight onto the right foot, and at the same time, separate the hands with the right hand going up to face level, palm facing in and the left hand going down to the left side of the body, palm facing down *(fig 78)*.

TAI CHI CHUAN - A COMPARATIVE STUDY

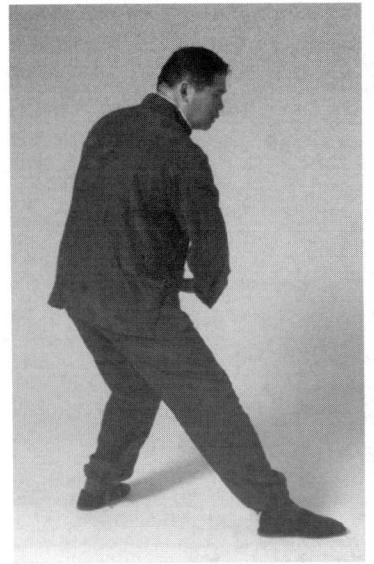

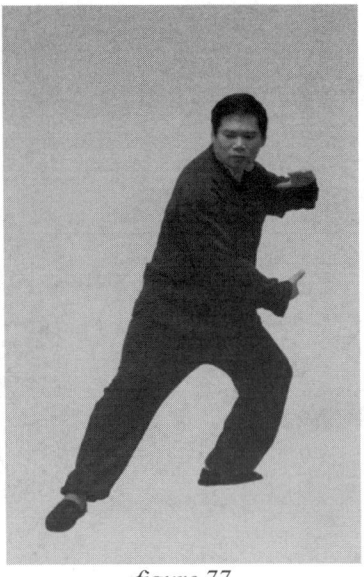

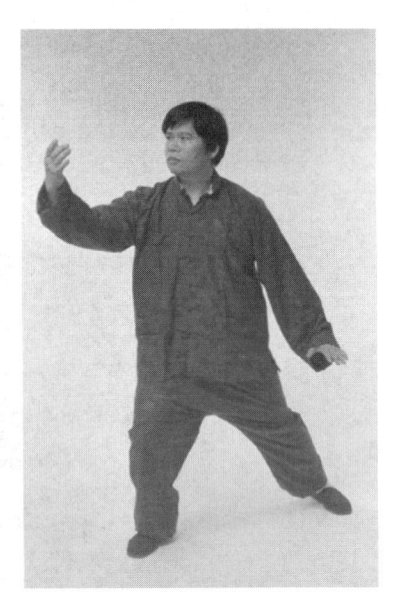

figure 76   *figure 77*   *figure 78*

13. Lift Hands

From the preceding movement, turn the left foot outward. Shift the body's weight onto the left foot, and bring the left hand up in front of the chest as the right palm turns to face down *(fig 79)*. With the body's weight on the left foot, pick up the right foot, and place it to the front on its heel. Then bring the two hands together with the left palm facing the right elbow and the right palm facing to the left *(fig 80)*.

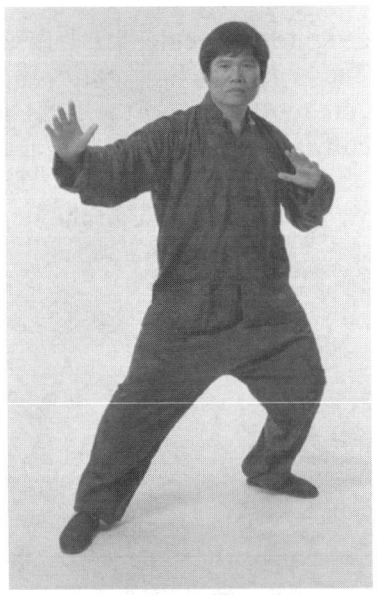

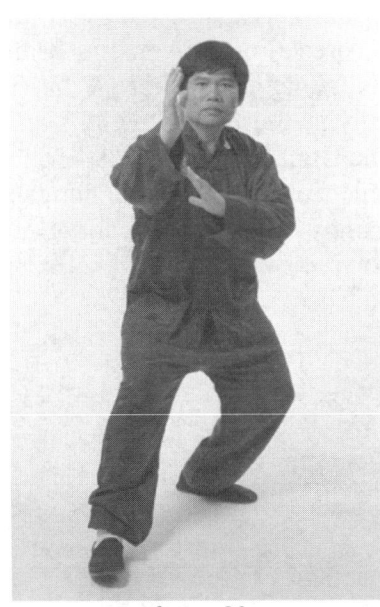

figure 79   *figure 80*

14. White Crane Spreads Its Wing

From the preceding movement, turn the left palm to face up and the right palm to face down. Pull the hands down to the left side of the body *(fig 81)*. Pick up the right foot, and step forward. Shift the body's weight onto the right foot. At the same time, the hands move forward with the left hand against the right elbow *(fig 82)*.

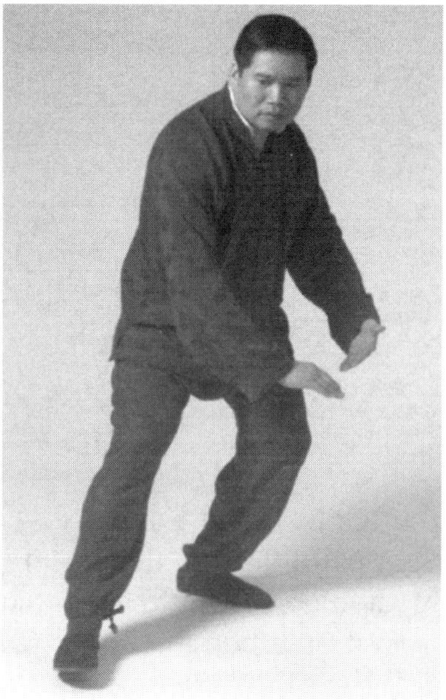

figure 81

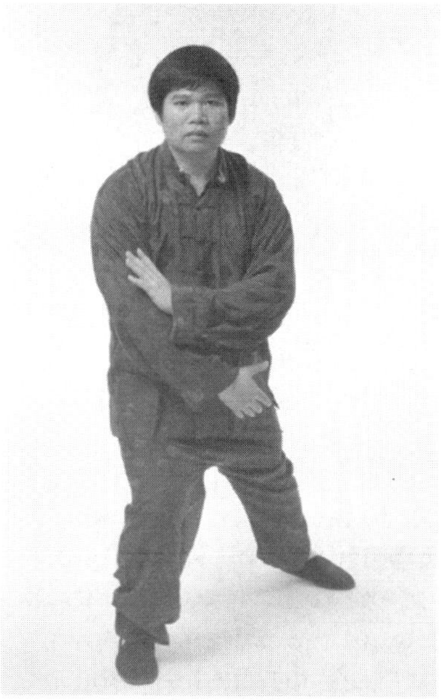

figure 82

Separate the hands with the right hand coming up to face level, palm facing in, and the left hand going down to the left side of the body, palm facing down *(fig 83)*. With the body's weight on the right foot, look out to the left; then pick up the left foot, and place it on the ground, toes only. Turn the right palm to face out, and bring it up in front of the forehead with the thumb pointing down; at the same time, rotate the waist to the left. The left hand remains on the left side of the body *(fig 84)*.

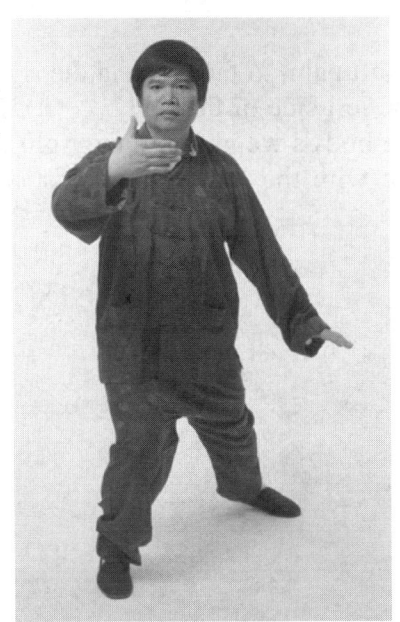

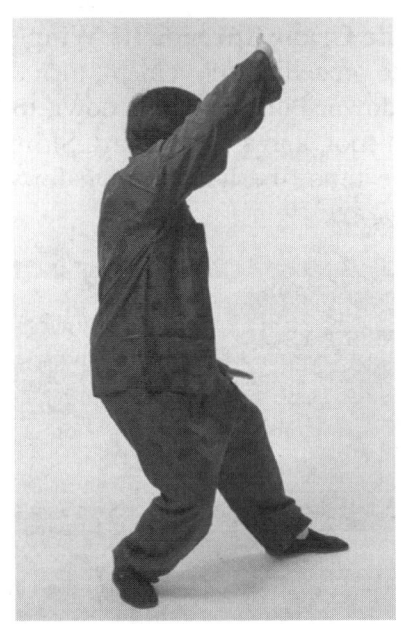

figure 83 *figure 84*

15. Brush Knee, Twist Step, and Push the Right Hand Forward

From the preceding movement, turn the right palm face in; then swing it down and out to the right side, level to the right shoulder. Bring the left hand up to the chest with the palm face down *(fig 85)*. With the body's weight still on the right foot, pick up the left foot, and step forward. While shifting the body's weight onto the left foot, brush the left hand down to the left side of the left knee with the palm face down, and bring the right hand in front of the right shoulder; then push it forward with the palm face forward *(figs 86 & 87)*.

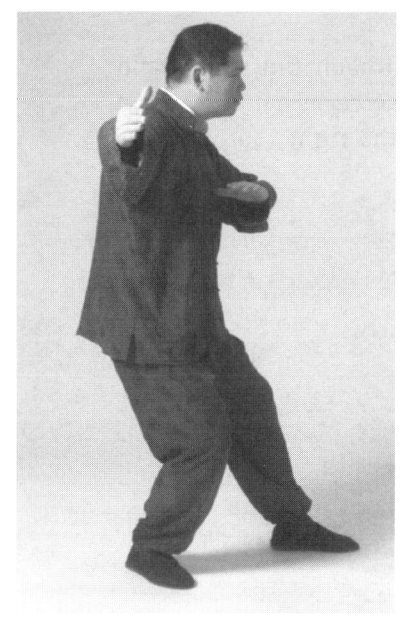

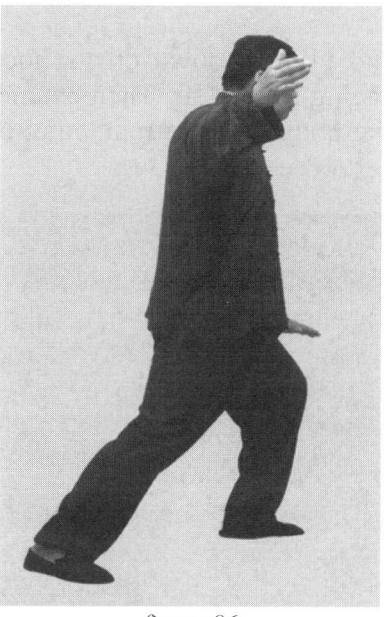

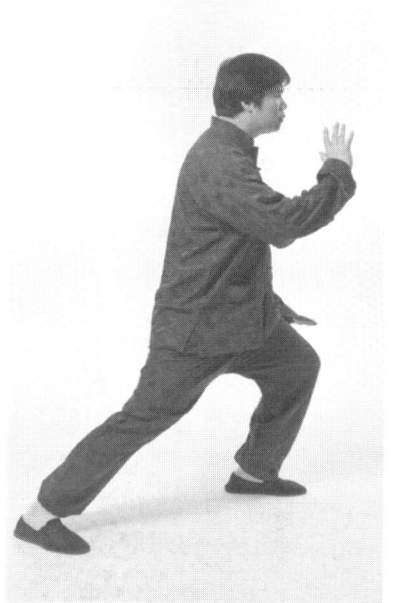

figure 85 *figure 86* *figure 87*

16. Pick Up Needle in Sea Bottom

From the preceding movement, step the right foot forward beside the left foot; then bring the right hand back in front of the shoulder as the body's weight shifts onto the right foot *(figs 88 & 89)*.

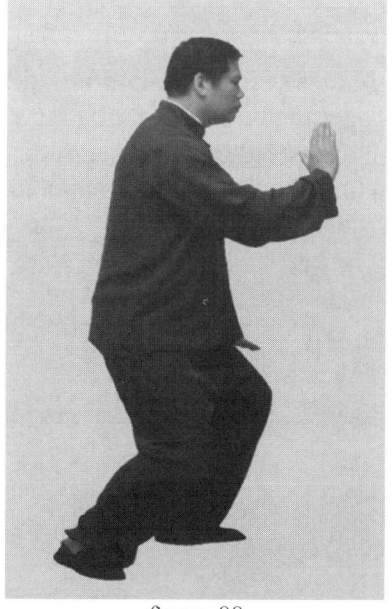

figure 88 *figure 89*

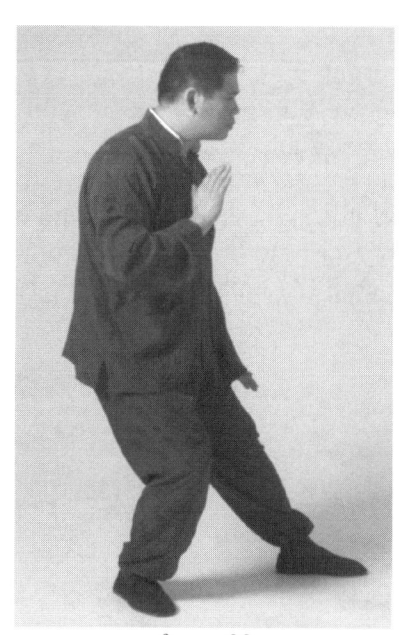

Pick up the left foot, and place it down on the toes. Reach the right hand forward with the palm facing to the left. Then extend the right hand down in front of the body with the body's weight remaining on the right foot, and the left hand outside of the left knee *(figs 90 & 91)*.

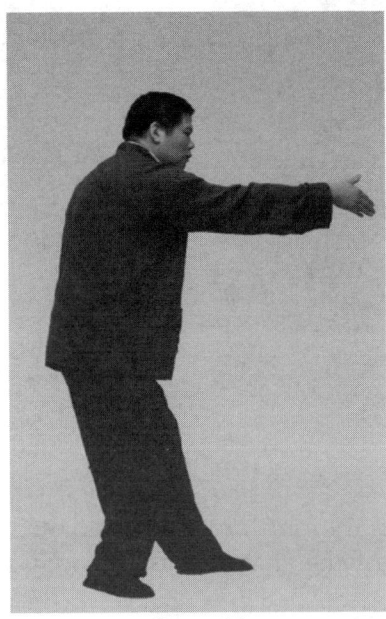

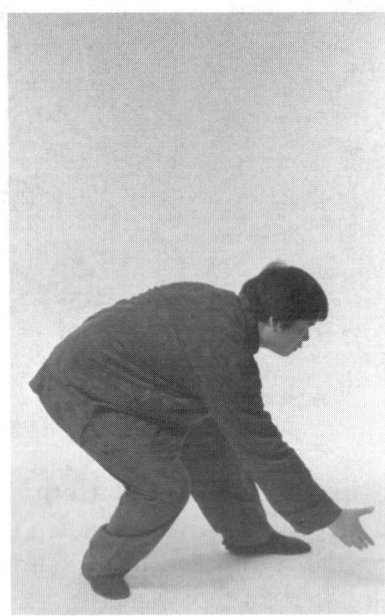

figure 90   *figure 91*

17. Fan Back

From the preceding movement, with the body's weight remaining on the right foot, the body and both hands come up together with the hands arriving near the chest area *(fig 92)*. Pick up the left foot, and step forward; set the right hand level with the right ear, palm facing out while the left hand remains in front of the chest. Shift the body's weight onto the left foot while pushing the left hand forward with the palm facing obliquely. The right hand remains near the right ear *(fig 93)*.

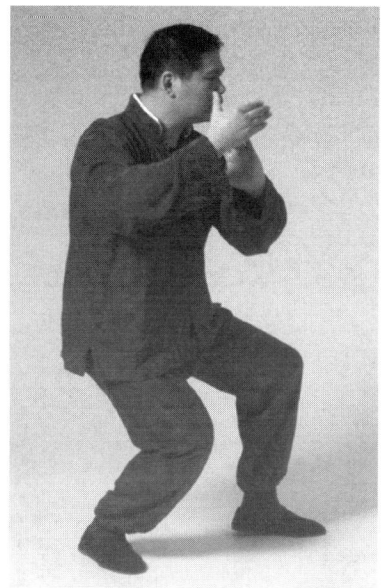

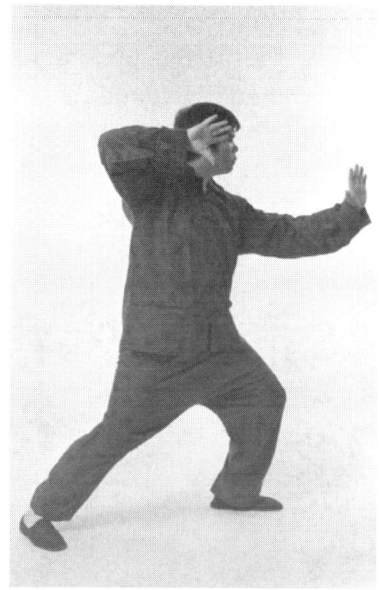

figure 92 *figure 93*

18. Turn Around and Punch

From the preceding movement, close the right hand into a fist, and bring it down to the chest *(fig 94)*. With the body's weight remaining on the left foot, rotate the waist to the right, and turn the body to face forward. At the same time, turn the left foot in, and bring the left hand in front of the face with the palm facing out *(fig 95)*.

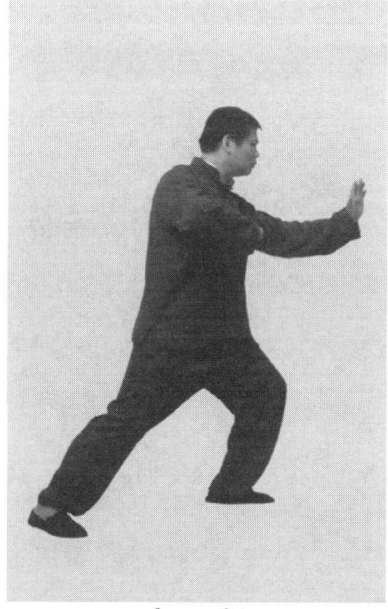

figure 94 *figure 95*

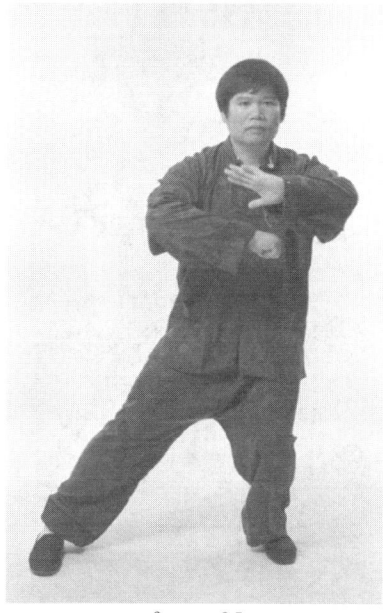

225

TAI CHI CHUAN - A COMPARATIVE STUDY

Turn the head, and look out to the right. Pick up the right foot, and step forward *(fig 96)*. Shift the body's weight onto the right foot as the right fist circles forward then down and the left hand arrives in front of the left shoulder *(fig 97)*. With the body's weight on the right foot, pull the right fist back onto the right side of the hip while the left palm pushes forward *(fig 98)*.

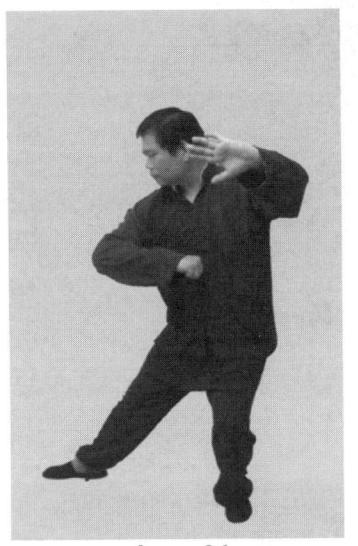

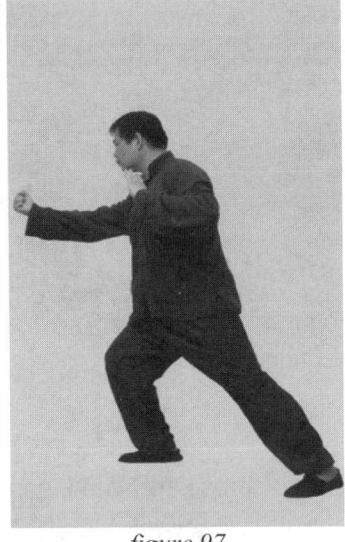

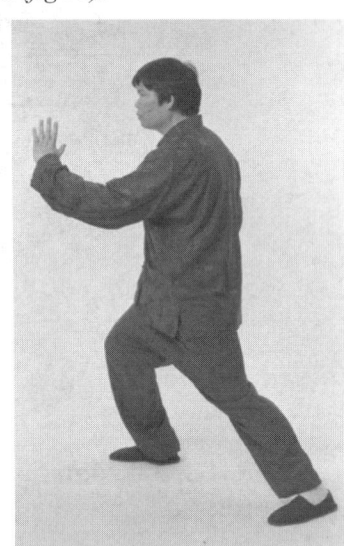

figure 96 *figure 97* *figure 98*

19. Right Part the Wild Horse's Mane
From the preceding movement, turn the left palm to face up, and reach the right fist out above the left palm *(figs 99 & 100)*.

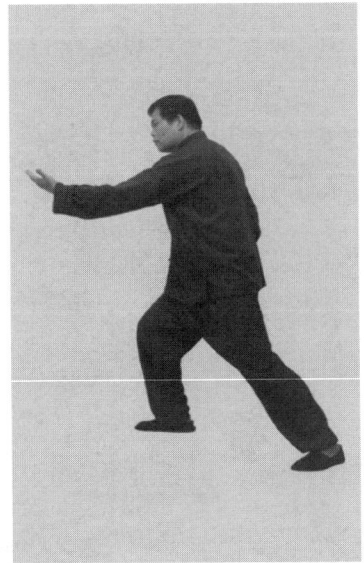

figure 99 *figure 100*

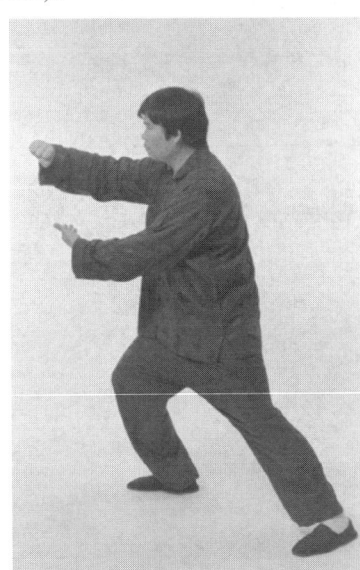

226

Shift the body's weight onto the left foot while opening the right hand and then pulling the hands back so the left is over the right and the palms face each other *(fig 101)*. Pick up the right foot, and step it to the right corner. Shift the body's weight onto the right foot while separating the hands, lifting the right to face level as the left goes down to the left side of the body with the palm facing down *(fig 102)*.

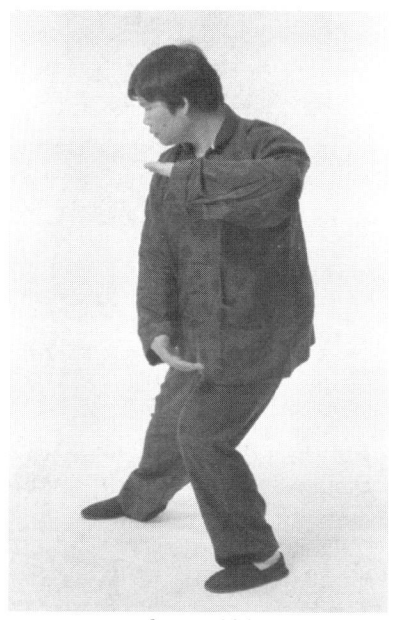

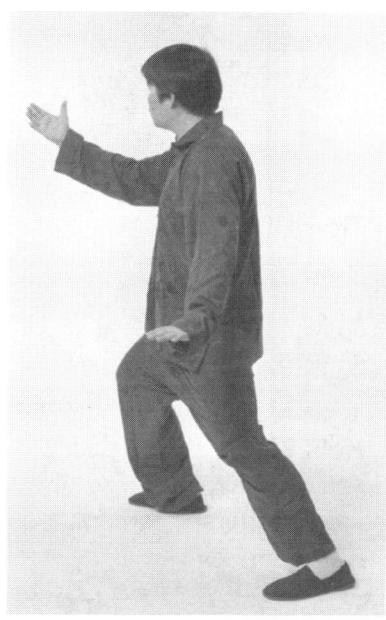

figure 101 *figure 102*

20. Left Warding Off

From the preceding movement, shift the body's weight onto the left foot while the hands remain the same *(fig 103)*. Rotate the body to the left with the right hand coming along and the right toes turning in *(fig 104)*.

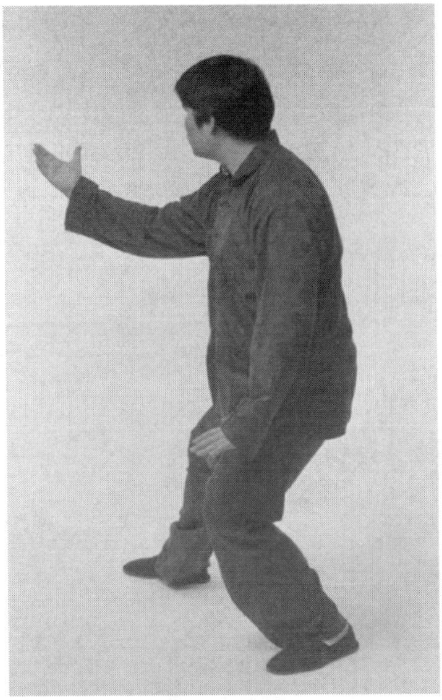

TAI CHI CHUAN - A COMPARATIVE STUDY

figure 103

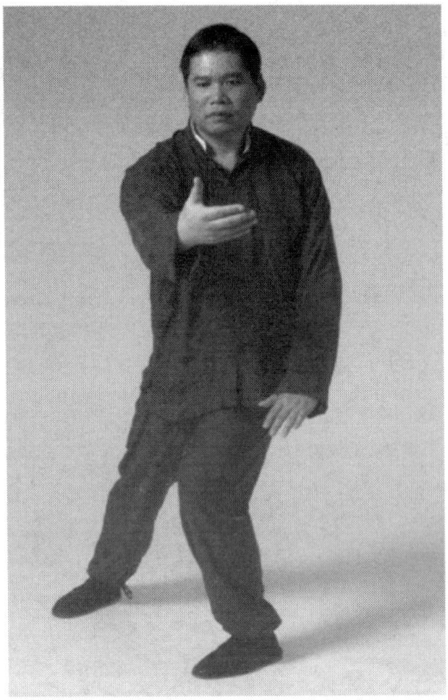

figure 104

Turn the right hand's palm to face down *(fig 105)*, and shift the body's weight back onto the right foot. The right hand comes up to the right shoulder, and the left hand remains the same in front of the abdomen *(fig 106)*.

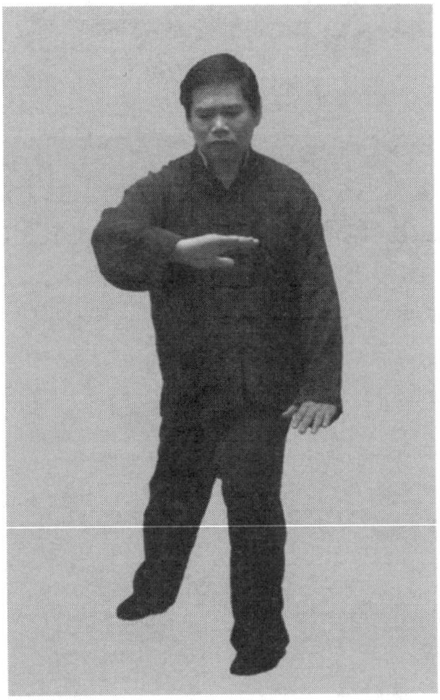

figure 105

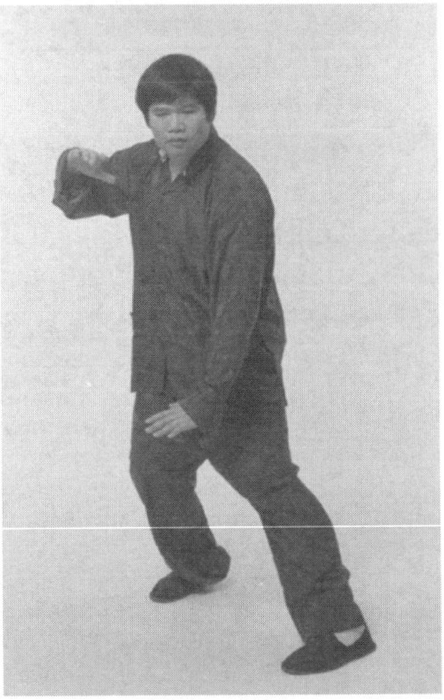

figure 106

With the body's weight on the right foot, pick up the left foot, and step forward *(fig 107)*. Shift the body's weight onto the left foot while separating the hands with the left hand coming up to face level and the right hand going down to the right side of the body, palm facing down *(fig 108)*.

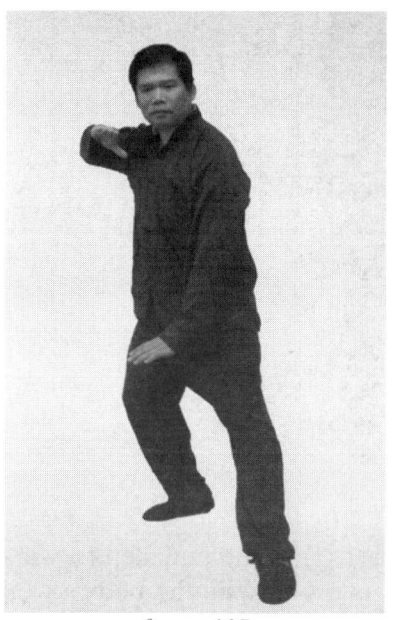

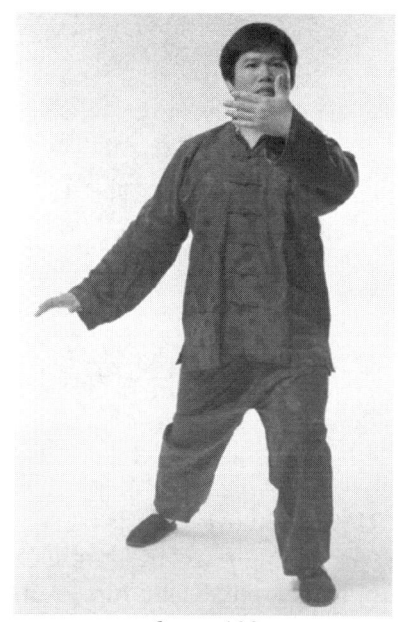

figure 107 *figure 108*

21. Waving Hands Like Clouds (7 times)
Part 1: Left Waving Hands

From the preceding movement, bring the right hand up to face level, palm facing in, and push the left hand down above the left knee, palm facing down *(fig 109)*.

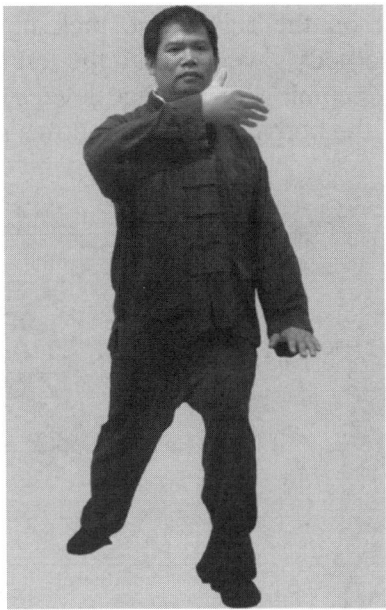

figure 109

Part 2: Right Waving Hands
From the preceding movement, pick up the right foot, and step forward next to the left foot; then rotate the hip to the right along with the body's weight. The hands follow the waist's rotation to the right *(figs 110 & 111)*.

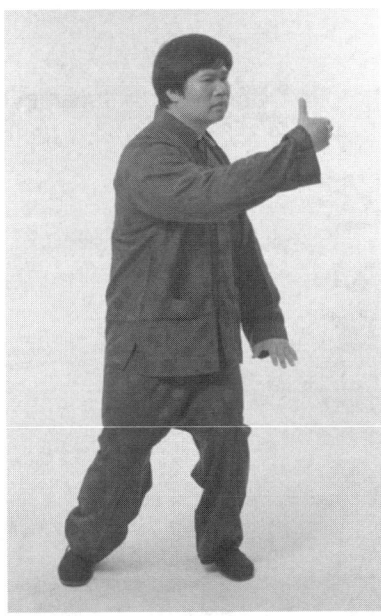

figure 110   *figure 111*

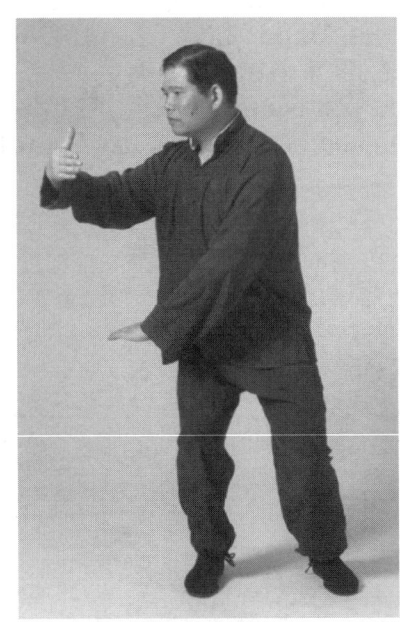

Part 3: Left Waving Hands

From the preceding movement, change hands by bringing the left hand up to face level with the palm facing in and pushing the right hand down above the right knee with the palm facing down *(fig 112)*. Pick up the left foot, and step out to the left *(fig 113)*. Rotate the hip to the left with the body's weight while the hands follow the waist's rotation to the left *(fig 114)*.

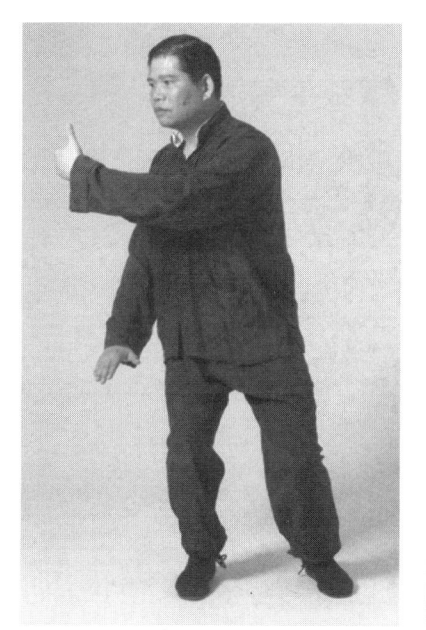

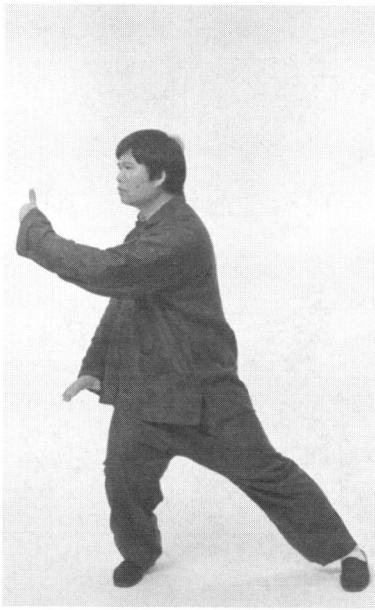

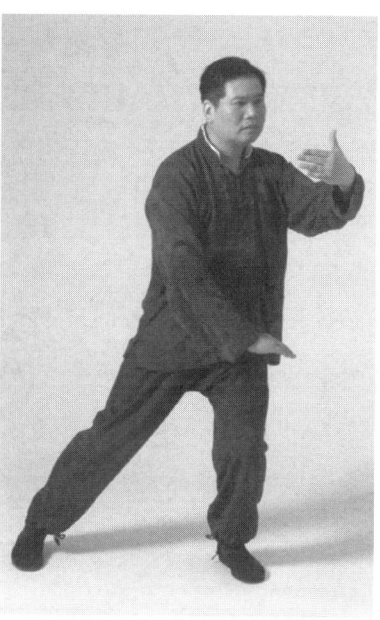

figure 112   *figure 113*   *figure 114*

Part 4: Right Waving Hands

From the preceding movement, change hands by bringing the right hand up to face level with the palm face in and pushing the left hand down above the left knee with the palm face down. Pick up the right foot, and step next to the left foot *(fig 115)*; then rotate the hip to the right with the body's weight while the hands follow the waist's rotation to the right *(fig 116)*.

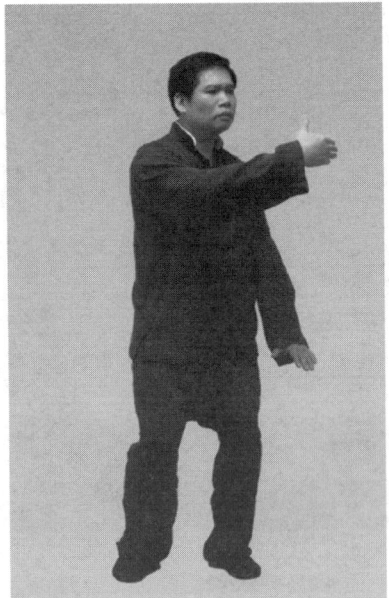

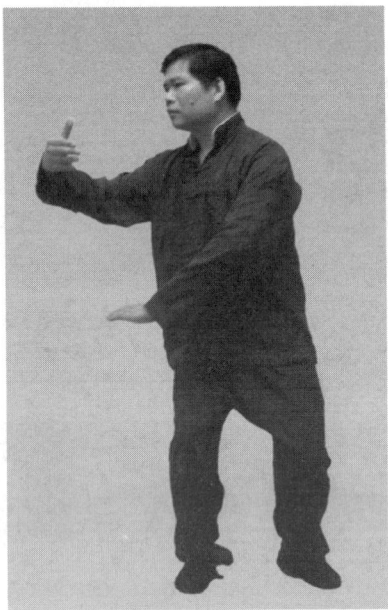

figure 115

figure 116

Part 5: Left Waving Hands

From the preceding movement, change hands by bringing the left hand up to face level with the palm face in and pushing the right hand down above the right knee with the palm face down *(fig 117)*. Pick up the left foot, and step out to the left *(fig 118)*. Rotate the hip to the left with the body's weight while the hands follow the waist's rotation to the left *(fig 119)*.

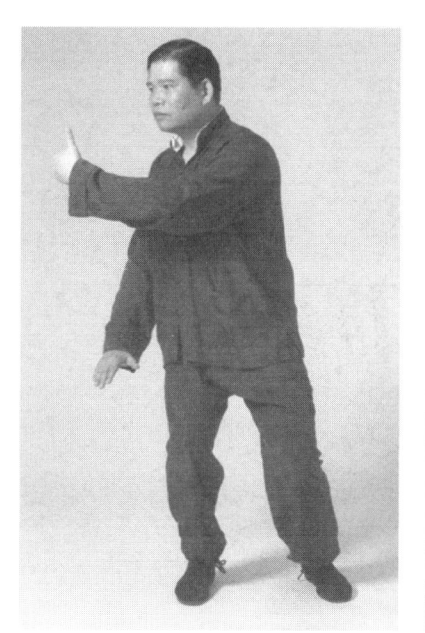

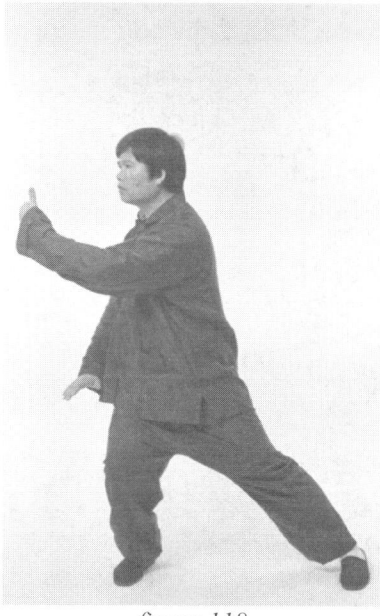

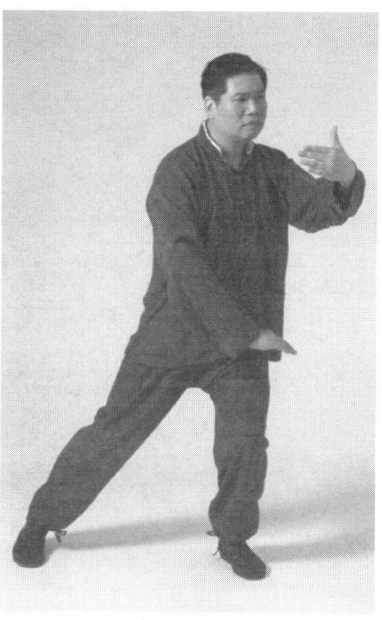

figure 117

figure 118

figure 119

Part 6: Right Waving Hands
From the preceding movement, change hands by bringing the right hand up to face level with the palm face in and pushing the left hand down above the left knee with the palm face down. Pick up the right foot, and step next to the left foot *(fig 120)*; then rotate the hip to the right with the body's weight while the hands follow the waist's rotation to the right *(fig 121)*.

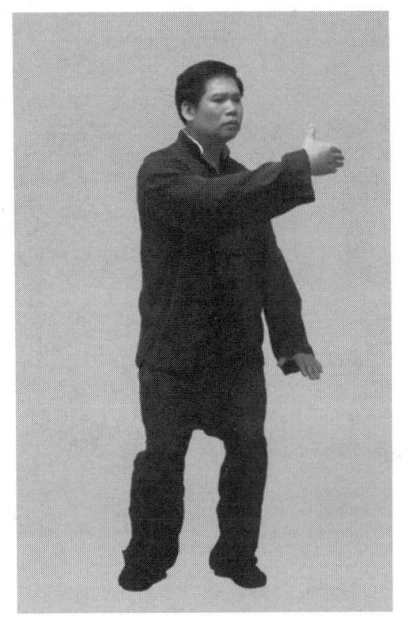

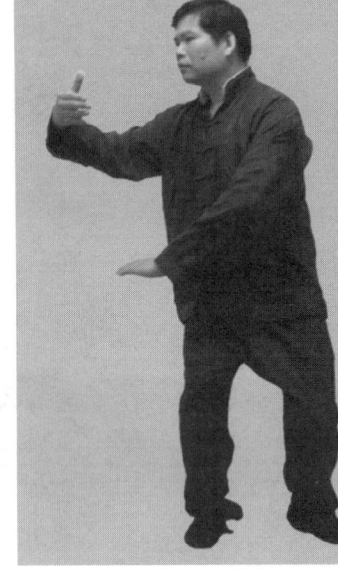

figure 120   *figure 121*

Part 7: Left Waving Hands

From the preceding movement, change hands by bringing the left hand up to face level with the palm face in and pushing the right hand down above the right knee with the palm face down *(fig 122)*. Pick up the left foot, and step out to the left *(fig 123)*. Rotate the hip to the left with the body's weight while the hands follow the waist's rotation to the left *(fig 124)*.

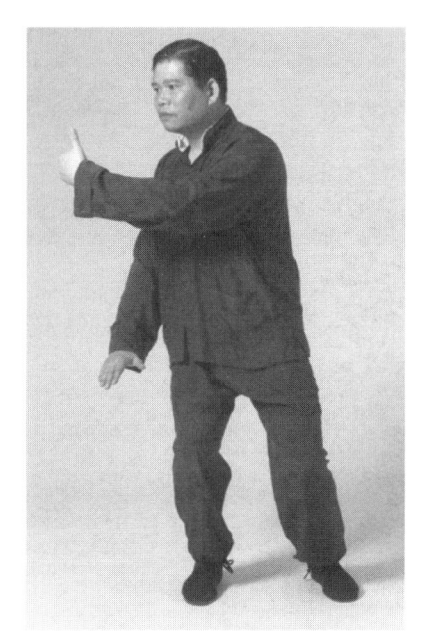

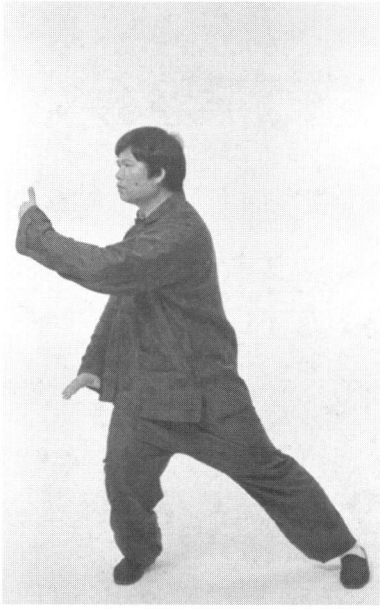

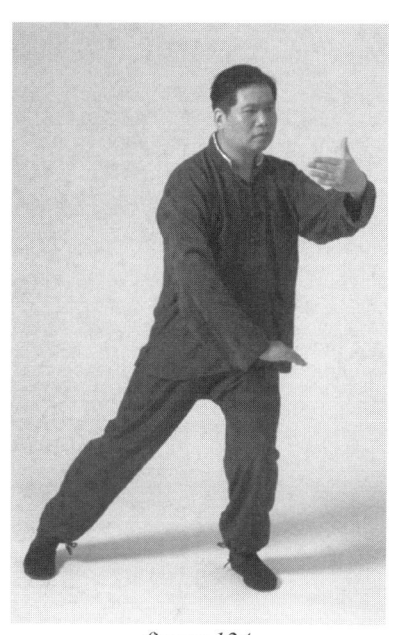

figure 122

figure 123

figure 124

Part 8: Right Waving Hands

From the preceding movement, change hands by bringing the right hand up to face level with the palm face in and pushing the left hand down above the left knee with the palm face down. Pick up the right foot, and step next to the left foot *(fig 125)*; then rotate the hip to the right with the body's weight while the hands follow the waist's rotation to the right *(fig 126)*.

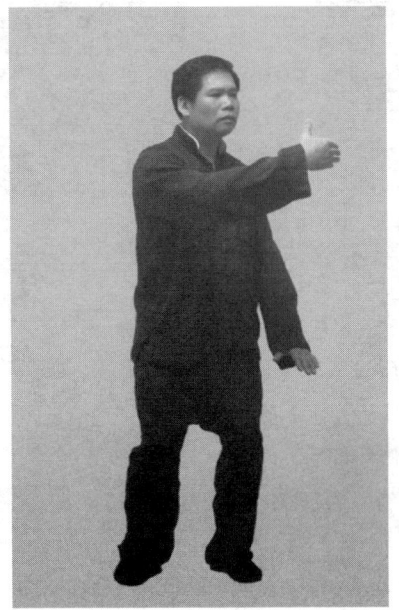

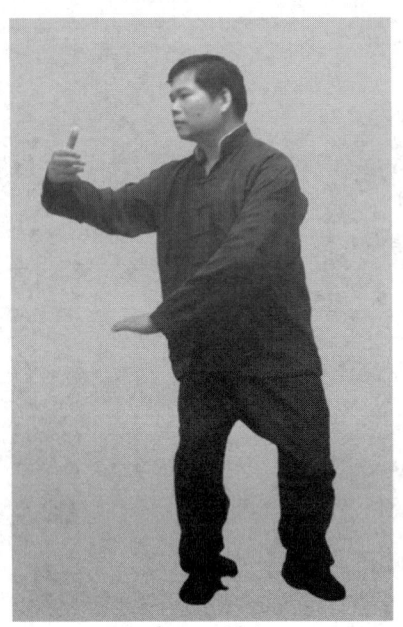

figure 125

figure 126

22. Single Whip

From the preceding movement, close the right hand's fingers together to form a beak, bend the wrist to form a hook; then extend the right arm, and set the left hand in front of the face with the palm facing in *(fig 127)*. Turn the head and look to the left; then pick up the left foot and step to the left *(fig 128)*. Shift the body's weight onto the left foot. Finally, turn the left palm to face forward while the right hand's hook remains the same *(fig 129)*.

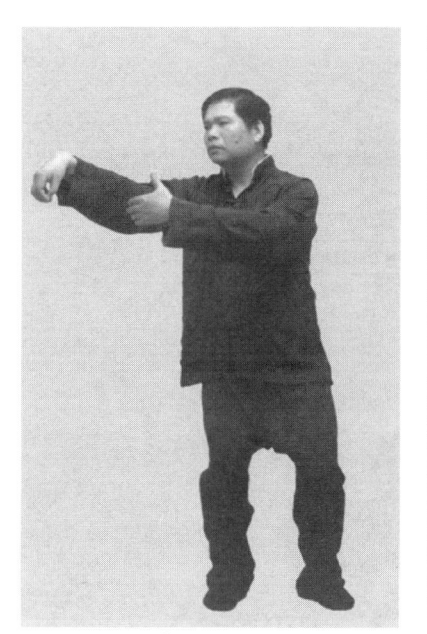

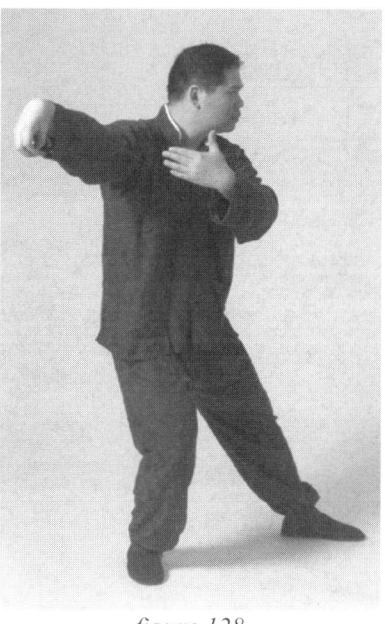

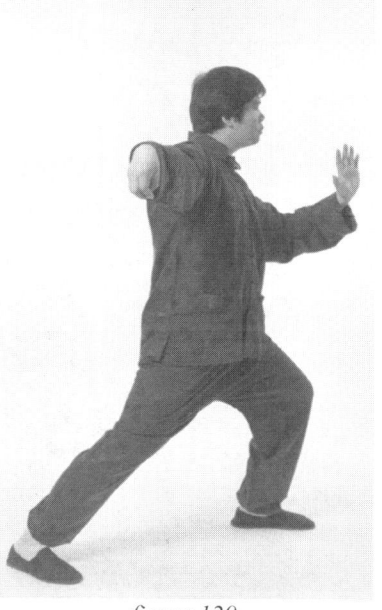

figure 127   *figure 128*   *figure 129*

23. High Pat Horse

From the preceding movement, with the body's weight on the left foot, turn the left palm to face up. Then shift the body's weight back onto the right foot; lift the left foot and place its toes on the ground *(fig 130)*. With the body's weight on the right foot, open the right hand, and put it on top of the left shoulder with the palm face down. Then push the right hand forward with the palm face out, thumb pointing down, and at the same time, bring the left hand back onto the left side of the waist *(fig 131)*.

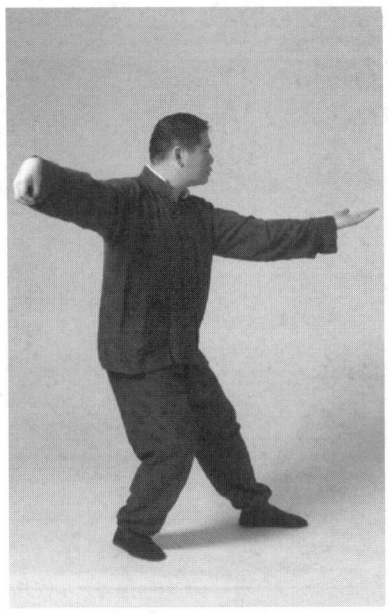

figure 130 *figure 131*

24. Left and Right Side Kicks
Part 1: Right Kick

From the preceding movement, bring the right hand back next to the left elbow *(fig 132)*. The left foot then steps to the left corner. The body's weight shifts onto the left foot, and the hands push out *(fig 133)*. Circulate the right hand to the outside of the left arm with both palms facing in upon arrival. Turn the palms face out, and separate the hands with the right hand going to the right corner and the left hand going to the back *(fig 134)*. The body remains facing forward.

THE 42 MOVEMENT MEDIUM FRAME SOLO FORM

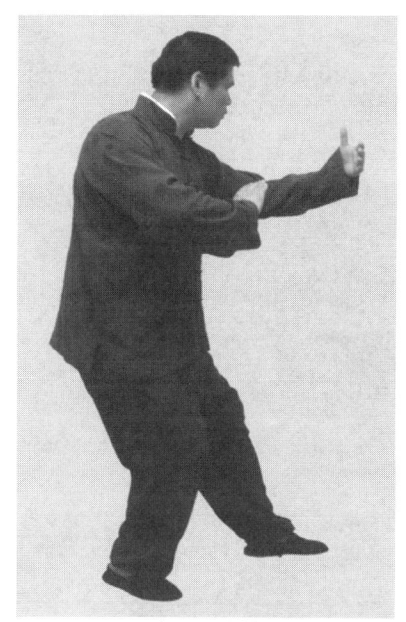

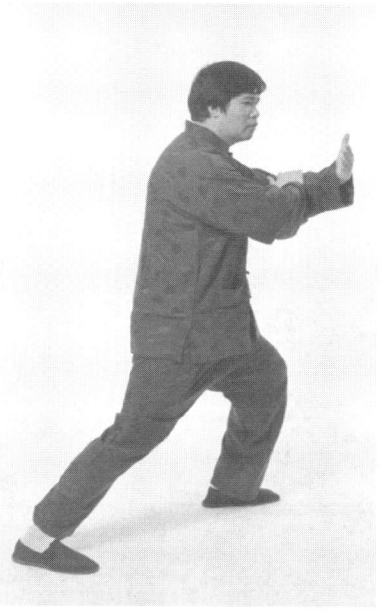

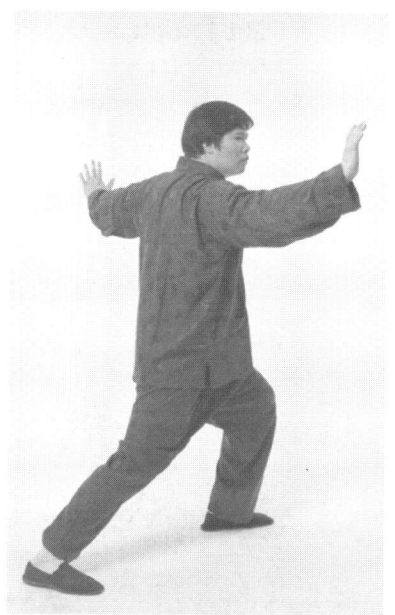

figure 132

figure 133

figure 134

With the body's weight on the left foot, raise the right leg up, and kick with the side of the foot to the right corner *(figs 135 & 136)*.

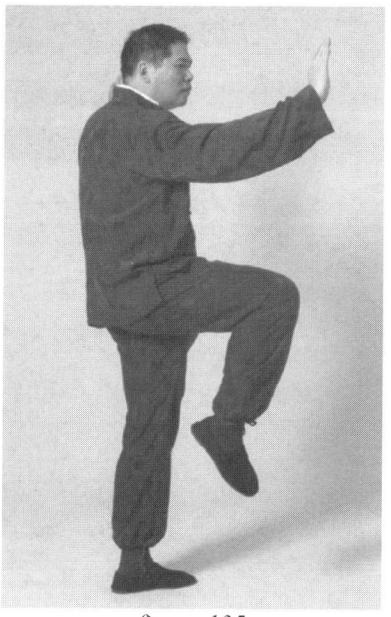

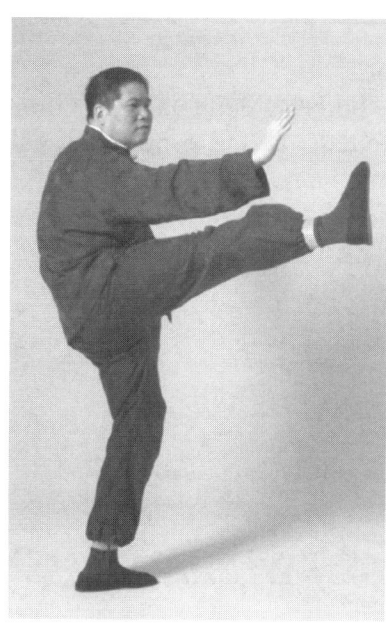

figure 135

figure 136

Part 2: Left Kick

From the preceding movement, bring the right foot back, and turn the right palm to face in *(fig 137)*. Set the right foot down, pointing to the corner, and bring the left hand forward next to the right elbow *(fig 138)*.

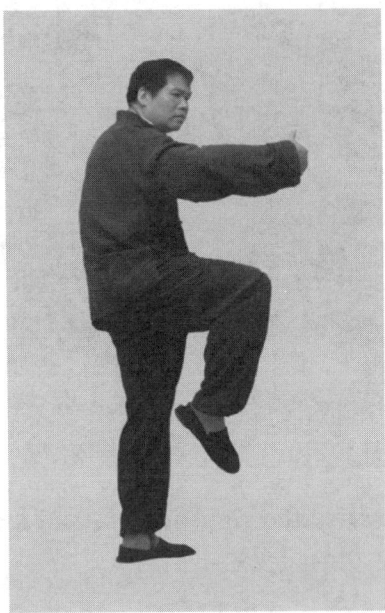

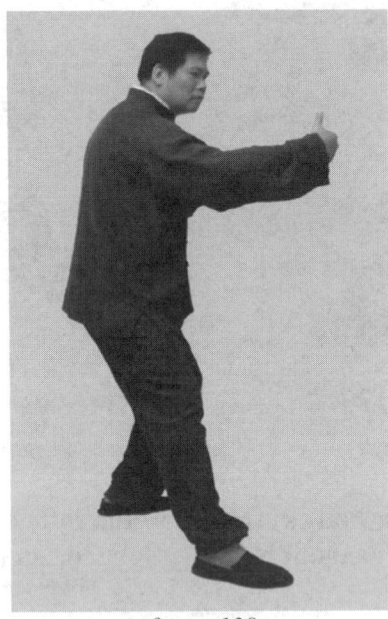

figure 137 *figure 138*

With the body's weight shifting onto the right foot, push the hands forward *(fig 139)*. Circulate the left hand to the outside of the right arm so the palms face in upon arrival *(fig 140)*.

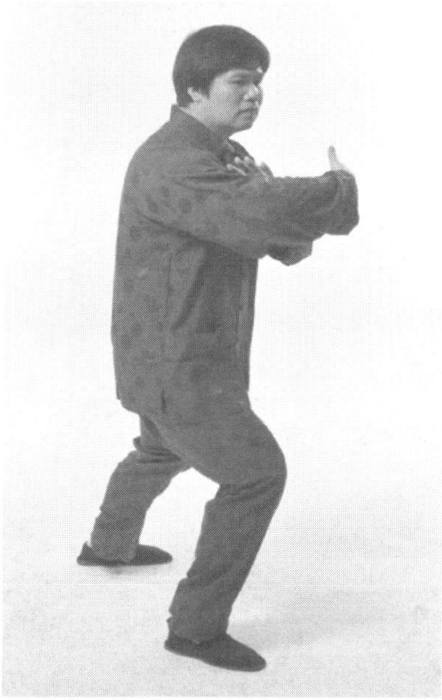

THE 42 MOVEMENT MEDIUM FRAME SOLO FORM

figure 139

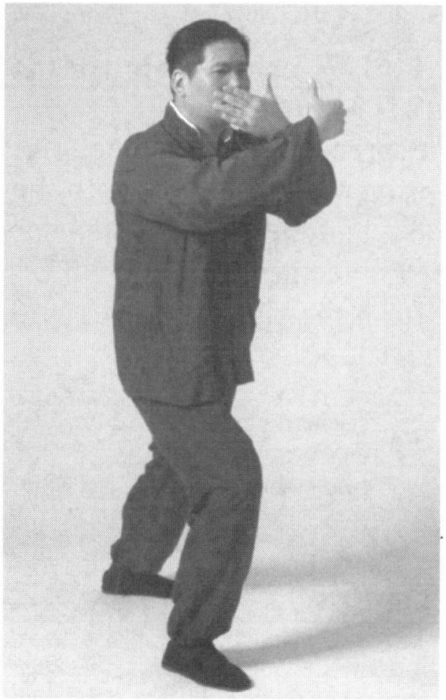

figure 140

Turn the palms face out, and separate the hands with the left hand going to the left corner and the right hand going to the back *(fig 141)*. With the body's weight on the right foot, raise the left leg up, and kick with the side of the foot to the left corner *(fig 142)*.

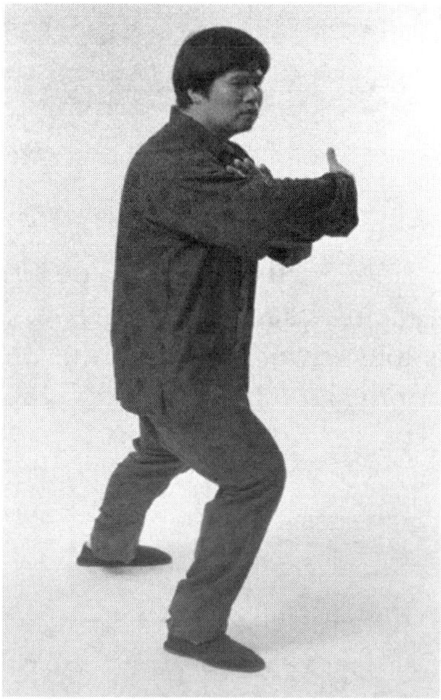

figure 141

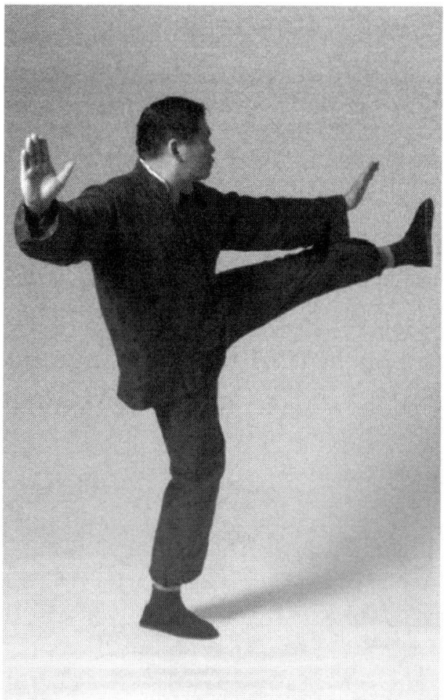

figure 142

25. Fair Lady Works on Shuttles (2 times)
Part 1: Left Shuttle

From the preceding movement, with the right foot supporting the body's weight, bring the left leg close to the body *(fig 143)*. The left hand comes close to the body, and the left foot steps down to the left corner *(fig 144)*. Lift the left hand up above the head with the palm face out, and push the right hand forward from the right shoulder with the body's weight shifting onto the left foot *(fig 145)*.

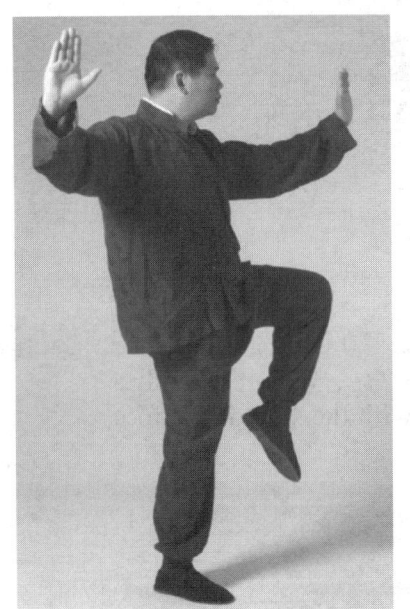

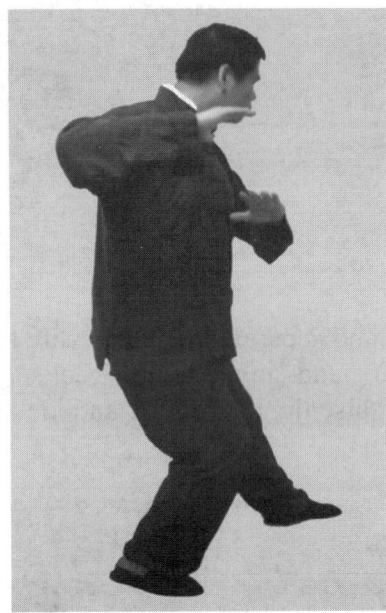

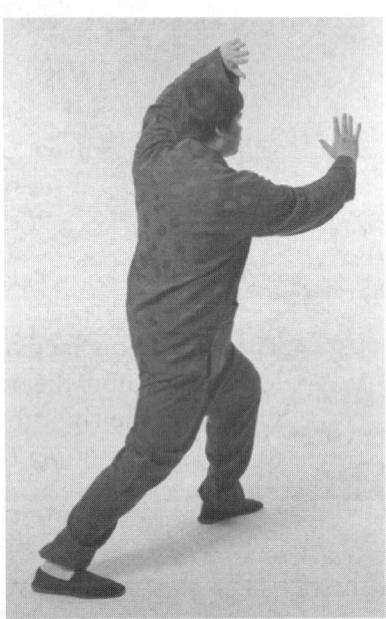

figure 143 *figure 144* *figure 145*

Part 2: Right Shuttle

From the preceding movement, turn the right palm face up, and bring both hands down to the chest with the palms facing each other *(fig 146)*. Turn the body to the right while bringing the left toes inward by pivoting on the left heel; the head looks out to the right corner *(fig 147)*.

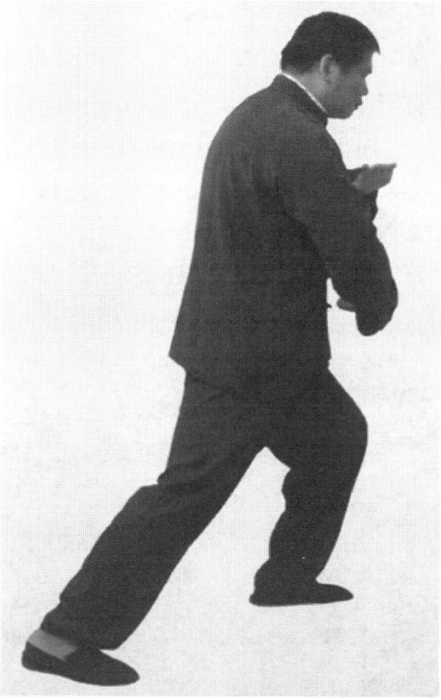

THE 42 MOVEMENT MEDIUM FRAME SOLO FORM

figure 146

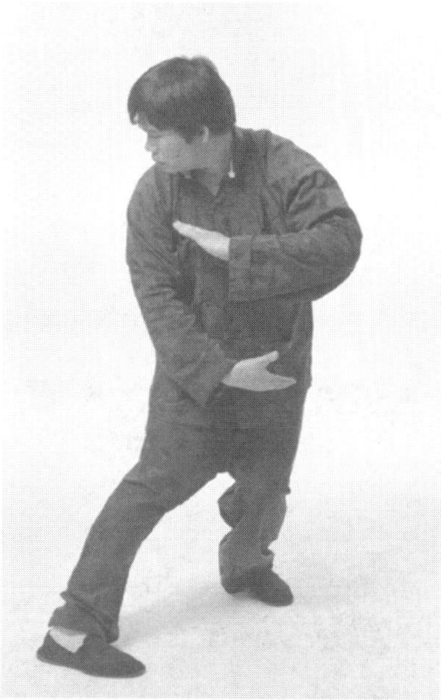

figure 147

Pick up the right foot, and step to the right corner *(fig 148)*. With the body's weight shifting onto the right foot, lift the right hand up above the head with the palm facing out, and push the left hand forward from the left shoulder *(fig 149)*.

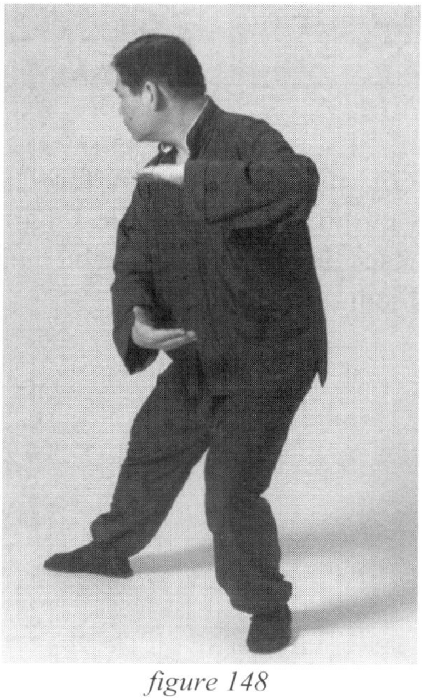

figure 148

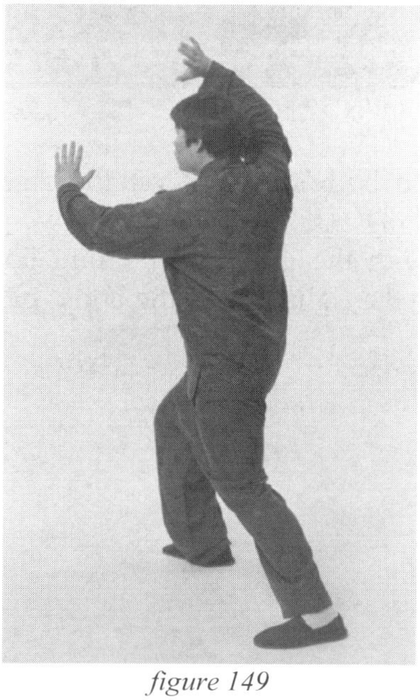

figure 149

26. Left Warding Off

From the preceding movement, bring the right hand down in front of the body with the left hand coming back next to the right elbow and the body's weight shifting onto the left foot *(fig 150)*. Rotate the waist and the right foot to the left with both hands face down *(fig 151)*. Rotate the waist to the right, and shift the body's weight back onto the right foot, bringing the right hand back to the right shoulder while the left hand goes down to the abdomen *(fig 152)*.

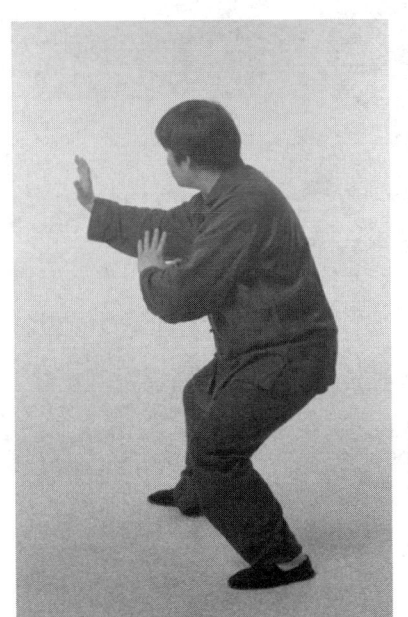

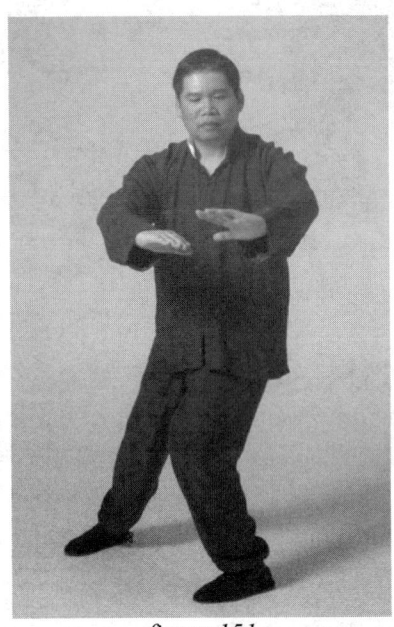

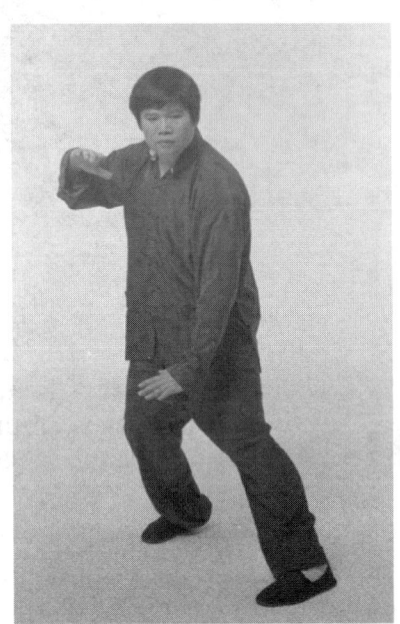

figure 150   *figure 151*   *figure 152*

With the body's weight on the right foot, pick up the left foot, and step forward *(fig 153)*. Shift the body's weight onto the left foot while separating the hands with the left hand coming up to face level and the right hand going down to the right side of the body, palm facing down *(fig 154)*.

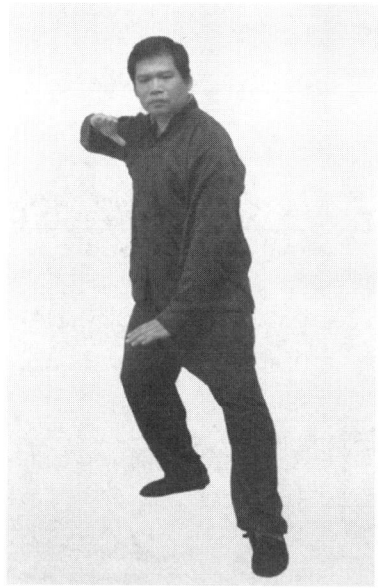

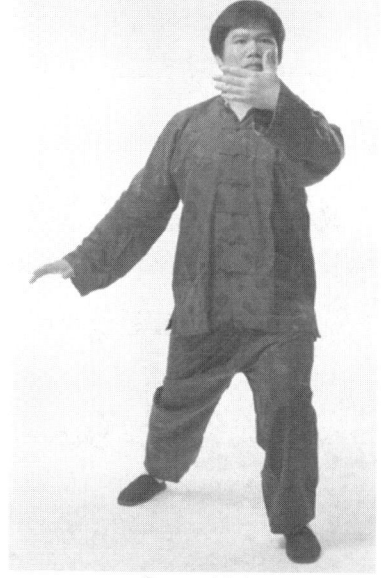

figure 153   *figure 154*

27. Right Foot Kick

From the preceding movement, bring the right wrist up across the left wrist with the palms facing in *(fig 155)*. Turn the palms to face out, and separate the hands with the right hand going right and the left hand going left *(figs 156 & 157)*. With the body's weight on the left foot, pick up the right foot, and kick with the heel *(fig 158)*.

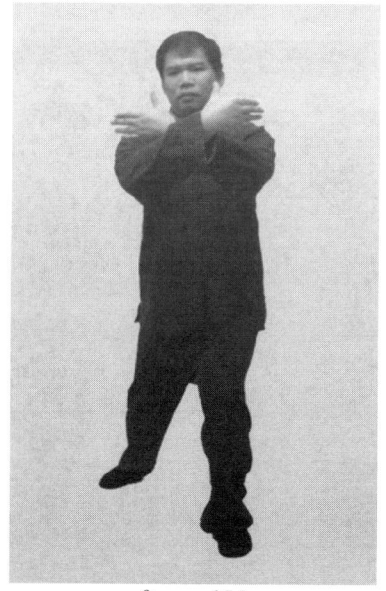

figure 155   *figure 156*

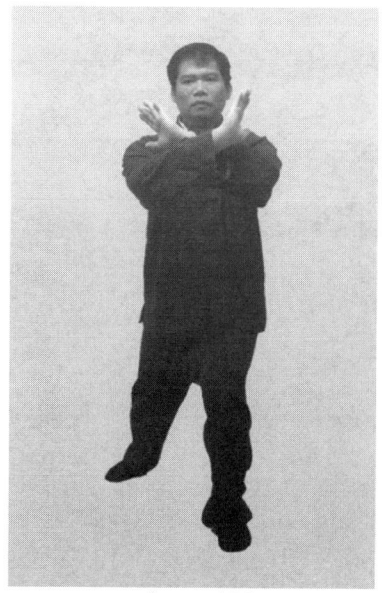

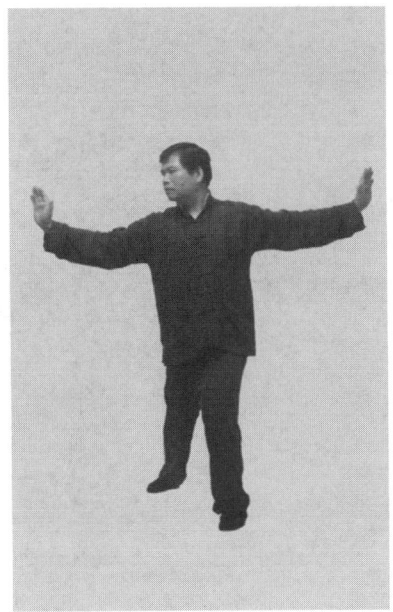

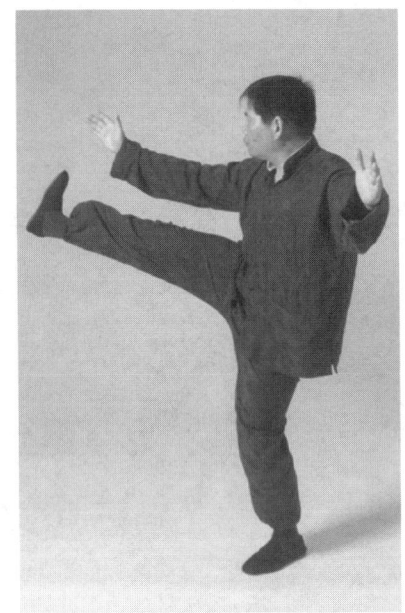

figure 157   *figure 158*

28. Left Hitting Tiger
From the preceding movement, bring the right foot close to the body *(fig 159)*. Bring the right hand to the chest. Set the right foot down with the toes pointing forward, and push both arms out above the right knee with the palms facing downward *(figs 160 & 161)*.

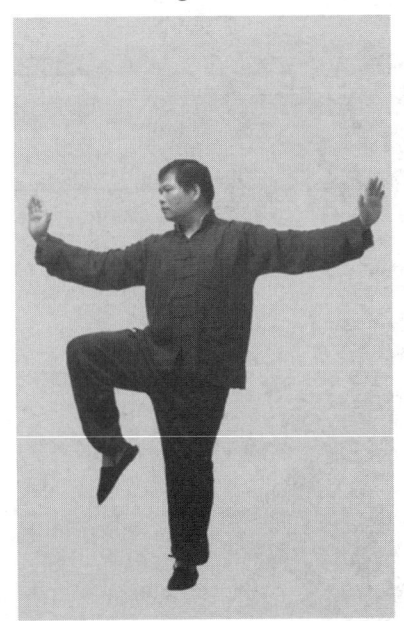

figure 159   *figure 160*   *figure 161*

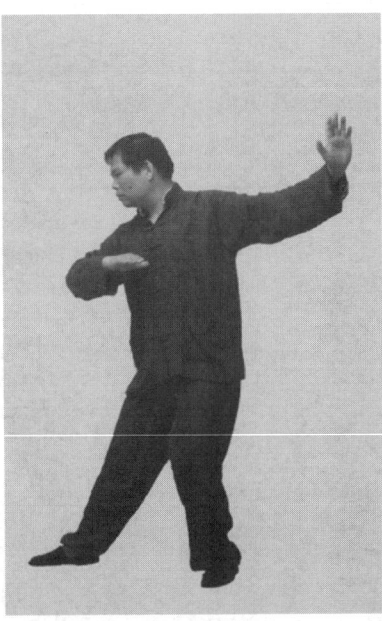

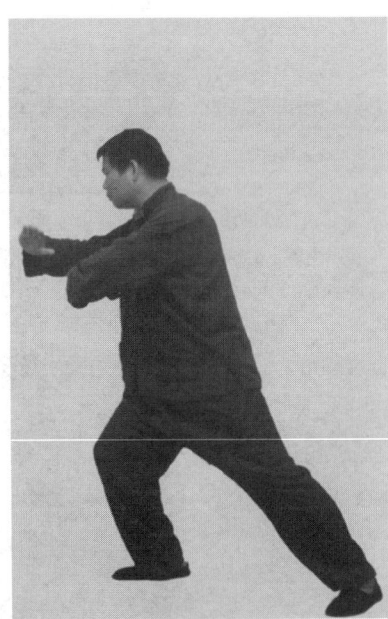

With the body's weight on the right foot, turn the right toes inward, and at the same time, rotate the left arm so the palm faces up under the right palm; the eyes look forward to the left *(fig 162)*. With the body's weight still on the right foot, pick up the left foot, and step forward with the hands closing into fists *(fig 163)*. Shift the body's weight onto the left foot while bringing the left fist out in a half circle to above the head and the right fist before the chest *(fig 164)*.

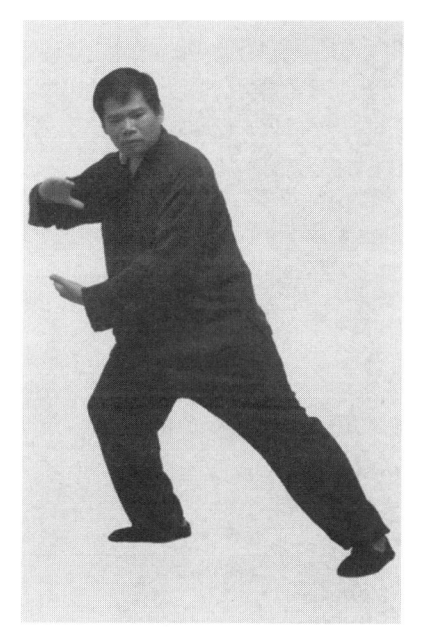

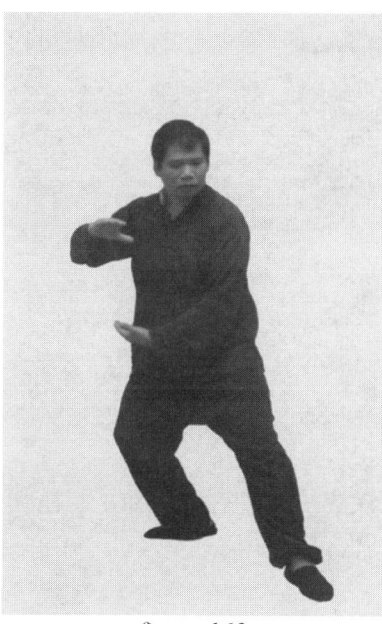

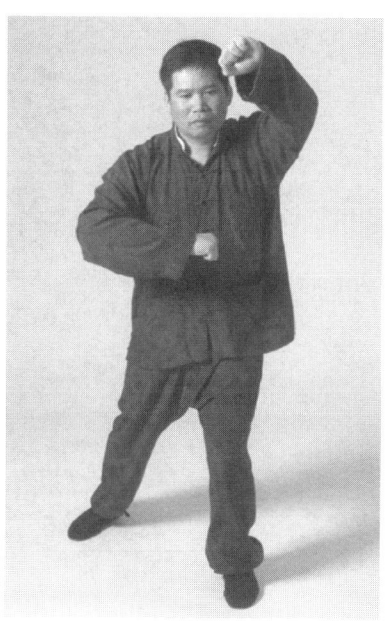

figure 162   *figure 163*   *figure 164*

29. Hit the Ears with Two Fists
From the preceding movement, turn the left foot in, and bring the two fists to the right corner, facing up at chest level. The body faces to the right corner *(fig 165)*. Open the fists with the palms face up. Pull the hands back while shifting the body's weight onto the left foot. Lift the right knee up to the chest with the palms resting on both sides of the right knee *(figs 166 -168)*.

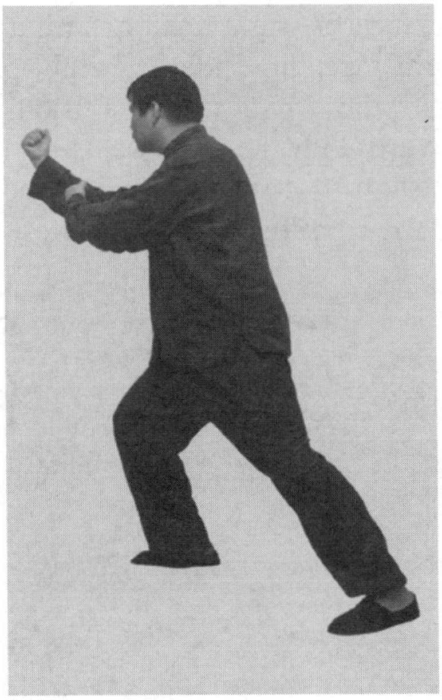

TAI CHI CHUAN - A COMPARATIVE STUDY

figure 165

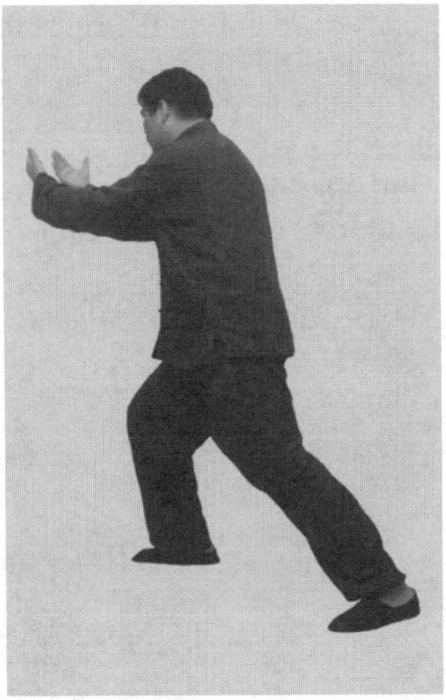

figure 166

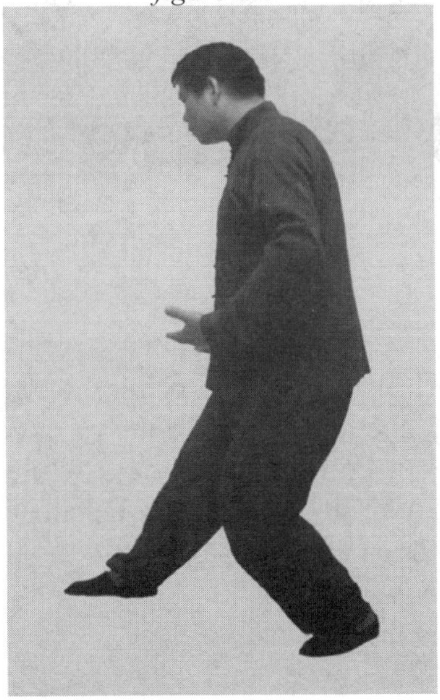

figure 167

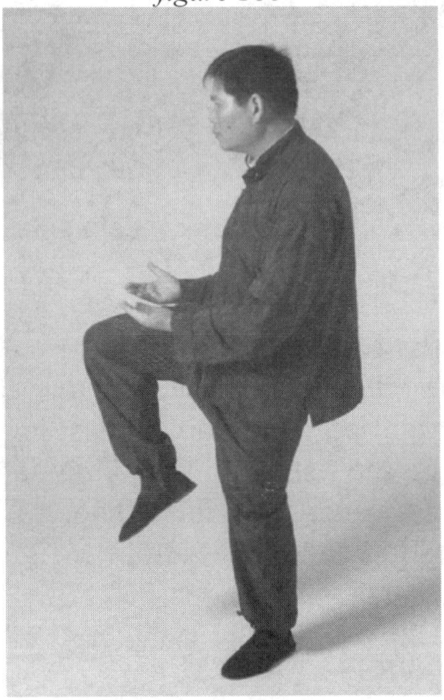

figure 168

With the right foot, step to the right corner *(fig 169)*. Bring the fists up to ear level while shifting the body's weight onto the right foot *(fig 170)*.

THE 42 MOVEMENT MEDIUM FRAME SOLO FORM

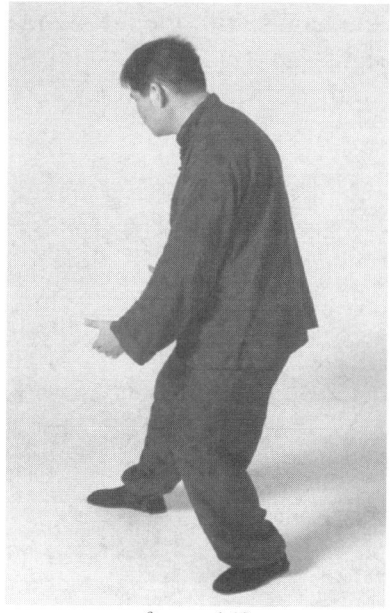

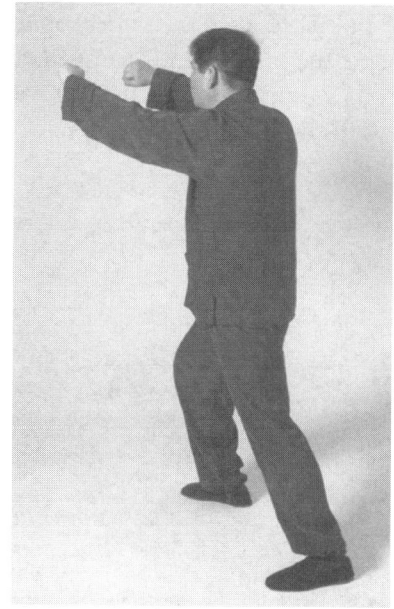

figure 169

figure 170

30. Left Foot Kick

From the preceding movement, open the fists, and bring the hands down, crossing them above the right knee with the palms face down, left wrist over right *(fig 171)*. Bring the hands up in front of the face, the right hand outside the left and the palms facing in *(fig 172)*.

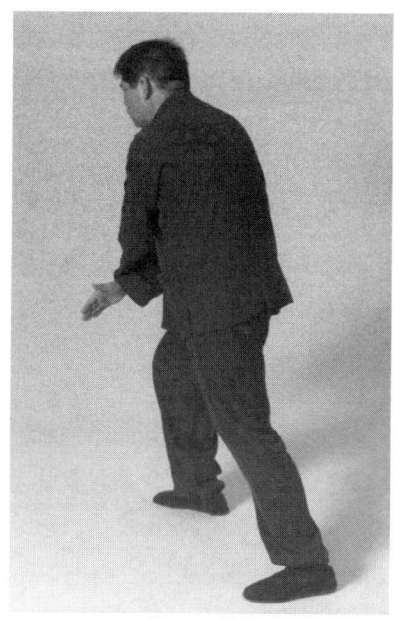

figure 171

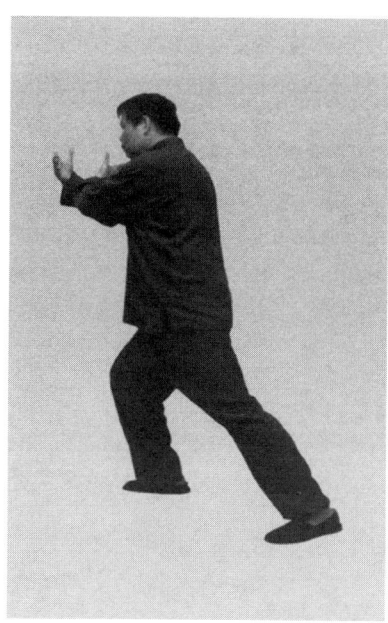

figure 172

Turn the palms to face out, and separate the hands with the left hand going to the left and the right hand going to the right *(figs 173 & 174)*. With the body's weight remaining on the right foot, pick up the left foot, and kick forward and upward with the heel *(fig 175)*.

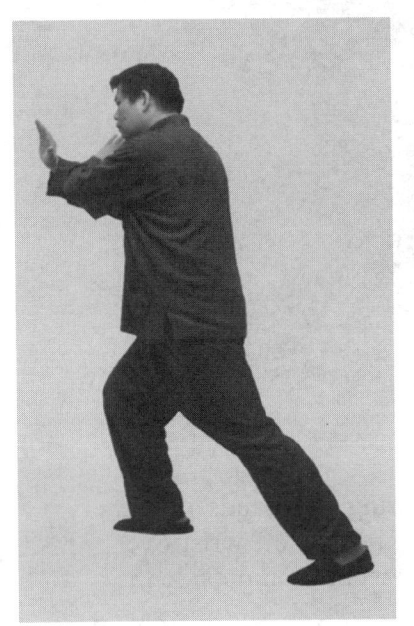

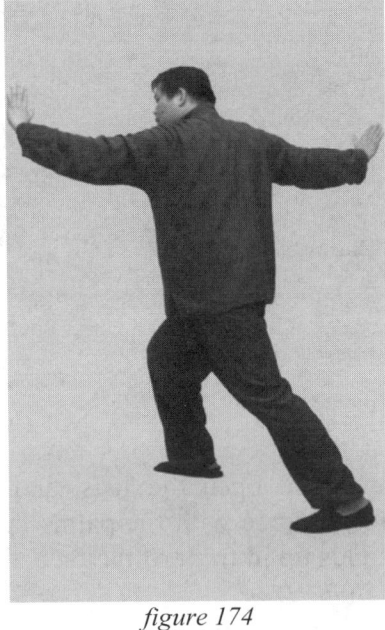

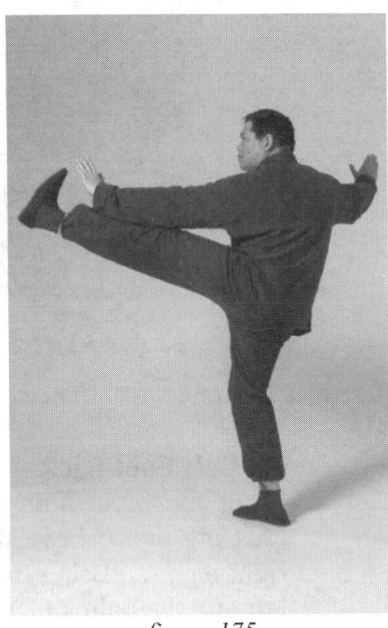

figure 173

figure 174

figure 175

31. Brush Knee with Twist Step (2 times)
Part 1: Left Hand Brush Knee

From the preceding movement, bring the left hand and left foot back to the body; the left palm faces down *(fig 176)*. With the left foot, step forward, brush the left hand down outside the left knee, and bring the right hand in to the right shoulder. Then push the right palm forward *(figs 177 & 178)*.

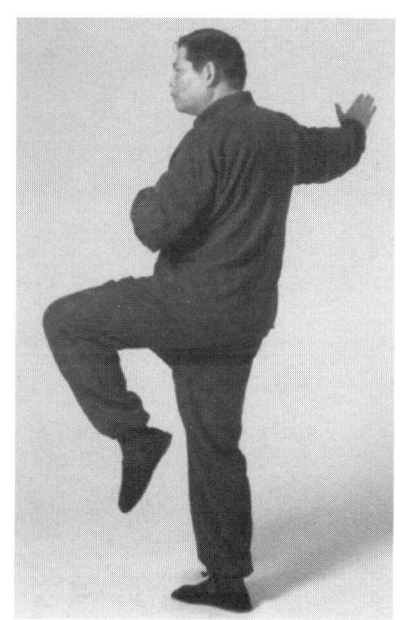

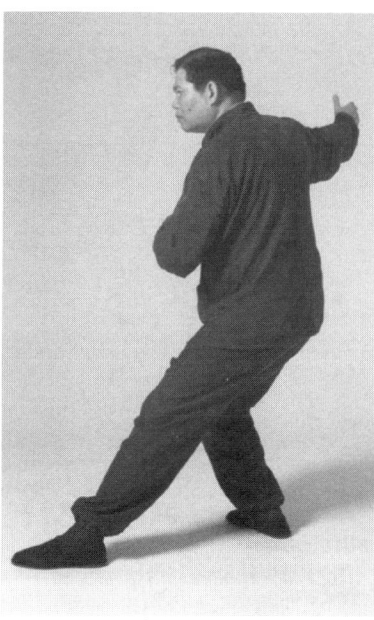

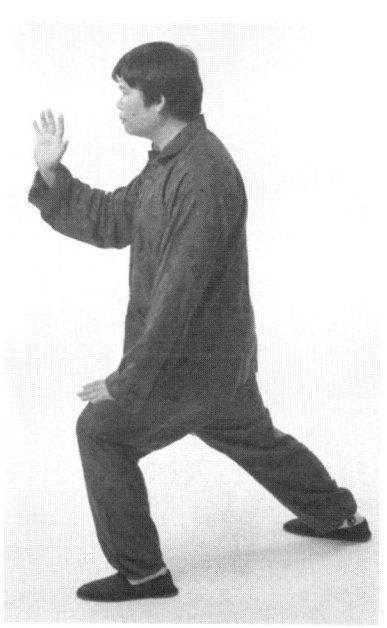

figure 176   *figure 177*   *figure 178*

Part 2: Right Hand Brush Knee

From the preceding movement, the left hand goes up to the left side level with the left shoulder, and the right hand comes back to the chest with the palm face down *(fig 179)*. Turn the left foot out, and step the right foot forward *(fig 180)*. Shift the weight onto the right foot with the right hand brushing down outside the right knee and the left palm coming in to the left shoulder, then pushing forward from the shoulder with the palm facing forward *(fig 181)*.

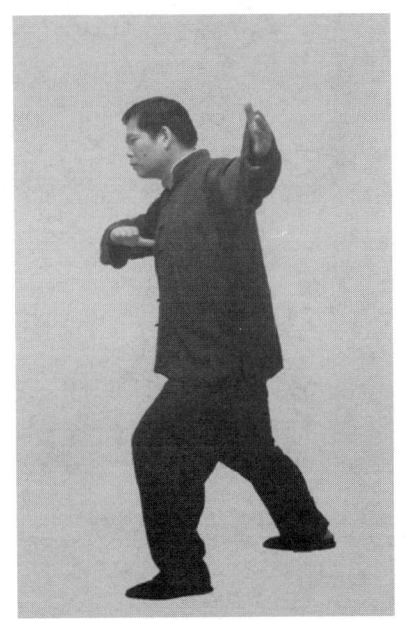

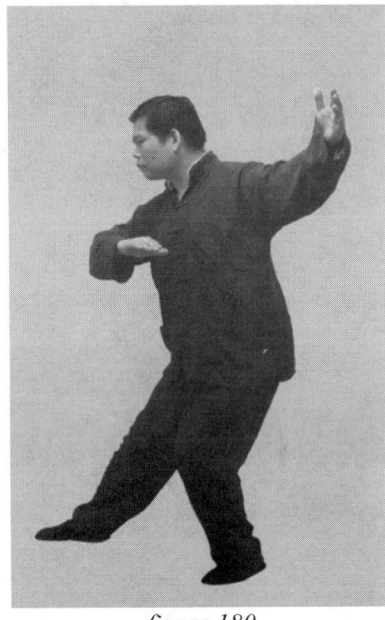

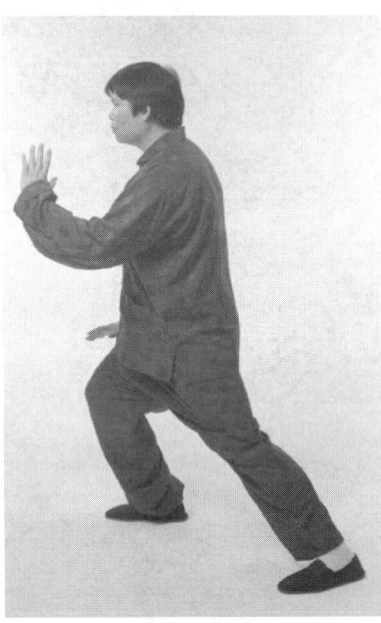

figure 179   *figure 180*   *figure 181*

32. Step Forward and Punch Down

From the preceding movement, the left hand comes back to the chest with the palm face down, and the right hand closes into a fist *(fig 182)*. The right fist comes up to the right side of the hip while the right foot turns outward. Pick up the left foot, and step forward. With the weight shifting onto the left foot, the left hand brushes down outside the left knee with the palm face down, and right hand punches forward and downward from the hip *(fig 183)*.

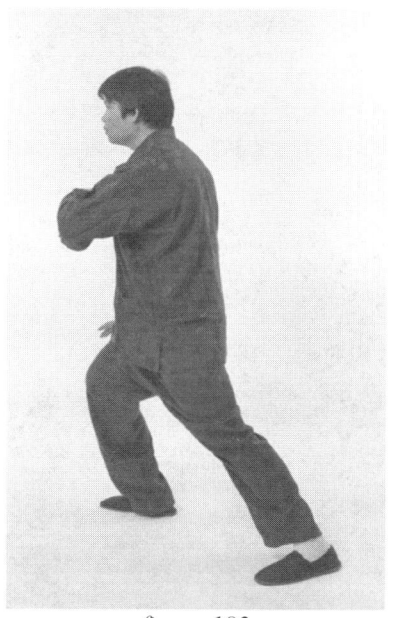

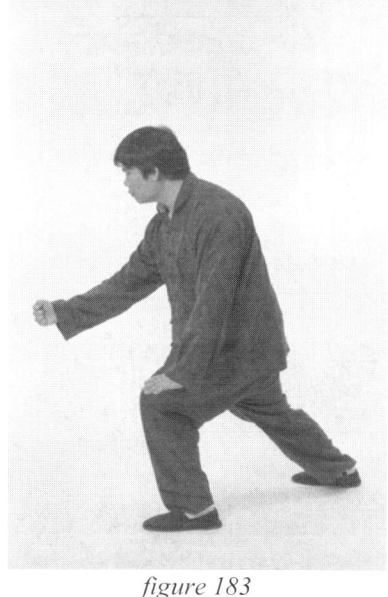

figure 182

figure 183

33. Step Forward Grasp Sparrow's Tail
Part 1: Left Part the Wild Horse's Mane

From the preceding movement, shift the body's weight onto the right foot, and draw the right fist back to the right shoulder while the left hand remains the same *(fig 184)*. Turn the left palm face up, and open the right fist with the palm face down. Turn the left foot out *(fig 185)*. As the body's weight shifts onto the left foot, lift the left hand up with the palm face up, and lower the right hand down next to the right leg with the palm face down *(fig 186)*.

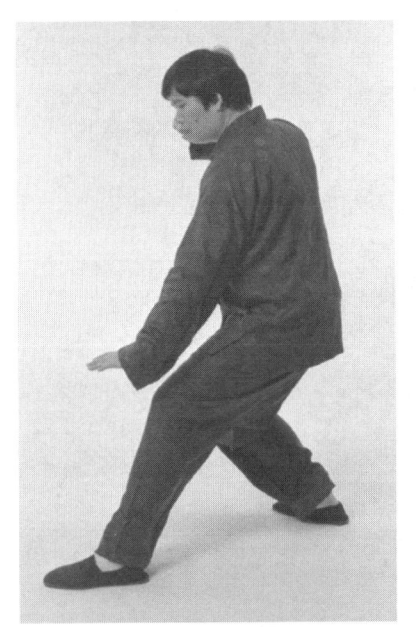

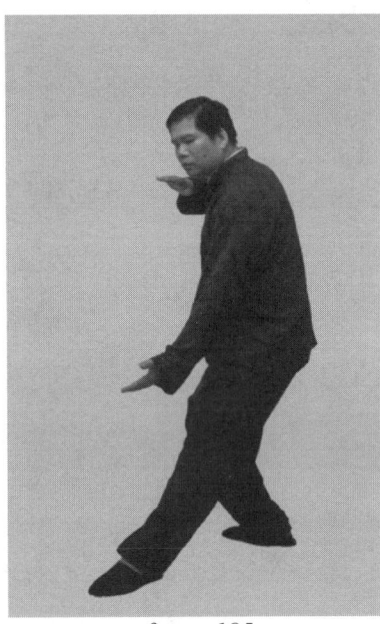

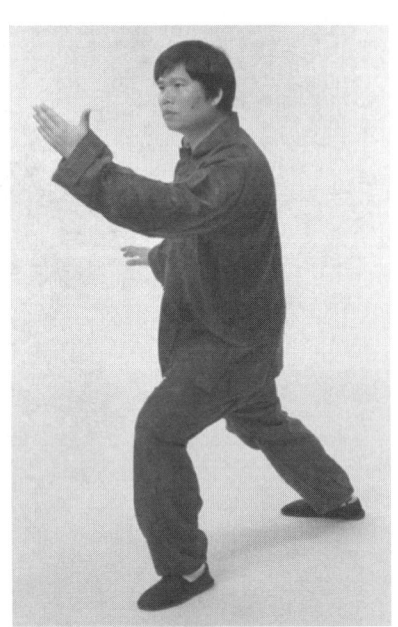

figure 184   *figure 185*   *figure 186*

Part 2: Right Warding Off

From the preceding movement, bring the right hand forward next to the left knee *(fig 187)*. With the body's weight still on the left foot, pick up the right foot, and step forward. Shift the body's weight onto the right foot, and bring both hands up to face level. The right palm faces in, and the left palm faces out *(fig 188)*.

THE 42 MOVEMENT MEDIUM FRAME SOLO FORM

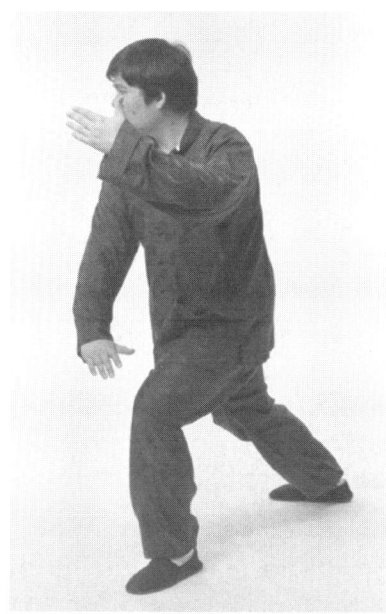

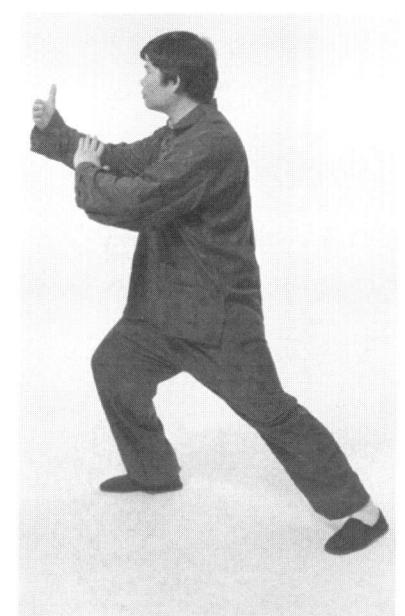

figure 187

figure 188

Part 3: Roll Back

From the preceding movement, turn both palms so the left palm faces up and the right palm faces down *(fig 189)*. Bring the hands back to the left side of the hip while shifting the body's weight onto the left foot *(figs 190 & 191)*.

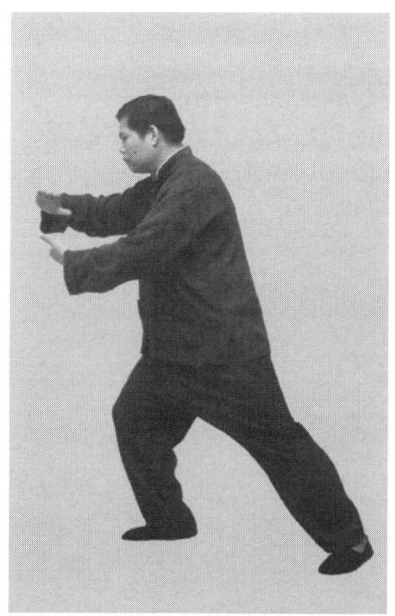

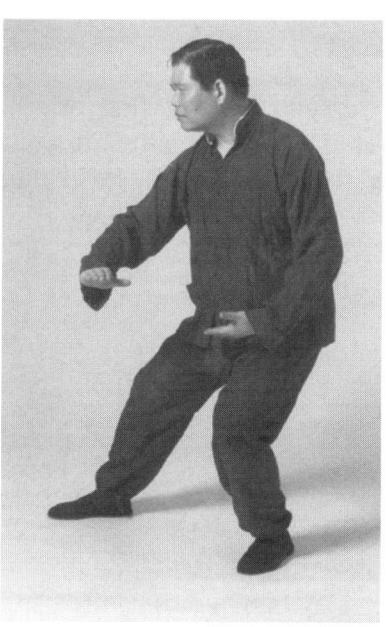

figure 189

figure 190

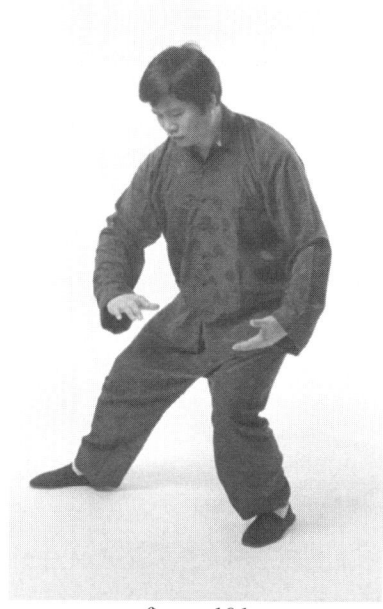

figure 191

Part 4: Press

From the preceding movement, turn the right palm face up and the left palm face down. The left hand then sticks to the right wrist *(fig 192)*. Press the hands forward with the body's weight shifting onto the right foot *(fig 193)*.

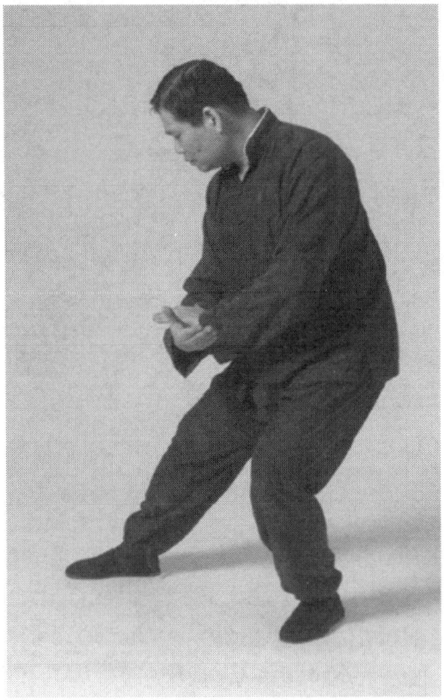

figure 192

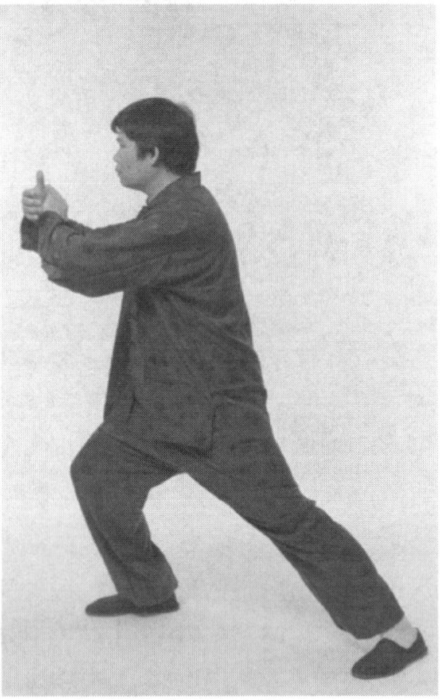

figure 193

Part 5: Push

From the preceding movement, separate the two hands *(fig 194)*. Bring the hands back to the chest as the body weight shifts onto the left foot. Bend the wrists so the palms face forward *(fig 195)*. Push the hands forward with the body's weight shifting onto the right foot *(fig 196)*.

THE 42 MOVEMENT MEDIUM FRAME SOLO FORM

figure 194 *figure 195* *figure 196*

34. Single Whip

From the preceding movement, bring the left hand back next to the right elbow as the body weight shifts onto the left foot *(fig 197)*. Rotate the waist to the left with the hands following along and the right toes turning in *(fig 198)*. Rotate the waist back to the right with the body weight shifting onto the right foot *(fig 199)*.

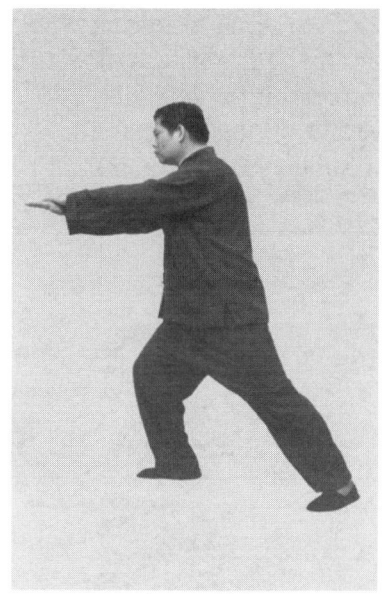

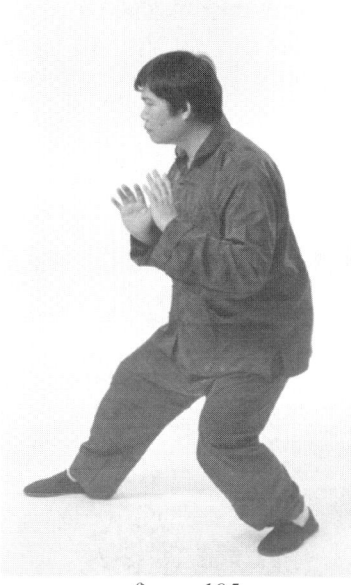

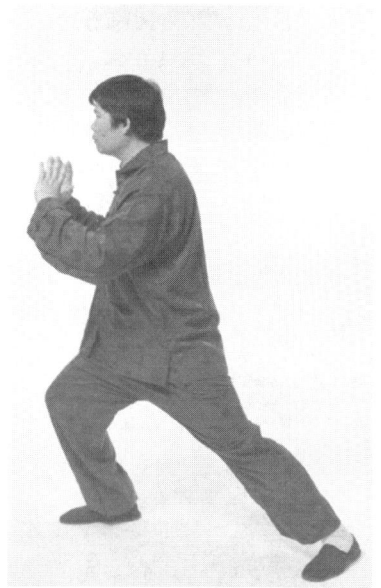

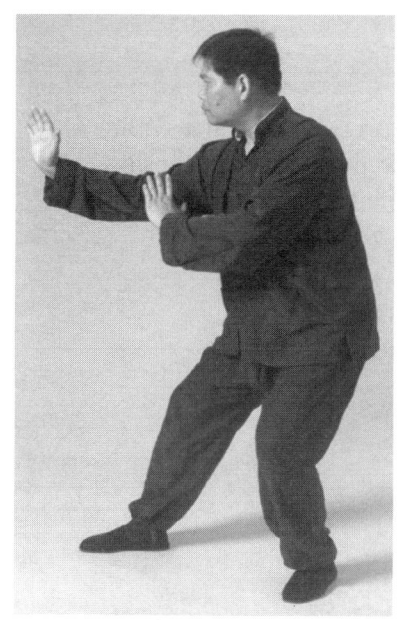

figure 197 *figure 198* *figure 199*

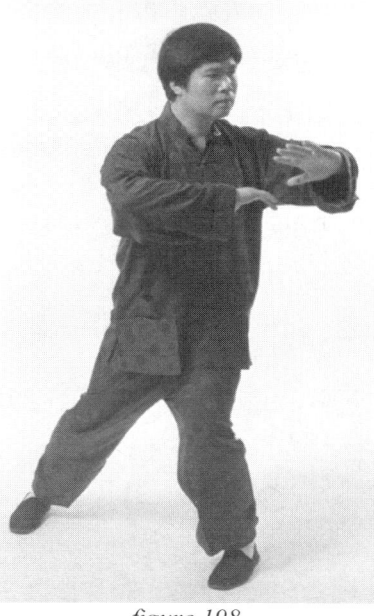

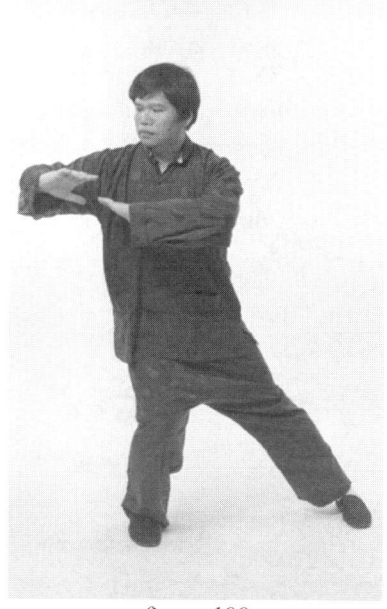

Bring the right hand's fingers together to form a beak, bend the wrist to form a hook; then extend the right arm, and set the left hand in front of the face with the palm facing in *(fig 200)*. Turn the head to the left; then pick up the left foot, and step forward to the left *(fig 201)*. With the body's weight shifted onto the left foot, turn the left palm face forward while the right hand's hook remains the same *(fig 202)*.

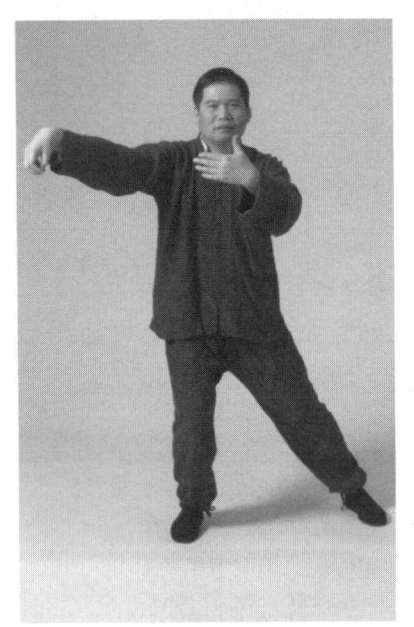

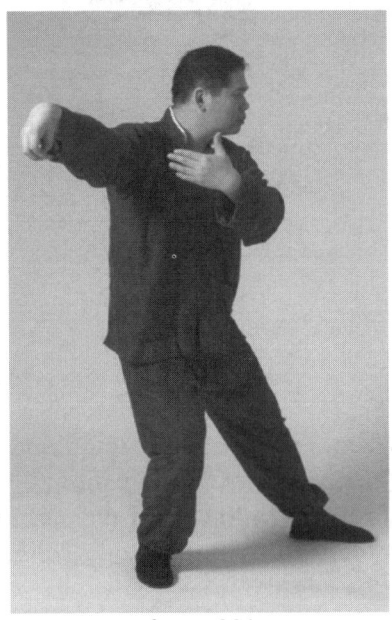

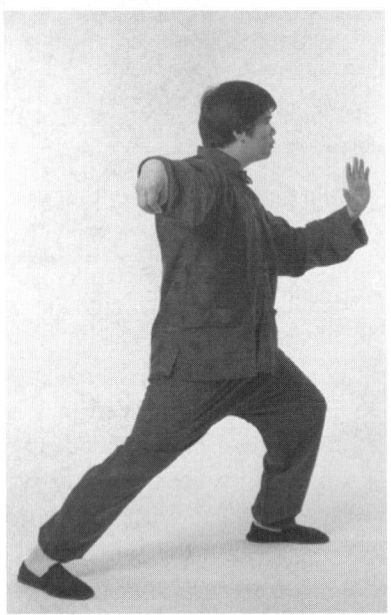

figure 200   *figure 201*   *figure 202*

35. Lower the Snake Body
From the preceding movement, turn the left palm face up, and turn the right toes out *(fig 203)*. Bring the left hand to the chest with the palm still facing up. Lower the body onto the right leg with the left toes turned in; extend the left hand along the left leg. The right hand remains the same *(fig 204)*.

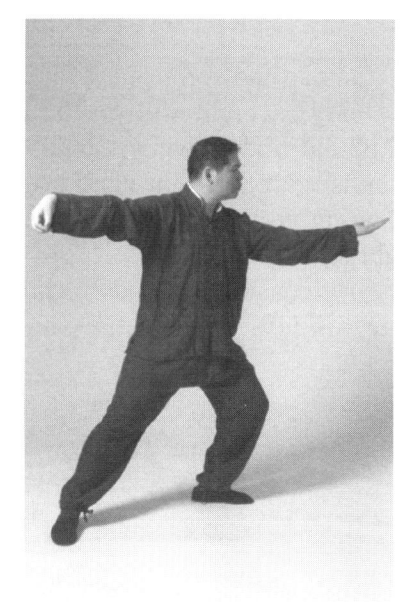

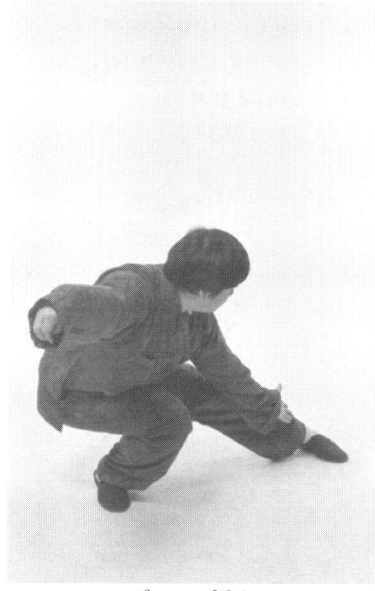

figure 203   *figure 204*

36. Step Forward to Become Seven Star

From the preceding movement, turn the left toes out, and shift the body's weight onto the left foot. Close the left hand into a fist in front of the chest *(fig 205)*. With the body's weight on the left foot, pick up the right foot, and step forward onto the toes. Close the right hand into a fist that then crosses under the left fist *(fig 206)*.

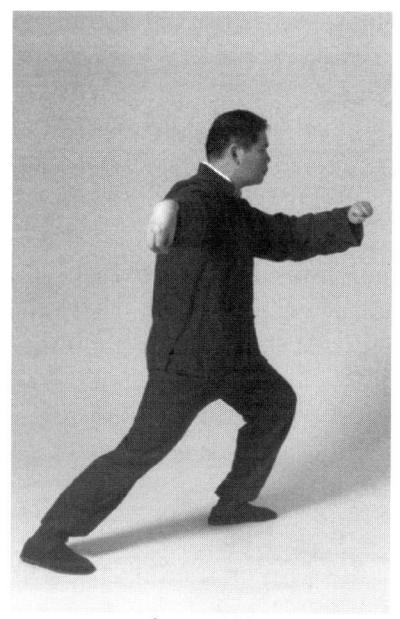

figure 205   *figure 206*

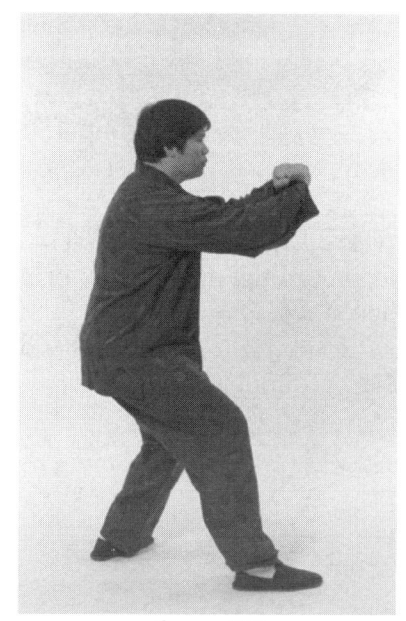

37. Retreat to Ride the Tiger

From the preceding movement, open the fists so the right palm faces in and the left palm faces out *(fig 207)*. With the body's weight still on the left foot, pick up the right foot, and step back. Shift the body's weight onto the right foot, and at the same time, separate the hands with the right hand going up to above the right shoulder and the left hand going down to level with the left hip *(fig 208)*. With the body's weight on the right foot, pick up the left foot and land it on the toes. At the same time, push the right hand forward from the right shoulder, and bring the left hand close to the left leg with the palm facing down *(fig 209)*.

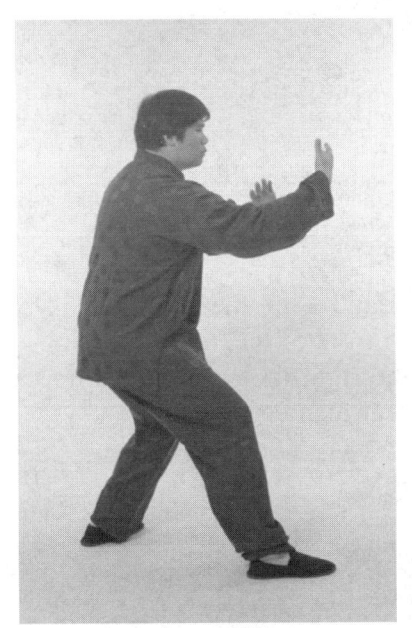

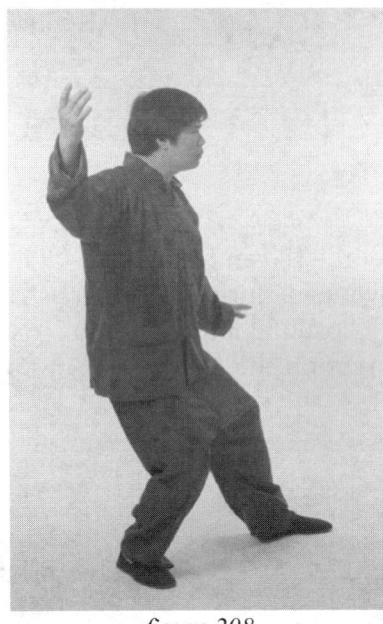

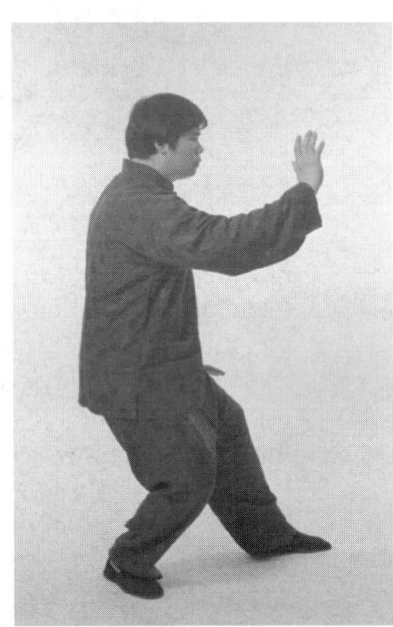

figure 207 *figure 208* *figure 209*

38. Turn Around with Lotus Kick

From the preceding movement, bring the hands back to the chest with the palms face down *(fig 210)*. With the body's weight on the right foot, pivot clockwise to the right on the right toes with the left foot sweeping around to behind the right foot *(fig 211)*.

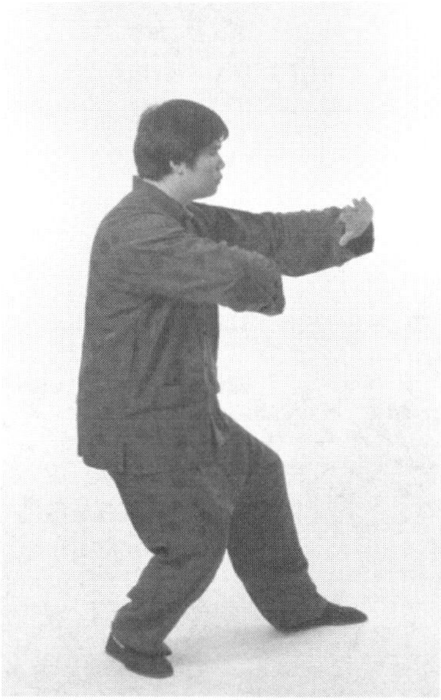

THE 42 MOVEMENT MEDIUM FRAME SOLO FORM

figure 210

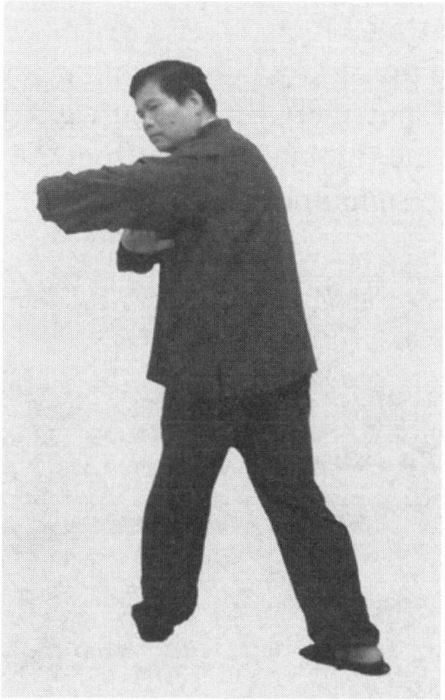

figure 211

With the body weight moving onto the left foot, pivot on the left heel to complete the turn. The hands come back to the chest again with the left hand inside the right elbow. The body has now turned 360 degrees *(fig 212)*. With the body's weight on the left foot, pick up the right foot and make a half circle kick in front of the body from left to right as the hands move from right to left, brushing over the kick *(fig 213)*.

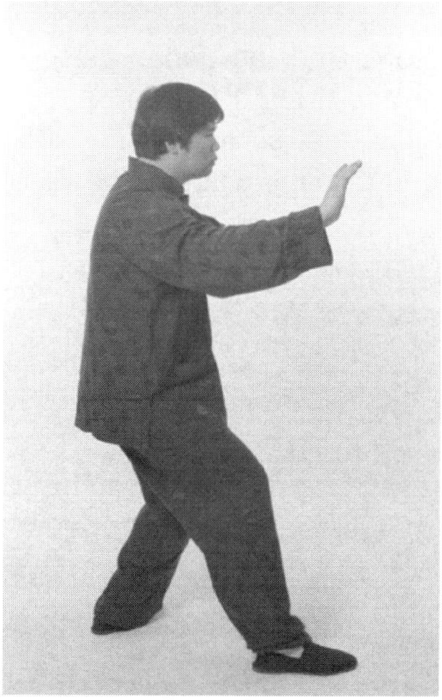

figure 212

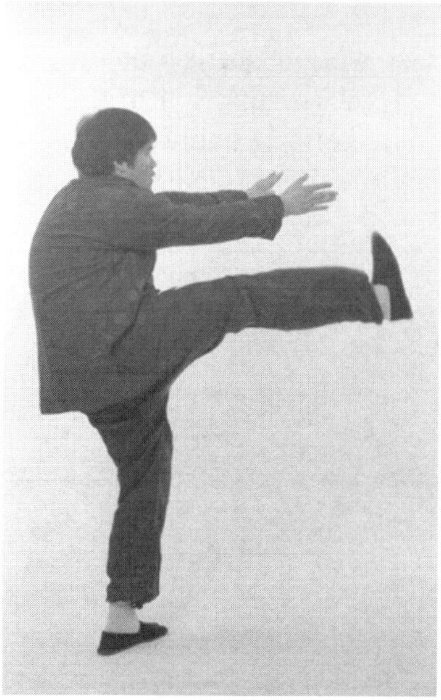

figure 213

39. Shooting Tiger

From the preceding movement, as the left and right hands arrive to the left and center respectively, bring the right leg in *(fig 214)*. Then place the right foot down to the right corner, shifting the weight onto it as the hands draw down to above the right knee *(figs 215 – 216)*.

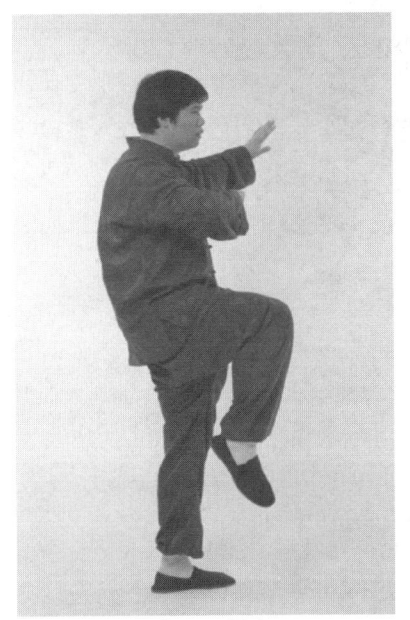

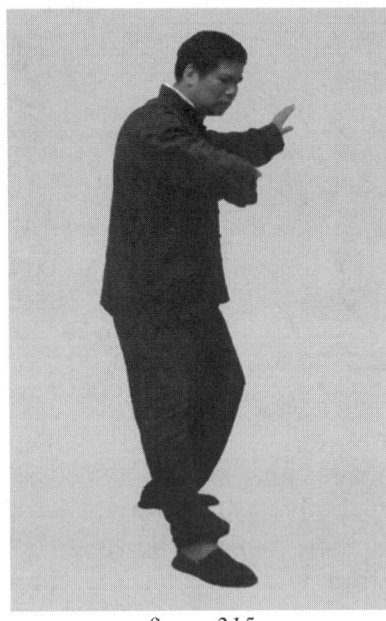

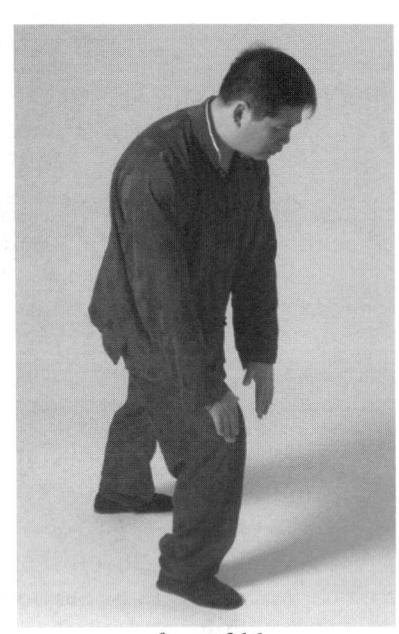

figure 214   *figure 215*   *figure 216*

The body's weight shifts onto the right foot, and the hands close into fists. Bring the right fist up next to the right ear and the left fist up by the chest *(fig 217)*. The left fist punches outward to the left corner level with the left shoulder while the right fist remains close to the right ear *(fig 218)*.

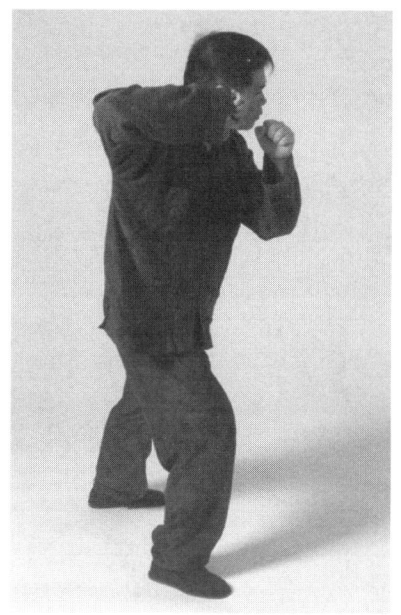

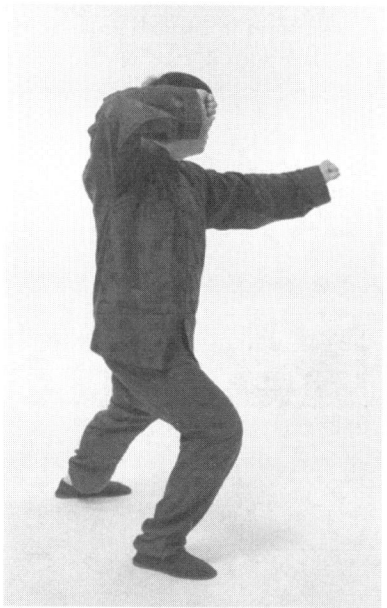

figure 217   *figure 218*

40. Step Forward, Parry, Intercept and Punch

From the preceding movement, open the left fist so the palm faces up *(fig 219)*. Reach the right fist out to the left palm, and then draw the hands back to the left side of the hip with the right fist above of the left palm. The weight shifts to the left *(fig 220)*.

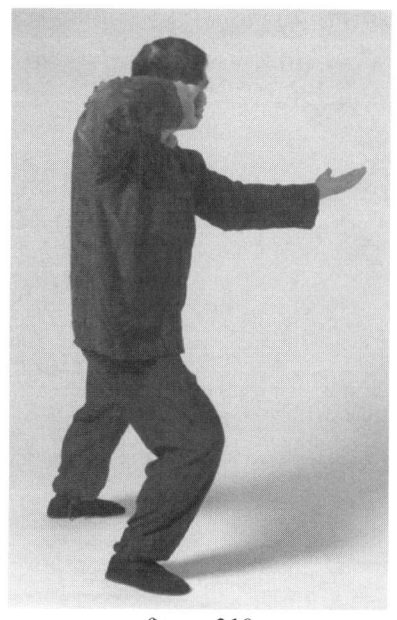

figure 219   *figure 220*

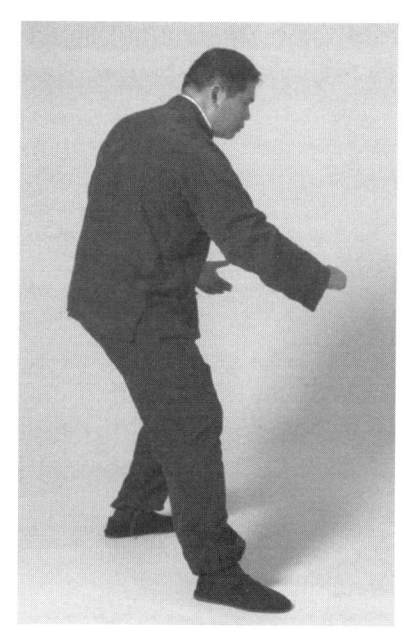

The right foot steps forward with the toes pointing to the corner. Bring the hands up in front of the left shoulder *(figs 221 & 222)*. With the body's weight shifting onto the right foot, the right hand fist circles forward then down *(fig 223)*.

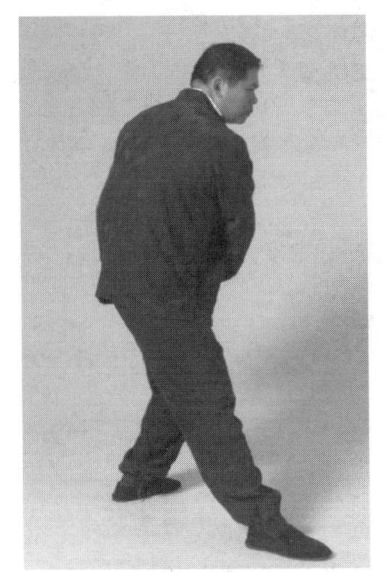

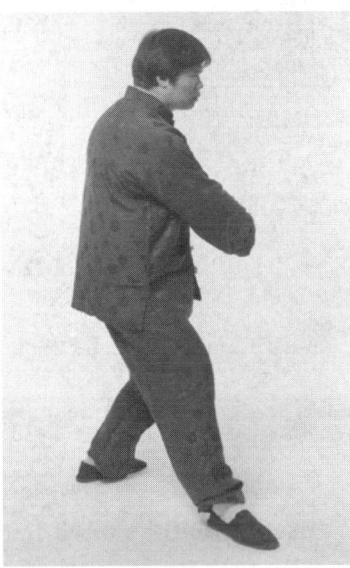

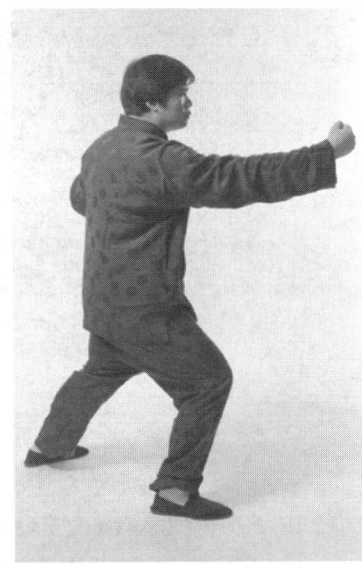

figure 221 *figure 222* *figure 223*

Bring the right fist back onto the right side of the hip, and push the left hand forward from the left shoulder *(fig 224)*. Pick up the left foot, and step forward *(fig 225)*. As the body's weight shifts onto the left foot, the right fist punches forward, and the left palm comes back next to the right elbow *(fig 226)*.

THE 42 MOVEMENT MEDIUM FRAME SOLO FORM

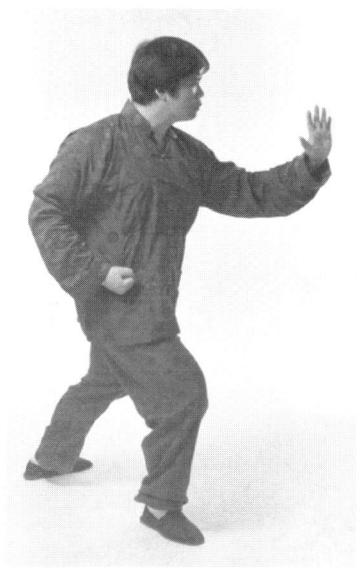

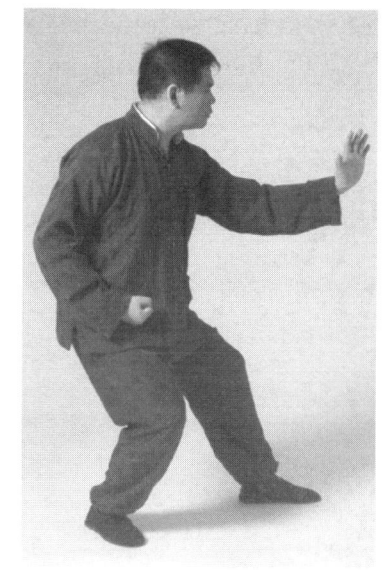

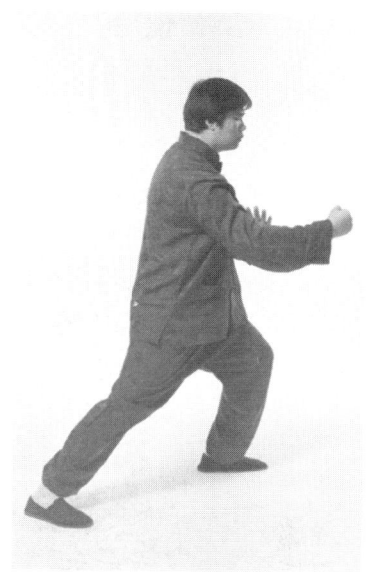

figure 224   *figure 225*   *figure 226*

41. Seal Tightly

From the preceding movement, put the left hand under the right elbow with the palm face up *(fig 227)*. Open the right fist, and bring it back to the right side of the hip with the body's weight shifting onto the right foot. Simultaneously, the left arm pushes forward with the palm facing in *(figs 228 & 229)*.

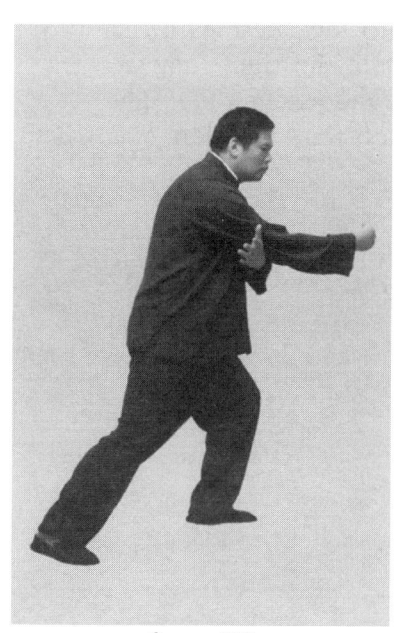

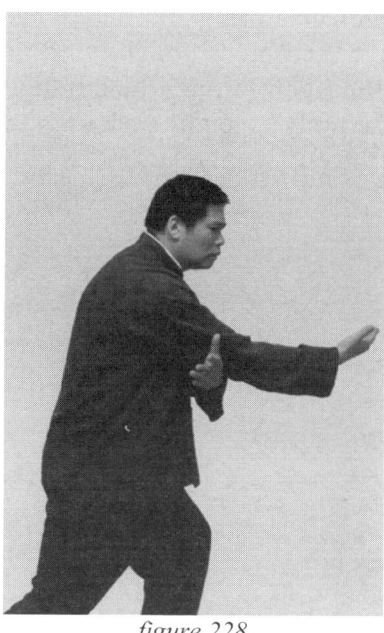

figure 227   *figure 228*   *figure 229*

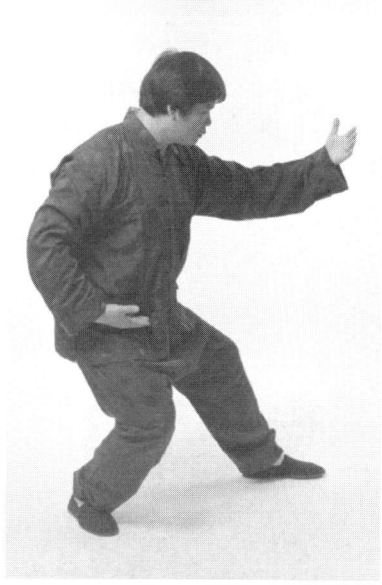

Bring the hands in front of the chest with the palms facing forward *(fig 230)*. Push the hands forward with the body's weight shifting onto the left foot *(fig 231)*.

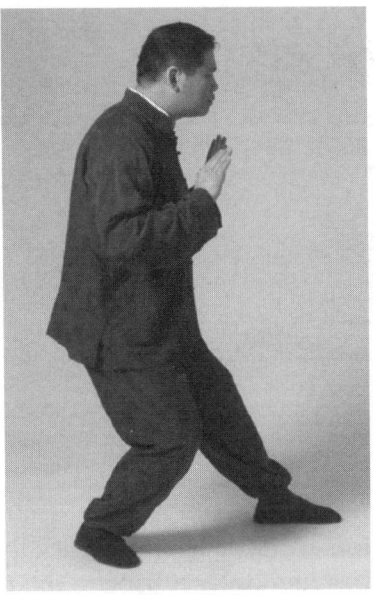

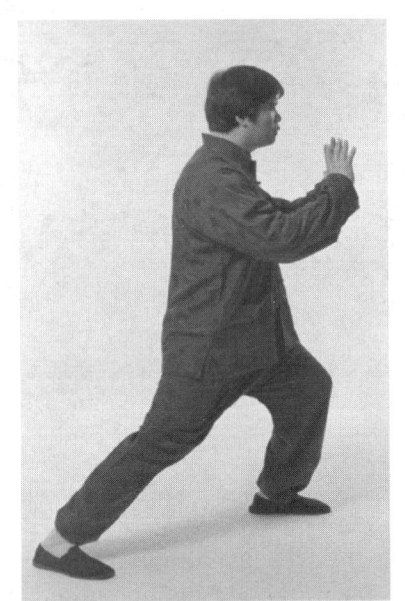

figure 230   *figure 231*

42. Closing Tai Chi Chuan

From the preceding movement, bring the hands back to the chest with the palms facing forward and the body's weight shifting onto the right foot *(fig 232)*. Rotate the body to the right, turning the left toes in and pushing the right hand out *(fig 233)*. Shift the body's weight back onto the left foot, look left, and push the left hand out to the left *(fig 234)*.

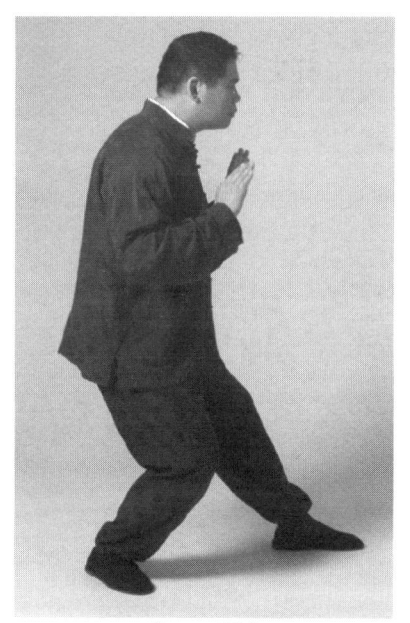

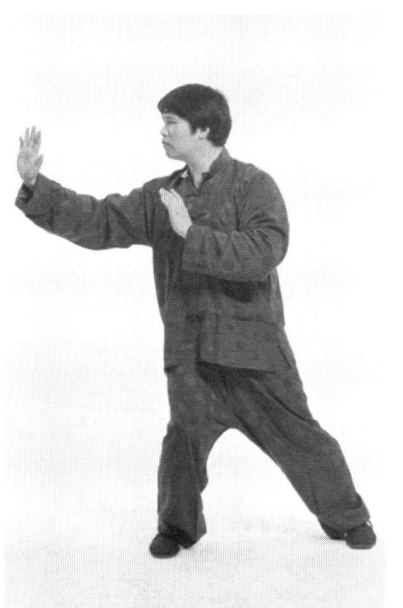

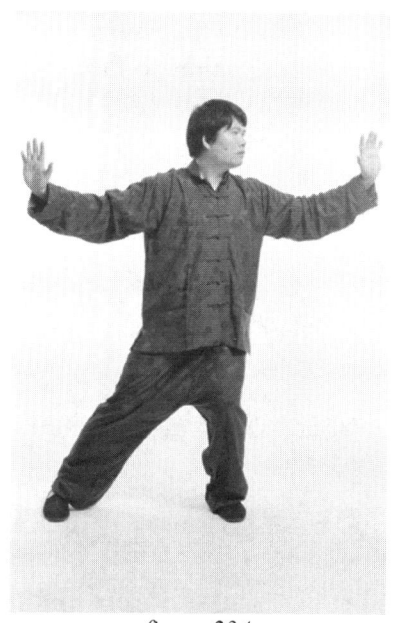

THE 42 MOVEMENT MEDIUM FRAME SOLO FORM

figure 232 *figure 233* *figure 234*

Place the right foot next to the left foot, and bring the hands down between the knees *(figs 235 & 236)*. Turn the hands to face up with the right hand under the left hand. Separate the hands to the same width as the shoulders *(fig 237)*.

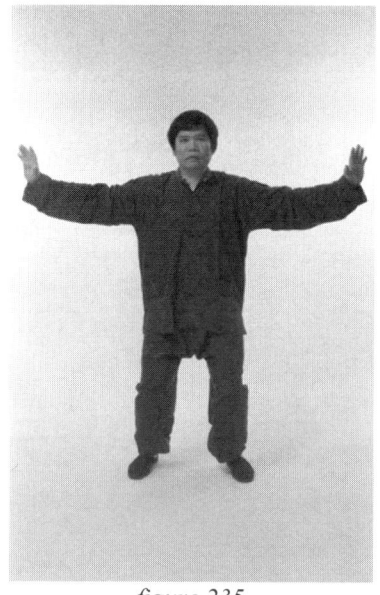

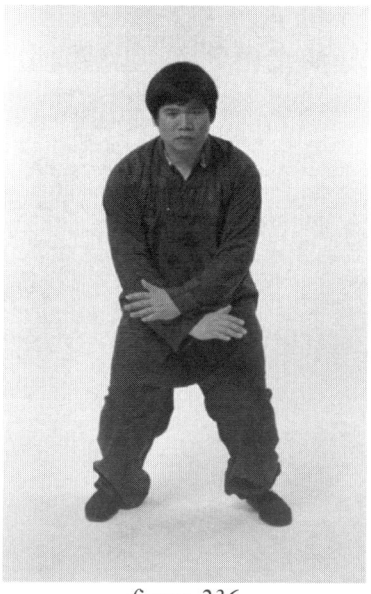

figure 235 *figure 236* *figure 237*

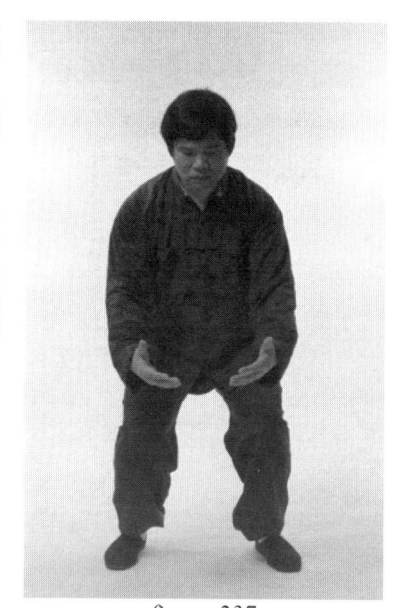

TAI CHI CHUAN - A COMPARATIVE STUDY

Bring the hands up to shoulder level while straightening the legs *(fig 238)*. Turn the palms to face down, and then bring the hands down to the sides of the legs *(figs 239 & 240)*.

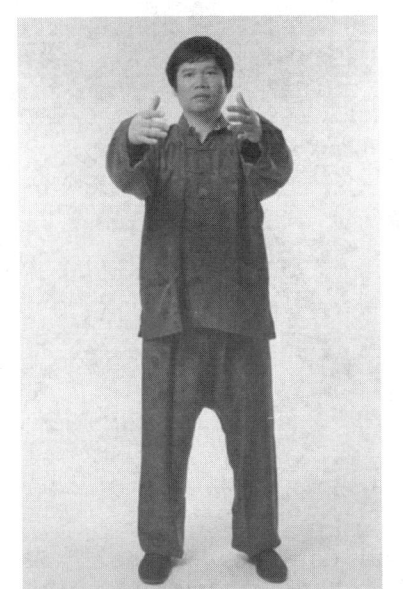

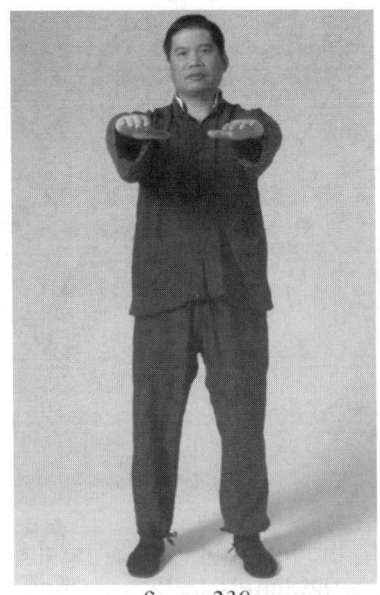

figure 238

figure 239

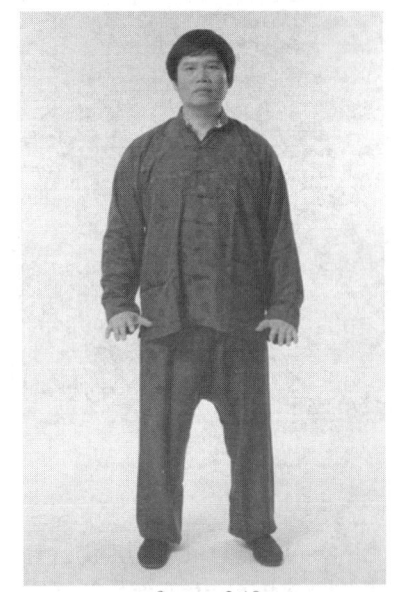

figure 240

Chapter 7
The 48 Movement Small Frame Solo Form

A. Introduction

Tai Chi Chuan is a close-quarter internal martial art. The movements are so compact that a spectator only sees a brief contact between practitioners before one of them is bounced back. The techniques and skills are profound and very difficult to master. The Yang Family members make the training easier by dividing the classical Tai Chi Chuan Solo Form into three levels, or frames, so that it is accessible to beginning students.

The Small Frame Solo Form introduced in this chapter is based on the original 108 Movement Solo Form. The stances are higher, and there are no obvious open and close movements compared to the Large and Medium Frame Solo Forms. Its compact movements work on the muscle groups to develop the internal power, *chi* circulation, and close quarter techniques. It focuses more on the trunk than on the limbs to emphasize training the vertebral column or the central nervous system, developing natural reflex. Therefore, it is said that the Small Frame Form appears to have smaller movements outside and larger movements inside.

Another characteristic of the Small Frame Form is that it loosens the body by stretching the muscle groups. In the beginning, the joints are usually hard and the limbs stiff. After one has practiced the Tai Chi Chuan Solo Form for many years, the body will be nimble and energetic, qualities demonstrated externally as well as internally. When one has reached this stage, conducting all physical activity is possible without injury to the body. This is what the *Tai Chi Chuan Classics* refer to when they say, "First seek out the softness. Later, it will become strong." Soft comes from elasticity. When one is truly soft, the soft spiral power will be developed, and all actions will be fueled by this power.

Yet another characteristic is *chi* circulation. When one practices the solo form slowly and softly, relaxing and stretching the muscle groups, the *chi* will circulate better and easier throughout the body. To be soft and relaxed is not enough; the body must have *chi*. When the body is permeated with *chi*, it is nimble and healthy. This is similar to a tire filled with air; it can support the car's weight and is able to move at the same time.

Practicing the Small Frame Solo Form trains the body completely, inside and outside. Internally the physiologic organs are massaged by the movement.

This action further improves their functions and regulates the central nervous system, *chi* and blood circulations. Externally, the muscular and skeletal systems are exercised by the movement to develop stronger bones and muscles. Based on its function, practitioners have referred to the Small Frame Solo Form as the advanced form in the Tai Chi Chuan system.

B. How to Practice *Chi* Cultivation in Tai Chi Chuan

Chinese martial arts and *chi* cultivation are inseparable. *Chi* cultivation is the fundamental building block of Chinese martial art training. If one is good in *chi* cultivation, one has good martial art skill.

All advanced Chinese martial art systems have *chi* cultivation exercise as part of their gong training. The function is to improve and better the body condition, which is necessary for martial art activity. Some people emphasize martial art skill in their training, and ignore *chi* cultivation. The result is that the martial art skill is excellent, but the body lacks energy.

All Chinese martial art systems follow the same guideline: 70% of one's effort is on *chi* cultivation, and 30% is on martial art skill training. If the body is not strong, the martial art technique is useless. This is like a tree without a root. It cannot last long.

Tai Chi Chuan is one of the advanced Chinese martial art systems. When one is practicing Tai Chi Chuan, one is practicing the *chi* cultivation exercise as well as training for Chinese martial art skill. Therefore, Tai Chi Chuan is often called an internal martial art health exercise. This is especially true when one is practicing the compact movements of the Tai Chi Chuan Small Frame Solo Form. Compared to the Medium Frame Solo Form and the Large Frame Solo Form, the Small Frame Solo Form movement is directly involved with the muscle groups in the trunk rather than with the hands.

The value of Tai Chi Chuan as a martial art has been proven over and over many times. Today, there are many Tai Chi Chuan practitioners who live well into their eighties and nineties. At the same time, there are many skillful practitioners who die young, sick and weak. Why does this happen? The reason lies in *chi* cultivation, or Tai Chi Chuan *Nei Gong*.

When one emphasizes the yin and yang interaction in martial art application, one tends to ignore the yin and yang harmony. Therefore, the *chi* in the yang meridians is circulating too quickly, and the *chi* in the yin meridians is circulating too slowly. If one does not fix this imbalance, disease will result later. Traditional Chinese Medicine indicates that yin and yang balance is the key to optimum health. A unique internal art, Tai Chi Chuan will develop martial art skill as well as improve one's health condition by harmonizing the *chi*. It is often said that a good healthy body without technique is not a practical body, and a technique without good health is an empty technique.

In order to have true Tai Chi Chuan skill, one has to pay close attention to posture, speed, breathing, and intent.

1. **Posture**
   Past practitioners concluded, "It is not easy to set rules and standards. However, without rules and standards, it is more difficult to draw a circle." Although all Tai Chi Chuan styles share the same philosophy and theory, they differ in the execution of the movements in the solo form. Therefore, each style has its distinctive fundamentals for solo form practice.

   Posture is the skeletal framework of Tai Chi Chuan. Movement is the soul. It is the execution of the Tai Chi Chuan Solo Form movements that differentiates the various Tai Chi Chuan styles. Over the years, such distinctions have resulted in the Large Frame Solo Form, the Medium Frame Solo Form, Middle Frame Solo Form, and the Small Frame Solo Form in the classical Yang Family style Tai Chi Chuan system.

2. **Speed**
   Tai Chi Chuan is practiced slowly, most of the time. Practicing Tai Chi Chuan slowly is to develop power and train martial art fundamentals. It is said that practicing Tai Chi Chuan movements slowly aims to train martial art fundamentals. Practicing Tai Chi Chuan movements fast is to train martial art skill. When one is practicing Tai Chi Chuan, one does it as a health maintenance exercise as well as a martial art discipline. Tai Chi Chuan can control and defeat an opponent's attack with its internal power. It is only when it is filled with internal power that the body becomes invincible to strikes and can discharge power. We know that in martial confrontation, nobody is guaranteed to go unhit. When the body is filled with internal power, it can repel the opponent's strike. This is similar to a basketball filled with air. It can easily bounce up and down when one hits it.

The second reason for doing slow movement is intent training. Combining Tai Chi Chuan Solo Form movements with intent is aimed at *chi* gathering. A body has *chi* in its natural state. This is similar to a mountain with creeks and streams. They are operating separately within the same mountain. Practicing Tai Chi Chuan slowly and with intent helps to bring the scattered *chi* together so that it becomes transformed into internal power. This is one of the criteria to determine one's Tai Chi Chuan skill. It functions better when it is drawn together and concentrated in a collected body. Therefore, Tai Chi Chuan training concentrates on the intensification of power more than the application of individual technique.

Chi is a type of energy and power. It has the ability to travel in space as well as penetrate through matter. It exists within matter or outside matter. It has characteristics similar to water. It can exist as a solid mass under certain conditions. When it does, the result is immeasurable.

Practicing *chi* gathering can maintain good health as well as heal disease. *Chi* is a very special type of energy. One has to train a long time with a knowledgeable instructor to be successful in bringing it together to function as a power source for martial art technique. It is said among practitioners that to cultivate *chi* is for health and to gather *chi* is for martial art.

When one is practicing Tai Chi Chuan slowly, it is under the guidance of the intent to gather *chi*. The mechanism combines breathing with Tai Chi Chuan Solo Form movements. The information of this combination must be obtained from a knowledgeable instructor. Many people spend decades practicing without any success in Tai Chi Chuan skill or improved health for lack of this information.

The third reason to practice Tai Chi Chuan slowly is to check and correct any mistakes. When a movement is done fast, a practitioner tends to gloss over it and neglects correcting errors. The slow meticulous execution of a technique allows the practitioner to see the proper trajectory and energetic composition of a movement.

A correct movement is not solely based on its physical movement. It is also based on *chi* circulation, physical vibration, and soundness when the body is aligning properly. Different ingredients, internal as well as external, physical as well as energetic, play an important role in making for a correct movement.

Another concept one has to know is that going slow does not mean stopping. When the execution of a movement seems to stop, it is actually in a transitional pause. This is what the *Tai Chi Chuan Classics* refer to when they say, "When the movement stops, the idea continues; if the idea does not stop, the *chi* does not stop." There is a continuation of the *chi* when the idea continues. It is the mind dictating the pace and extent of the *chi*.

3. **Breathing**

    Tai Chi Chuan also functions as an advanced *chi kung* technique. It follows the same principles and concepts of all *chi kung* exercises. The rhythm of breathing is small, long, slow and even so that one can easily manipulate the movement with the breathing.

    Practicing *chi kung* is working on three areas: regulating the *chi*, regulating the mind, and regulating the body. In its natural state, the body has *chi*, weak and strong. If one practices Tai Chi Chuan following all the principles and concepts correctly, one can easily transform the weak *chi* into stronger *chi*.

    Everyone needs oxygen for survival, and one's oxygen consumption differs based on differing physical activities and behaviors. In Tai Chi Chuan practices, I advise that breathing be natural. It is best if we are able to incorporate the intent while breathing. It does not matter if one has incorporated breathing into Tai Chi Chuan movement or not; the breathing itself is not under one's control. It is an involuntary activity. The *Tai Chi Chuan Classics* say, "If one can breathe, one is alive." This means inhale when you should and exhale when you should.

4. **Intent**

    Intent means the purpose and goal of the mind in a particular movement or series of movements. Practicing Tai Chi Chuan is the same as practicing the intent. When one practices Tai Chi Chuan, one should apply the intent to guide the *chi* to circulate inside the body. The physical movement is the result of *chi* circulation.

Besides its function in *chi* circulation, practicing the intent in Tai Chi Chuan should also include the understanding and awareness of the offensive and defensive techniques within the Tai Chi Chuan Solo Form. As the *chi* circulates through the intent, the practitioner is likewise conscious of the martial purpose of the movement.

a. The Role of Intent in Tai Chi Chuan

Tai Chi Chuan practitioners often emphasize the importance of using the intent in training. The *Tai Chi Chuan Classics* say, "Every movement is based on the intent." "When the intent and *chi* come, the bone and flesh are secondary." "First on the mind, later on the body." "First, the intent moves, later, the power follows." "All of them are based on the intent; it is not based on the external movement." "When the *chi* is not there yet, the intent is already there." "When practicing the solo form and push hand exercises, one should pay attention to the intent."

These quotations clearly define the priority and relationships among the intent, the *chi*, and the body. In every Tai Chi Chuan form, a movement is initiated by the intent, continues with the *chi* and ends with the body movement. It does not matter whether it is *chi* circulation or body movement; it is directed by the intent.

Intent creativity, *chi* circulation, and body movement are the disciplines that Tai Chi Chuan incorporates to work on the three subjects of intent, *chi*, and body. This is based on the ancient Chinese philosophy that the body is the basic matter of life, the mind is life's controller, and the *chi* is life's communicator. The objective of the *chi* is to have the body and mind in unison. A body is considered alive because of the mind. The intent manages the body based on the function of the *chi*. These three components joined together are the key to Tai Chi Chuan training.

Intent initiates and activates the physiological organ functions. Intent, or its power, is a special kind of conscious behavior of the brain which carries a coded message to function inside the body as well as outside the body. In other words, intent controls all physiological functions.

b. **The Nature of Intent**
   Since intent is so important in Tai Chi Chuan training, it is necessary for one to fully understand and define it. There are two approaches to its understanding: intent guides the body movement, and intent guides the *chi* circulation.

   i. The Intent Guides the Body Movement
      When the intent moves, the body follows. Intent guiding the body movement means that all movements are controlled by the intent.

      Intent's movement means creativity. The body following means the body is moving according to the intent's instruction. In Tai Chi Chuan training, all movements are initiated from the intent, and then follow with the body movement. Therefore, the body movement is the outward expression of intent's creativity. If one is able to follow this expectation throughout the Tai Chi Chuan training, one's skill will progress quickly.

   ii. The Intent Guides the *Chi* Circulation
       When the intent moves, the *chi* circulates. The intent guiding the *chi* to circulate means all *chi* circulation follows the intent's instruction. Intent movement means intent creativity. *Chi* circulation means that the *chi* circulates inside the body following the intent's instruction. Intent creativity and *chi* circulation are internal. To find out what is inside, one has to begin from outside. What is internal will be expressed outwardly. Although the intent creativity and *chi* circulation are intangible, the posture and movement a practitioner demonstrates in Tai Chi Chuan is the outward expression of intent creativity and *chi* circulation. From observing the change in a movement, one can tell the condition of the intent creativity and *chi* circulation.

       The highest form of Tai Chi Chuan training is to have the intent creativity and *chi* circulation inside the body combined with outside physical movement. Therefore, if there is no movement inside the body, there should be no movement outside. When there is movement, the components of outside and inside move together in unity.

Although intent is an important factor to determine the outcome of Tai Chi Chuan skill, it is abstract and difficult to understand. However, it has the following meanings and characteristics:

a. It means attention.
b. It has a meaning similar to *chi*. It is a form of energy and power.
c. It is a form of thinking and imagination.
d. It has many levels. A student emphasizes the intent differently according to his or her skill.
e. It is repeatable. At each time, however, the meaning and fulfillment are different.
f. It can be understood from observing physical movement, feeling and sensation. A student may not be able to understand it in the beginning. After much practice, the understanding becomes better.
g. Since its essence is abstract and intangible, it can be interpreted in many different ways according to one's experience. Therefore, its grasping does not have a set priority or order.
h. It is a state of mental condition.
i. It is a mental activity and creativity.
j. It is an objective and goal.
k. Although it has many meanings, each meaning contributes to achieve a complete and united whole.

iii. Intent and Creativity
To increase the intent creativity, one must cultivate it daily and incorporate it throughout the Tai Chi Chuan training. This includes practical experiences and daily activity.

From psychological experimentation, we understand that intent has a very close association with one's emotion and experience. Whenever we have a good and positive experience, the emotion is positive, and the intent creativity is not restricted. When the emotion is negative, the intent creativity is limited. Therefore, it is necessary to have good experiences and positive emotions that can be generated and supported in tranquil environments. Serenity is a condition that allows one to concentrate and focus, and the creativity to flow and cohere. The result is quite miraculous.

c. Intent and Tai Chi Chuan

From a martial art perspective, intent emphasizes technique and strategy, but most importantly, the opponent's weaknesses.

Tai Chi Chuan is a relaxed, soft, internal and external physical activity. Its movements are stable, circular, and continuous, and the body is upright. Based on these principles, Tai Chi Chuan movement works under a set of rules. When one is engaging in Tai Chi Chuan training, one is consciously controlling the body to function under these rules.

How does one incorporate the intent into Tai Chi Chuan training? The following are some of the common practices.

When one is practicing the Tai Chi Chuan Solo Form, one should assume that one is involved with an opponent in an offensive and defensive maneuver. It is only when the intent is true that the power gets to the target and the movement is effective. One develops confidence in each movement by understanding its application and variations. Believing in oneself during confrontation is important for the technique to be applied freely without any hesitation or restriction. The *Tai Chi Chuan Classics* say, "When the *chi* is not yet there, the intent is already there." When people say, "confidence is half of success," it refers to the power of intent.

One should understand the mechanism and application of a movement, the power and variation involved in each technique, and where and when to deliver the power. This is what the *Tai Chi Chuan Classics* refer to in the saying, "One should pay attention to each movement." One should pay close attention to each movement so the power can get to the target. One should clearly understand the power in each movement and the fist, palm, or finger strike in a movement. How to move the fingers to correctly apply the seize technique to easily control the opponent must also be understood.

In any particular posture, the head should have the intent of supporting an object upward. The body is sinking. The hands push forward. The arms move to the sides. The toes are pointing forward. The knees are bent like a nutcracker. The buttock is tucked in. The hip has roundness like a "U" shape.

The *Tai Chi Chuan Classics* say that one should walk like a cat. In practice, one can imagine that the stepping in advance or retreat, to empty or full, should be very quiet, spontaneous, and light. It is stable and continuous like running water.

The *Tai Chi Chuan Classics* say that mobilizing the *jin* is like pulling silk from a cocoon. In practice, one can imagine that the movement is gentle, circular, smooth, even, and continuous. Otherwise, the silk thread will break. Intent is a very important step in Tai Chi Chuan training. If one can incorporate it into daily practice as described above, one will definitely develop the Tai Chi Chuan skill and power quickly. When the body is nimble and every part a weapon, this is an outward expression of the intent, *chi*, and body united.

C. Fundamentals

The Tai Chi Chuan Small Frame Solo Form conjoins compact movements of the body with the rotation of the waist and pelvis. The movement appears very small externally but very large internally, working on and massaging the internal organs and promoting *chi* circulation. Therefore, in order for one to master this art, to have better health through *chi* cultivation and higher martial skill and to attain an understanding of Tai Chi Chuan, one must spend time practicing the fundamentals to build a stronger foundation.

Tai Chi Chuan fundamentals include movements of the hands and eyes, body position, stance, and stepping. It is often said that when one executes a hand technique without moving the feet, one is looking for trouble. When one is executing a movement, if the head is looking down like a dog and the body is stretching like a cat, one's skill is very poor. To avoid such shortcomings, one must spend time practicing the fundamentals.

1. **Basic Hands Techniques and Positions**

    Tai Chi Chuan involves many hand techniques. It is necessary to get them right so that a movement will be performed properly and executed correctly in martial application. The hand methods are divided into the fist *(fig 1)*, the palm *(fig 2)*, and the hook *(fig 3)*. The common Tai Chi Chuan techniques are ward off, roll back, press, push, pull down, split, elbow strike, shoulder strike, palm strike, punch, kick, and hook.

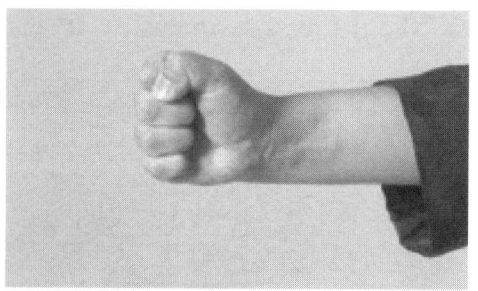

figure 1

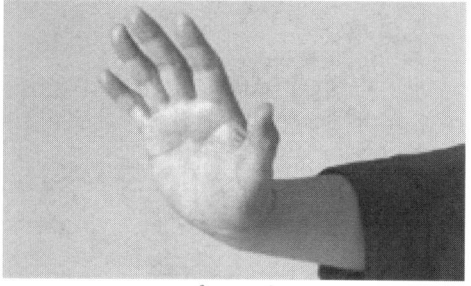

figure 2

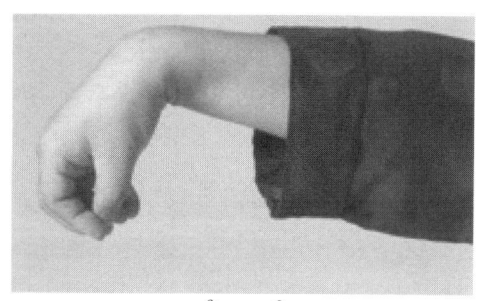

figure 3

When closing the fingers into a fist, the fingers should not be too tight. When forming a palm strike, bend the wrist so that the power will go directly into the center of the palm.

a. The Fists

The fist is a most important weapon in bare hand combat. There are several techniques involving the fist in Tai Chi Chuan. Here is the list.

i. Hidden Fist: The fist rests by the waist. It faces up.

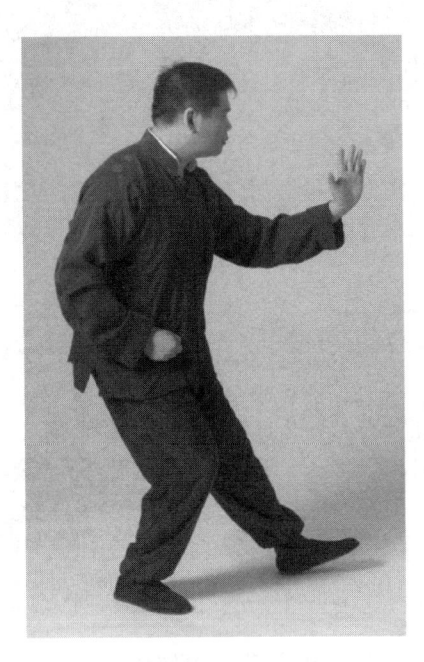

ii. Thrusting Fist: The fist rests by the waist then goes forward. Its position is not higher than the shoulder and not lower than the chest.

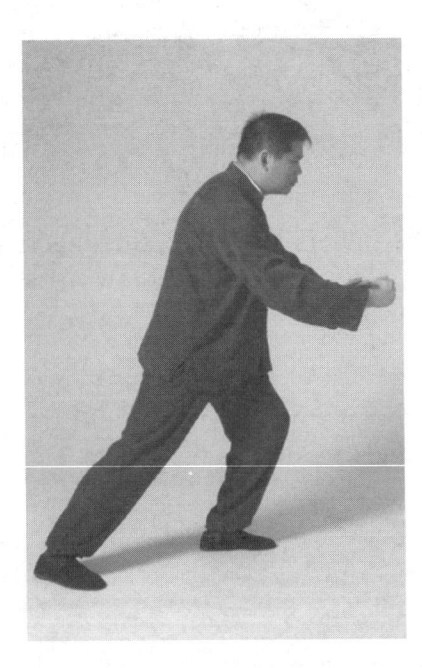

iii. Downward Fist: The fist rests by the waist then goes downward. It faces either to the left or right. It arrives level to the front knee.

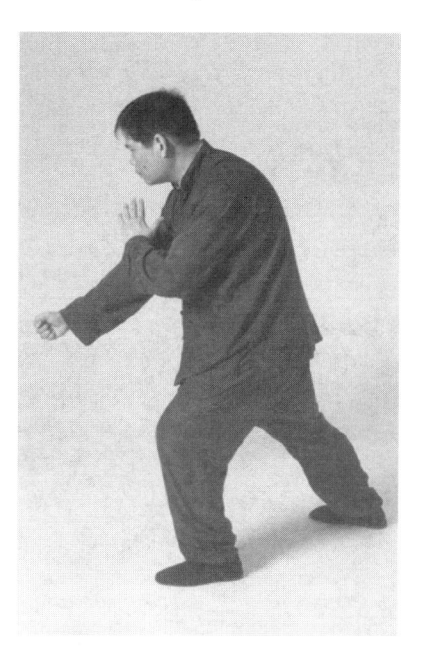

iv. Parry Fist: The fist comes up in an arc. It begins with the fist facing down and ends with the fist facing up to the front or side.

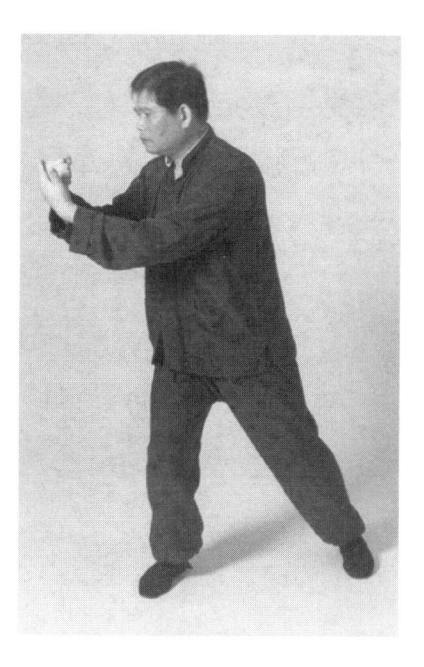

v. Back Fist: The fist moves upward then downward in an arc. It begins with the fist face down and ends with the fist face up.

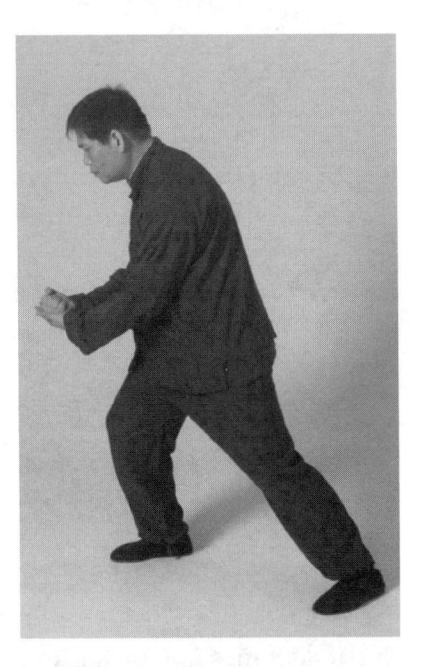

vi. Double Fist: The two fists go upward to ear level.

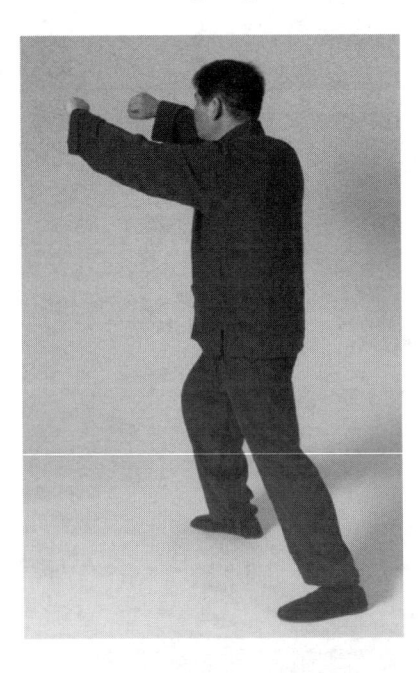

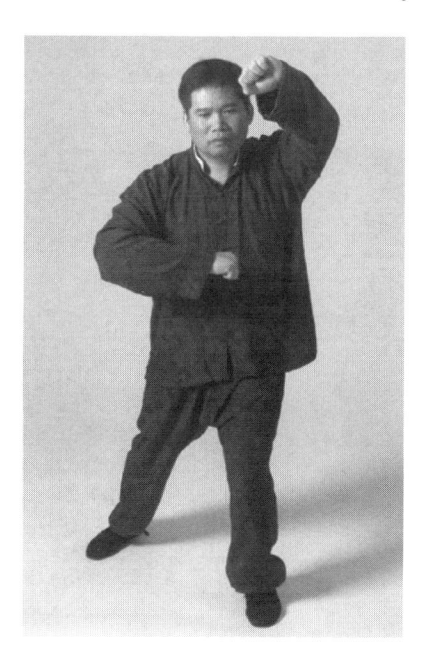

vii. Horizontal Fist: The fists move horizontally to the left or right.

b. **The Palms**

Although the name Tai Chi Chuan implies the use of the fist, most of the hand techniques in Tai Chi Chuan prefer the palm. Internal martial art practitioners recognize that a palm can easily be transformed into more options than the fist. Here is the list of common techniques involving the palm:

i. Single Palm Push: Bend the elbow and wrist with the fingers pointing up. The palm pushes forward on level with the shoulder.

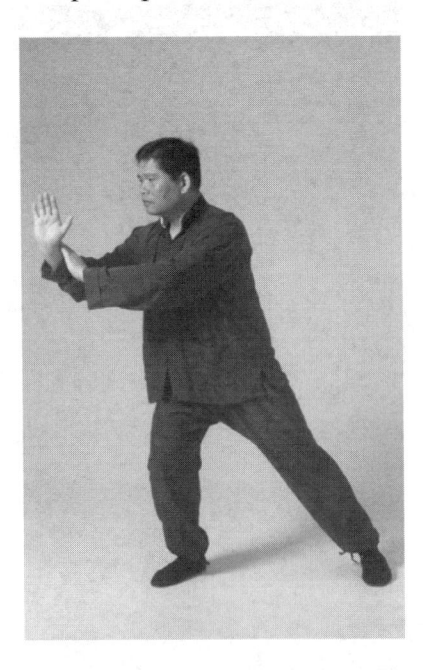

ii. Double Palm Push: The two palms push forward or downward from the shoulders with the fingers pointing straight ahead.

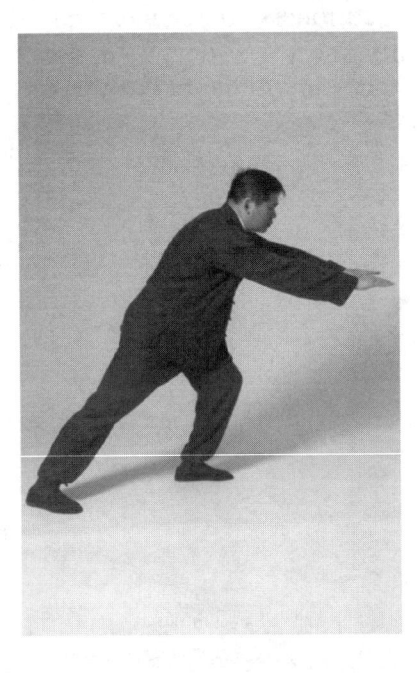

iii. Brush Palm: The palm brushes downward from the center of the body to the side of the body.

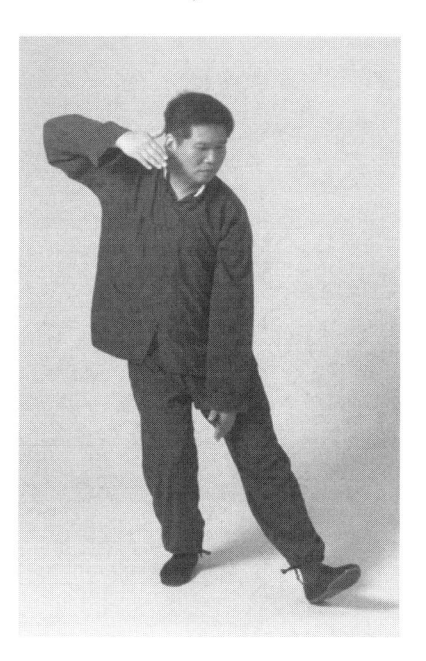

iv. Intercepting Palm: The palm comes from the side of the body to the chest with the palm facing down and forward. The fingers are pointing to the side.

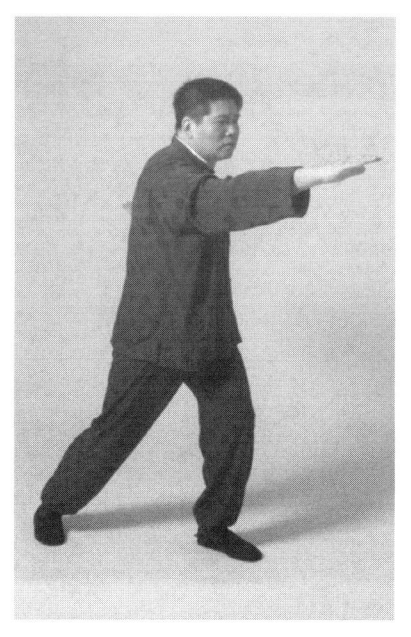

v. Separating Palm: The two palms begin from the center of the body, separating into two sides with the palms facing away from the body and the fingers pointing outward.

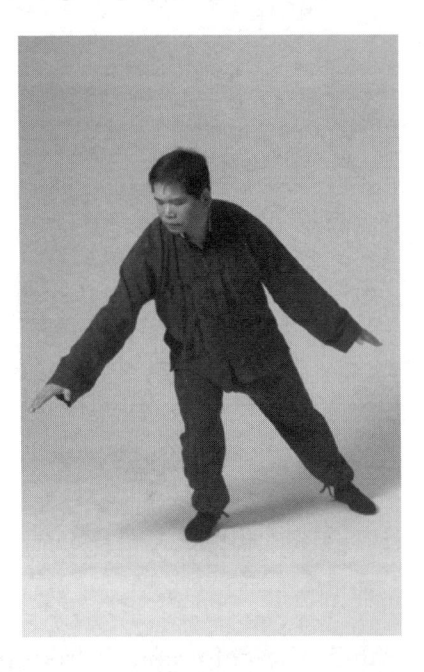

vi. Diagonal Separating Palm: The two palms begin from the center of the body, separating into top and bottom.

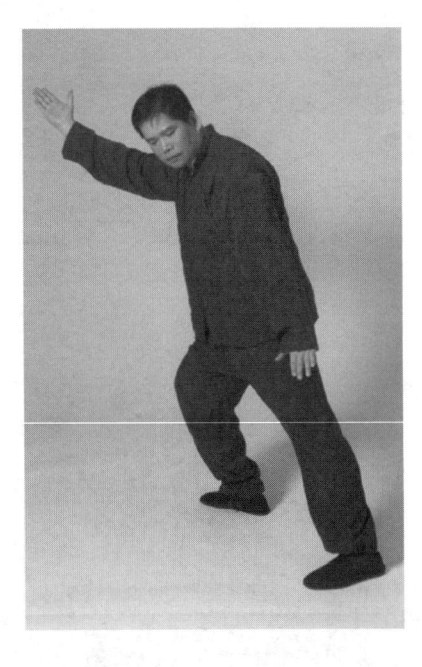

vii. Vertical Cloud Palm: The palms go up and down.

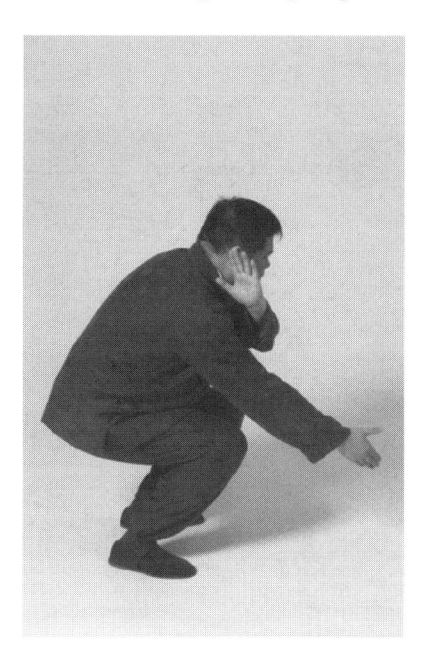

viii. Horizontal Cloud Palm: The palms move to left and right horizontally.

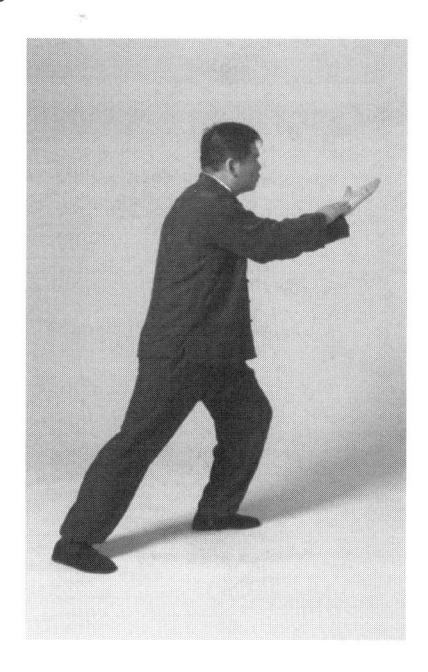

ix. Thrusting Palm: The palm goes forward with the fingers pointing upward.

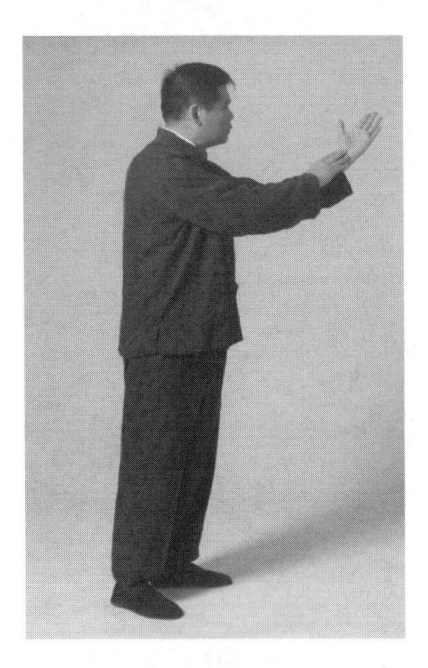

x. Blocking Palm: The palm goes upward above the head.

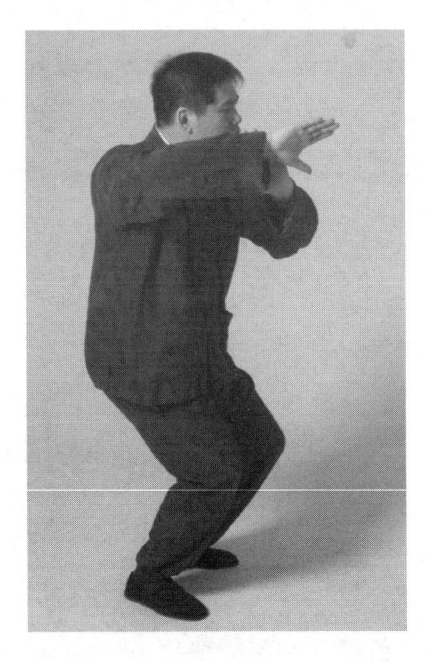

xi. Embracing Palm: The palms face inward with the fingers pointing up.

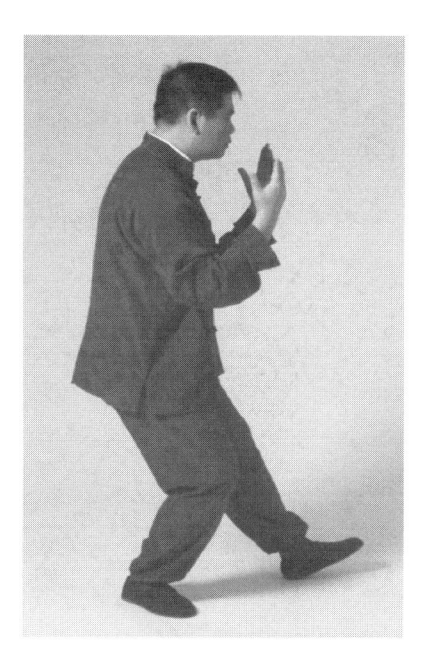

xii. Downward Palm: The palm goes down with the fingers pointing downward.

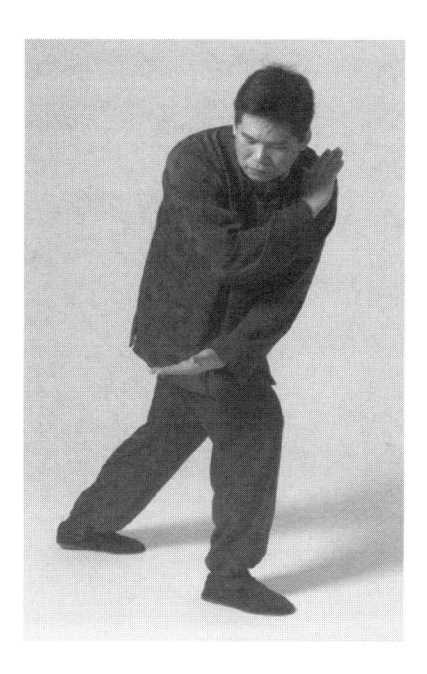

xiii. Lift Palm: The palm goes upward with the fingers pointing up.

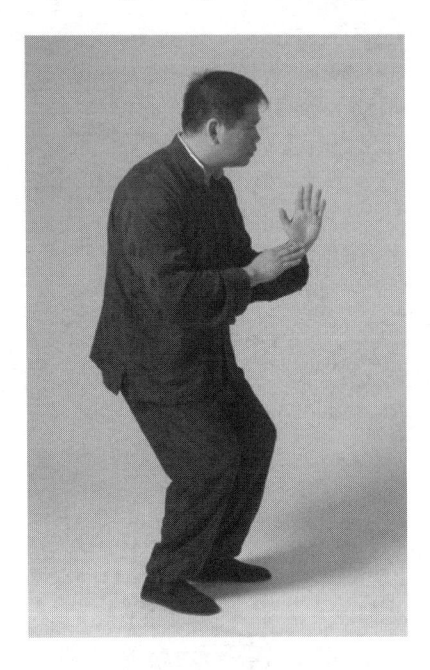

xiv. Yin Yang Palm: One palm faces up and the other palm faces down.

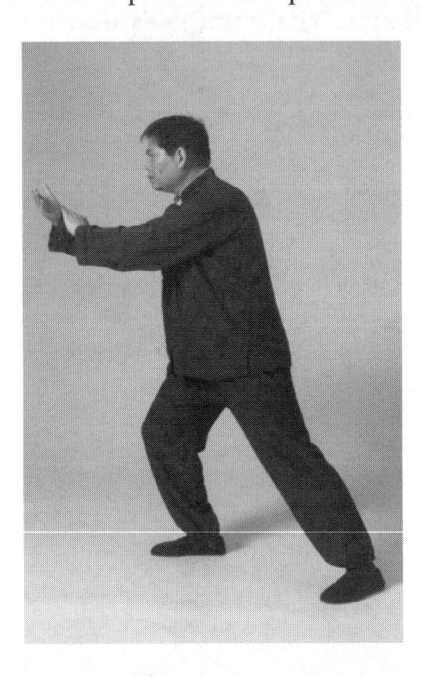

c. **The Arms**

In Tai Chi Chuan, the arm movements are often incorporated to execute the techniques of split, shoulder strike, and elbow strike. Here are some of the common arm movements.

i. Embracing: The palms face inward.

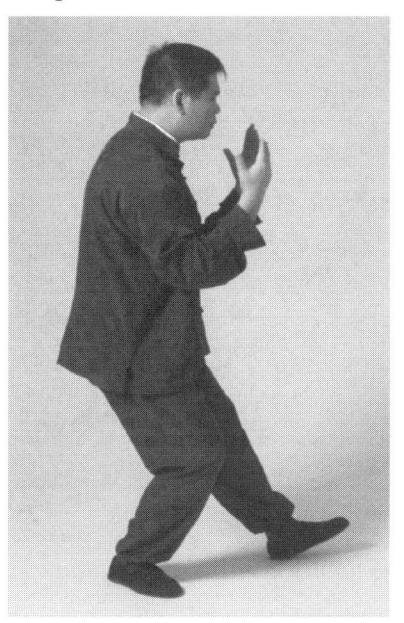

ii. Push: The two arms come together in front of the chest to push.

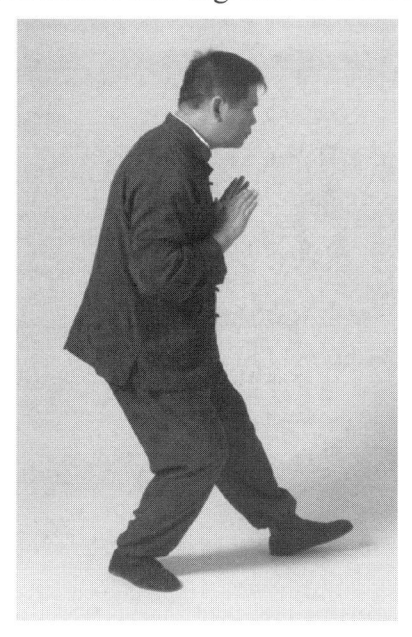

iii. Separating: The two hands separate into front and back.

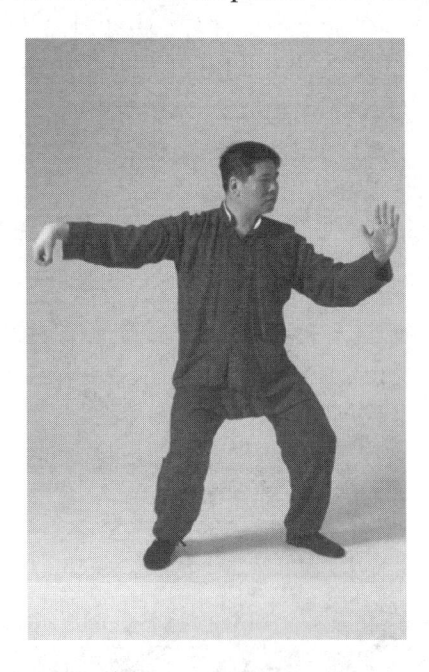

iv. Split: The two hands come together then separate to the sides.

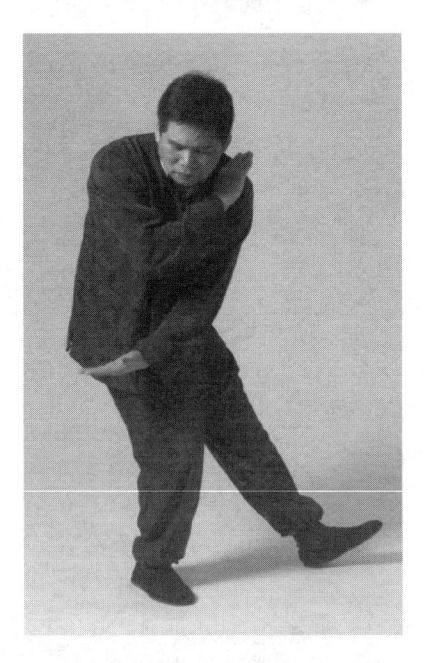

2. Eye and Body Techniques and Positions

a. Eye Position

As in all Chinese martial art systems, the eyes are very important in Tai Chi Chuan. They are related to the expression of *chi* and spirit in power delivery. In practice, it is necessary to concentrate the spirit and mind to project the full potential of a posture. The eyes follow each movement with the coordination from the intent, hands, and feet.

b. Body Position
  i. The head always remains upright with the eyes looking forward and far off so the spirit can reach to the top of the head. This means the head remains upright following the intent. When the top of the head is slightly lifted upward, the jaw tilts inward, and the tongue touches the hard palate. The trunk leans forward. This appears to be a vulnerable position, but actually it is not, for Tai Chi Chuan is a close quarter martial art. It is so close that the trunk contacts the opponent more often than the hands. Since the Tai Chi Chuan Small Frame Solo Form movement is based on the waist rotation, far less so than on the hands; each and every movement involves stretching the body. This action promotes better *chi* circulation throughout the body.
 ii. The neck is relaxed and straight. There is no tension on the neck muscles so that it is easy to rotate the neck to either side without stiffness. The head movement is like a dragon in the Tai Chi Chuan Small Frame Solo Form. It has many movements and is unpredictable. This action requires many neck muscles for support.
iii. The shoulders are relaxed and sunk. If the shoulders do not sink, blood flow is inhibited, and the *chi* will rise. This will inhibit the whole body from sinking downward to a better rooting. All the movements in the Tai Chi Chuan Small Frame Solo Form are guided by the shoulders, and this action reinforces the rotation of the waist and pelvic and body stretching.
 iv. The elbows should sink and point downward. Otherwise, they cause the same problem as the shoulders.
  v. The chest should be relaxed and natural so that the *chi* can sink to the *dan tien*, an area three inches below the navel. Make sure the chest does not thrust outward or sink inward.

vi. The back should be spread evenly so that the *chi* will be able to penetrate into the bones. It is said that as long as one has the chest relaxed, the back is automatically raised.
vii. The waist should be relaxed so that it is flexible. All Tai Chi Chuan movements are initially based on the rotation of the waist. Therefore, the more flexible and loose the waist, the better and more efficiently one will be able to execute the solo form movements.
viii. The hip and buttocks must tuck under so that all the postures are connected. Otherwise, if the posture is not properly connected, issuing power is difficult. Therefore, the hip should relax and sink to get a better balance, and the buttock should not protrude to the sides. Overall, the body should be relaxed and natural, and the sacrum in a straight and upright position so that all the movements are nimble and start from the waist.

3. **Step and Stance**

   Step and stance comprise some important areas in Tai Chi Chuan training. Stance training refers to stationary postures in the solo form, and step training refers to the movements involved with body weight transition in the solo form. Stance is the lower-body posture, and step is the movement of the lower-body posture. In Tai Chi Chuan training, when a beginner is unable to master the stance and step training, it is difficult to maintain body balance, correctly execute the movement, and progress in training. Therefore, stance and step skills are the basic requirements for body balance and mobility. They are so vital that all martial art systems require beginning students to spend many years on stance and step skill training before one is allowed to learn any routine. In the high standard of Tai Chi Chuan practices, principles such as walk like a cat and pulling silk from a cocoon require a lot of control and coordination. If the stance and step skills are not strong and correct, one cannot practice the principles properly.

   a. **Stance Position**

   In the Tai Chi Chuan Small Frame Solo Form, the feet are closer to each other and parallel. The trunk leans forward. The front knee is aligned to the toes, and the back leg is straight. It has several different types of stances. A list of the common stances follows:

i. Forward Bow Stance:
   Bend the front leg with the foot flat on the floor and the knee aligned to the toes. The back leg is straight, and the toes point forward so the feet are parallel. Generally, 60% of the body's weight is on the front leg, and 40% of the body's weight is on the back leg.

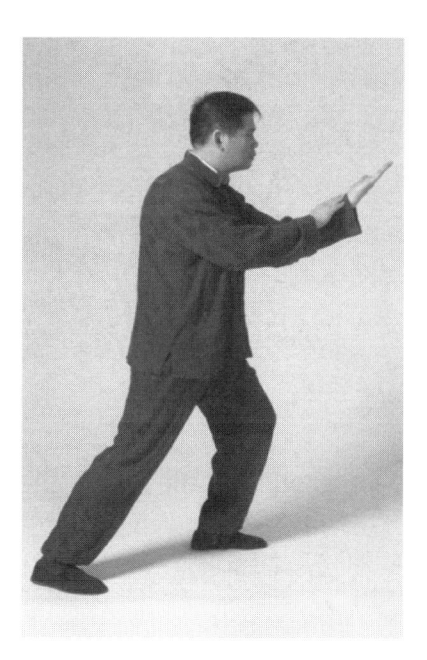

ii. Backward Bow Stance:
   Bend the back leg with the foot flat on the floor and the knee pointing to the same direction as the toes. The front leg is straight with the toes lifted off the ground. Generally, 60% of the body's weight is on the back foot, and 40% of the body's weight is on the front foot.

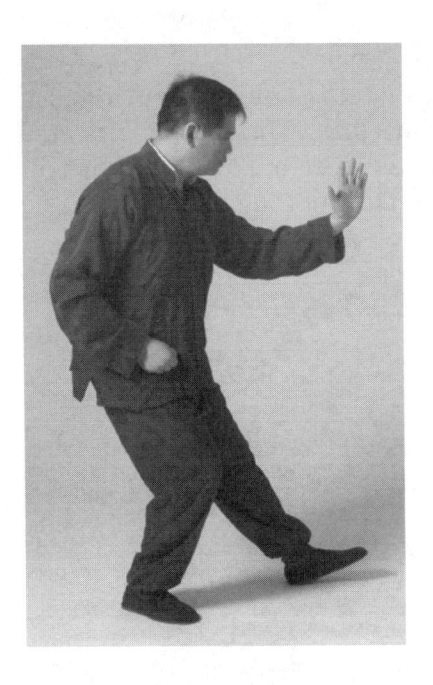

iii. Horse Stance:
Separate the feet as wide as the shoulders. Bend the legs, and line up the knees with the toes.

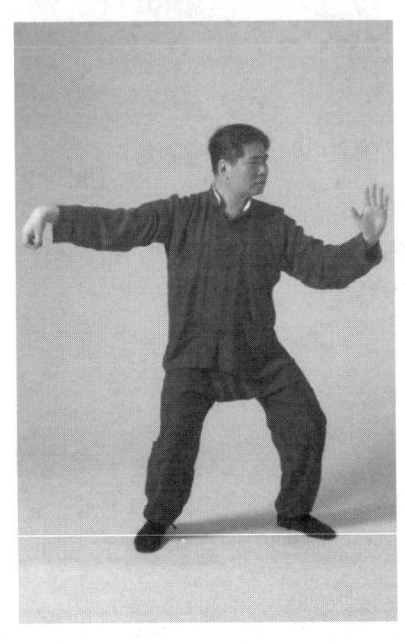

iv. Stand Up on One Leg:
   As the name implies, the body's weight is supported on one leg with the other leg suspended.

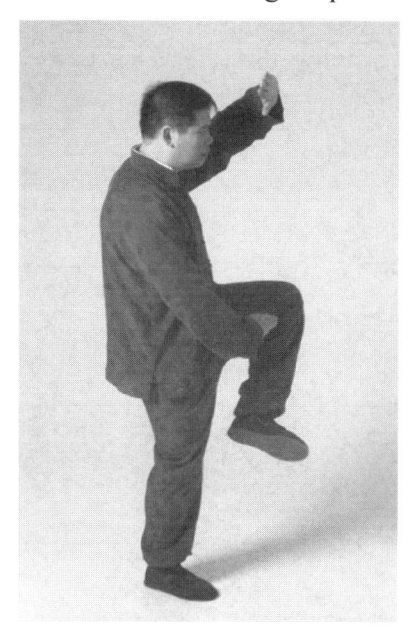

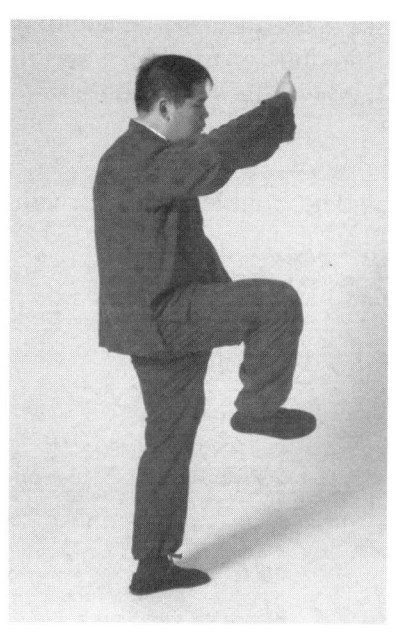

v. Low Stance:
   One leg supports the body weight lower to the ground. The other leg is extended straight forward.

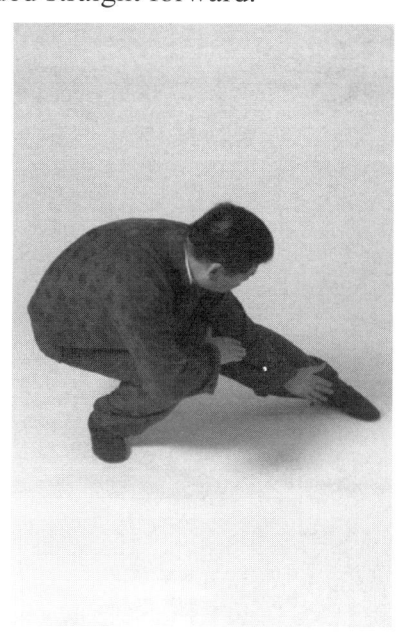

b. **Step Techniques**

Mobility is very important in all Chinese martial art systems. It is the ability for one to get close to or away from the opponent. It is often said that if one is launching a strike without moving the feet, one is looking for trouble. Therefore, moving the feet is very important. It is the soul of martial art.

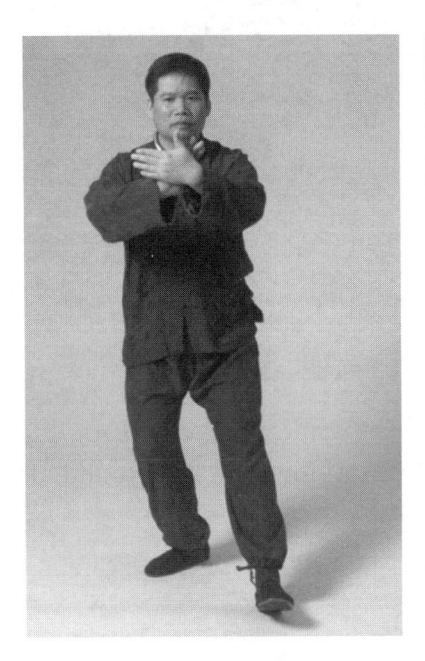

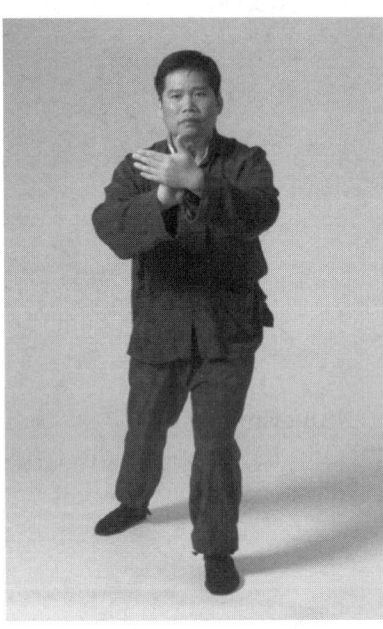

i. Forward Step:
The front leg steps forward.

ii. Backward Step:
   The front leg steps backward.

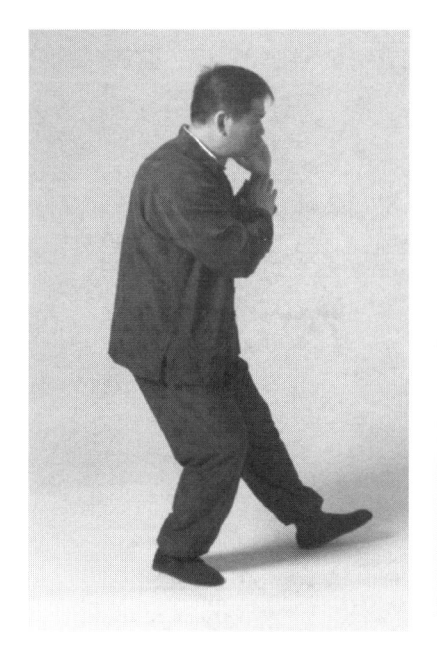

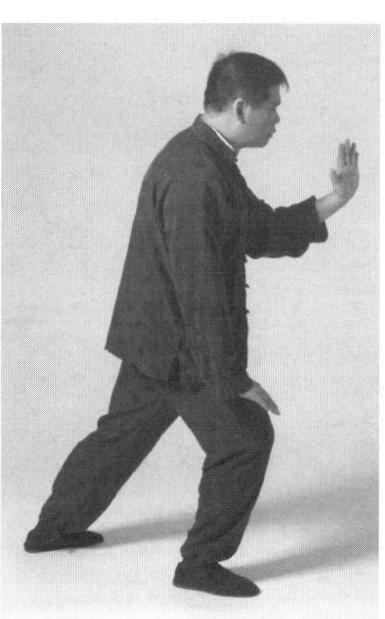

iii. Retreating Step:
   The front or back leg takes a half step back.

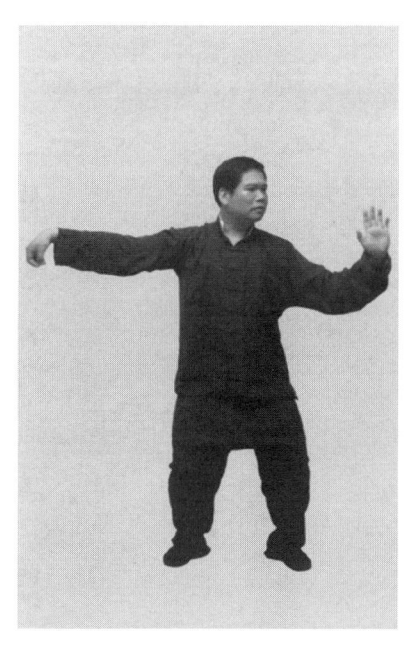

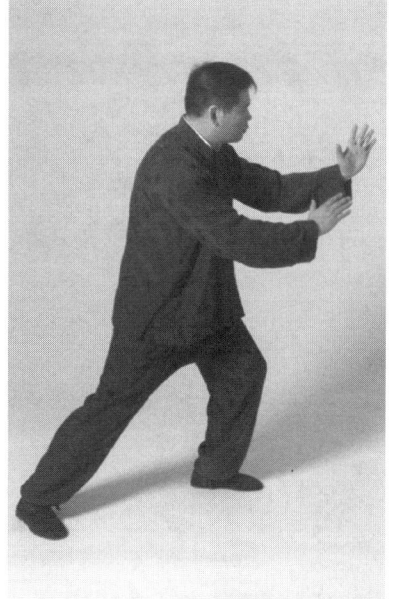

iv. Following Step:
   The back leg takes a half step forward.

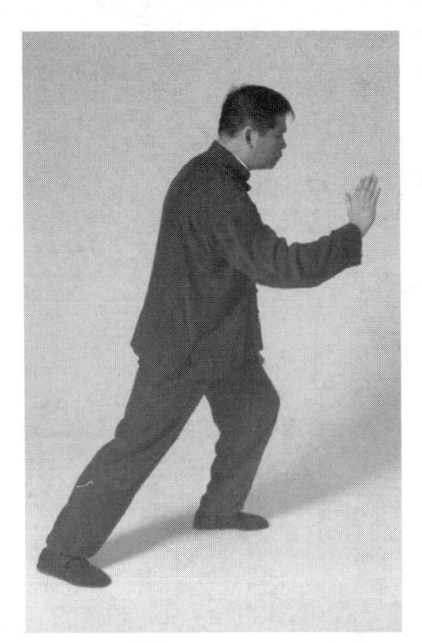

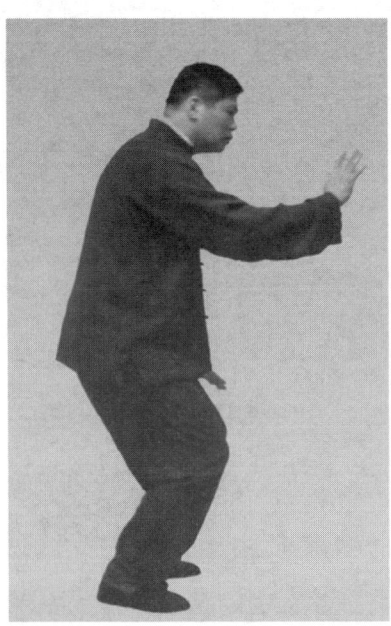

v. Side Step:
   Either foot steps to the side.

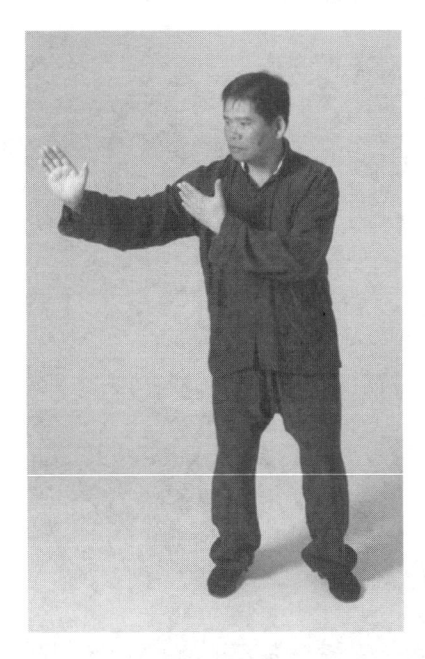

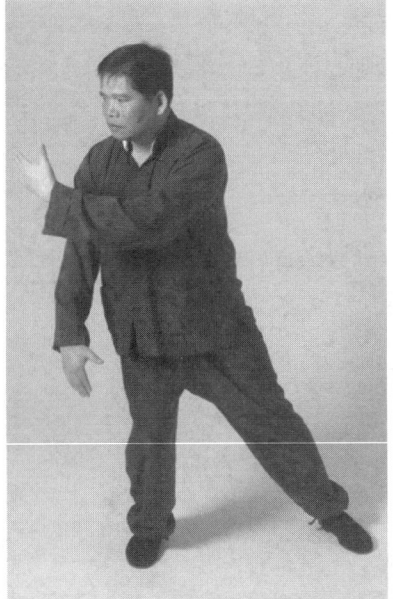

These are the common steps in Tai Chi Chuan. They must be executed slowly and evenly, distinguishing empty and full. When stepping forward, the front heel touches the ground first. When stepping backward, the toes touch the ground first. When shifting the body weight from one foot to another, do it slowly and maintain balance. The distance between the two feet generally corresponds to the width of the shoulders. If the distance is too wide, it affects mobility. If it is too narrow, it will not develop any skill. The rotations on the heels and the toes have to be right.

c. Kicking

In Tai Chi Chuan practice, the body is often supported by one leg. Therefore, there are many hidden low kicks in the solo form. The common kicks that one can see in the Tai Chi Chuan Solo Form follow.

i. Separation Kick:
It is a kick with the side of the foot. It targets the foe's rib cage.

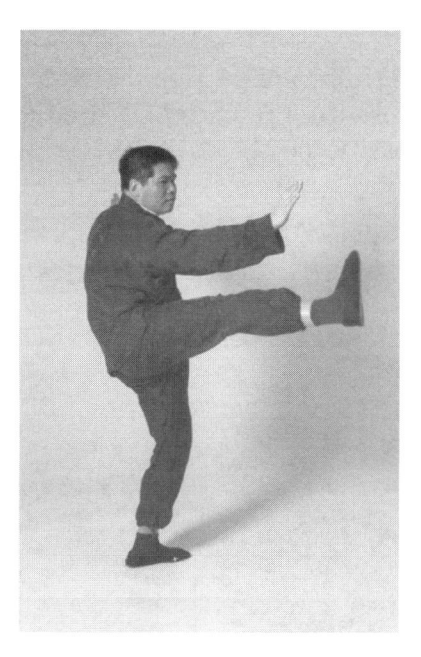

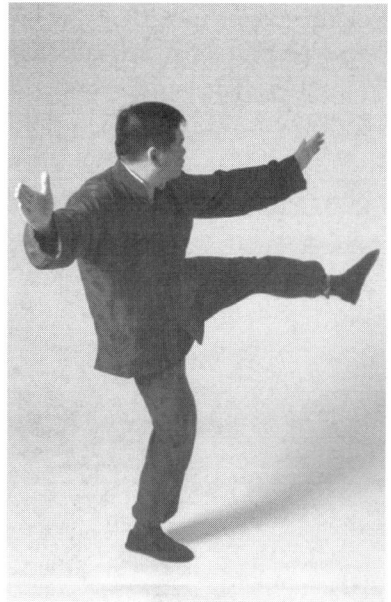

ii. Heel Kick:
As its name indicates, it is a kick with the heel. One should try to pull the toes inward so that the heel is exposed for kicking.

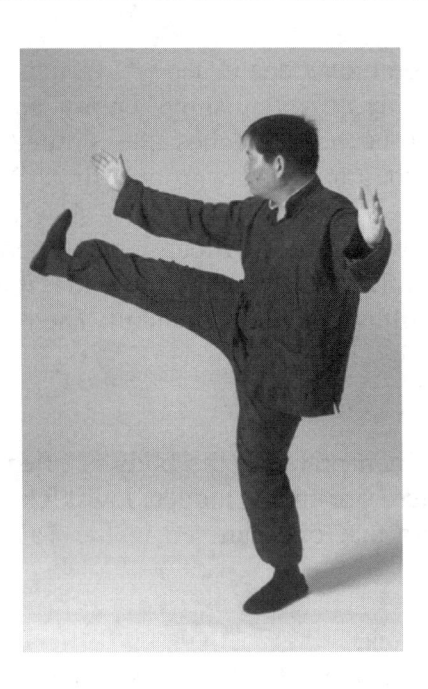

iii. Round Kick:
This is a kick in a half circle motion by the right leg and foot, sweeping upward and across from left to right at chest level or higher. The hands sweep across from right to left, striking the top of the right foot when they meet at the body's centerline.

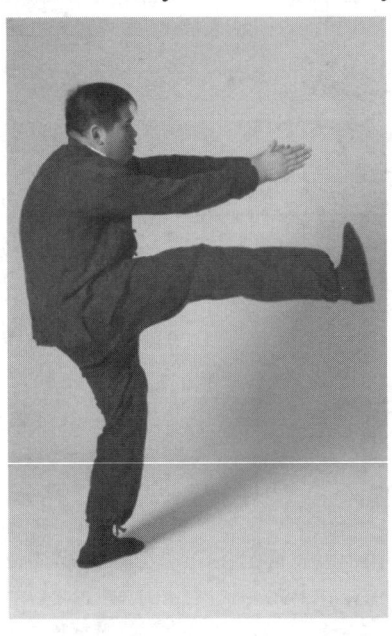

The 48 Movement Tai Chi Chuan Small Frame Solo Form

This condensed form follows the previous two forms with a similar sequence. The nature of these three condensed forms is the same: to teach the student the different characteristics and functions of each solo form without learning the complete long form. Although the condensed form has fewer movements than the long form, the condensed form has all the major movements of the long form so it is easy for one to complete the long form in the future if one decides to do so.

1. Beginning Tai Chi Chuan
2. Grasp the Sparrow's Tail
3. Single Whip
4. Play Guitar
5. Step Forward, Parry, Intercept, and Punch
6. Seal Tightly
7. Cross Hands
8. Embrace Tiger, Return to Mountain
9. Grasp the Sparrow's Tail
10. Single Whip
11. Fist under Elbow
12. Step Backward and Drive Away Monkey (three times)
13. Diagonal Flying
14. Right Hand Warding Off
15. Lift Hands
16. White Crane Spread Its Wings
17. Left Brush Knee, Twist Step, and Push Right Hand Forward
18. Pick up Needle in Sea Bottom
19. Fan Back
20. Turn Around and Hit Downward
21. Retreat Step, Parry, and Punch
22. Part the Wild Horse's Mane
23. Left Warding Off
24. Waving Hands Like Clouds (seven times)
25. Single Whip
26. Right High Pat Horse
27. Right Foot Side Kicks
28. Left High Pat Horse
29. Left Foot Side Kick
30. Fair Lady Works on Shuttles (two times)
31. Left Warding Off

32. Right Foot Kick
33. Left Hit Tiger
34. Hit the Ears with Two Fists
35. Left Foot Kick
36. Left Brush Knee, Twist Step, and Push Hand (two times)
37. Step Forward and Punch Downward
38. Step Forward and Grasp Sparrow's Tail
39. Single Whip
40. Lower the Snake Body
41. Step Forward to Become Seven Star
42. Retreat to Ride Tiger
43. Turn around Hit the Face
44. Lotus Kick
45. Shooting Tiger
46. Step Forward, Parry, Intercept, and Punch
47. Seal Tightly
48. Closing Tai Chi Chuan

THE 48 MOVEMENT SMALL FRAME SOLO FORM

1. Beginning Tai Chi Chuan

Begin with the feet standing parallel to the shoulders and the body facing forward *(fig 1)*. Slowly raise the hands up to level with the shoulders *(fig 2)*; then turn the palms down and lower the hands to the sides of the hip with the palms facing down *(figs 3 & 4)*.

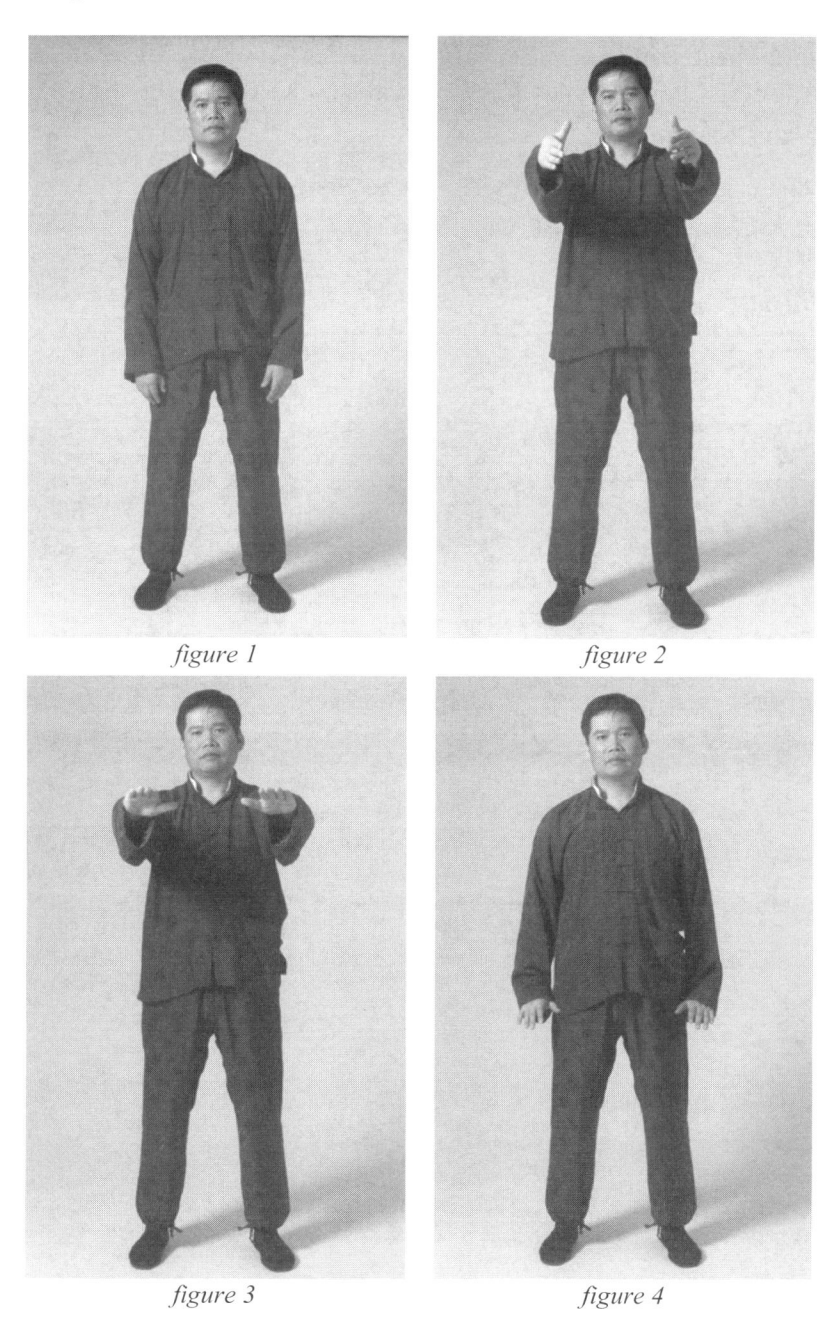

figure 1

figure 2

figure 3

figure 4

2. Grasp the Sparrow's Tail
Part 1: Left Hand Ward Off

From the preceding movement, shift the body weight onto the right foot, and bring the right hand up to the chest. The body turns to the right corner, and the left hand moves in front of the abdomen *(fig 5)*. Pick up the left foot, step forward, and land it on the heel. The eyes follow the left hand coming up in front of the chest with the palm face in *(fig 6)*. The right hand joins the left hand on the wrist, then pushes forward with the body weight shifting onto the left foot *(figs 7 & 8)*.

figure 5

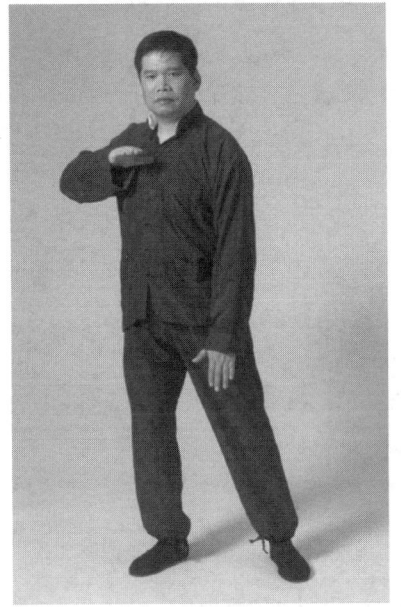

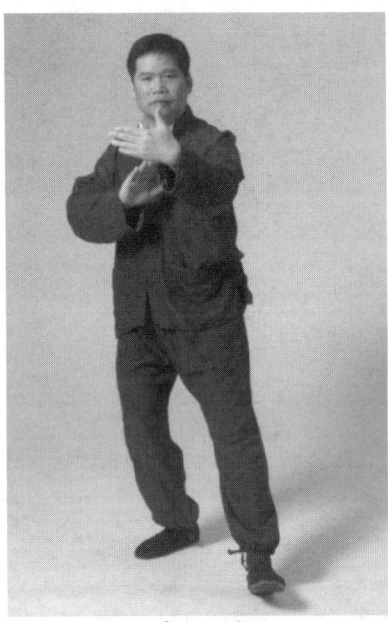

figure 6

figure 7 *figure 8*

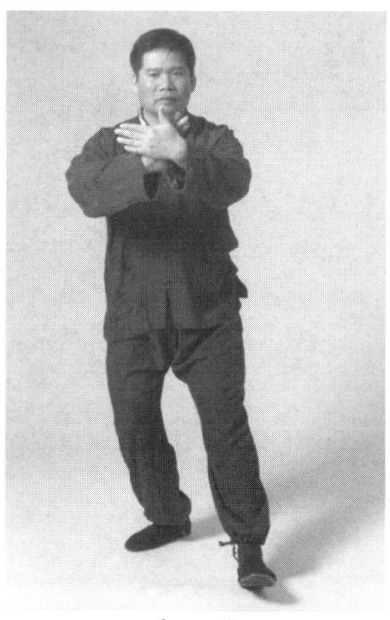

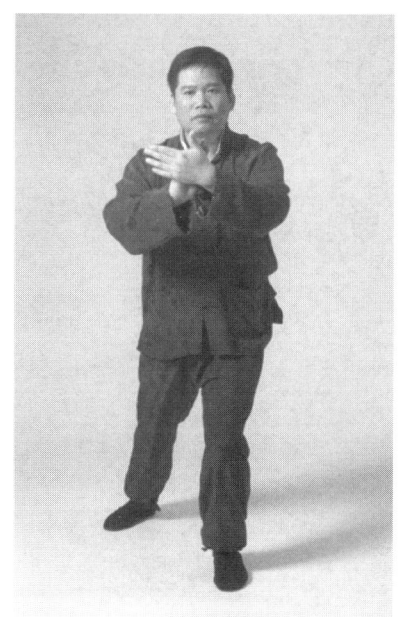

Part 2: Right Hand Warding Off

From the preceding movement, turn the left foot a little inward. The two hands make a small clockwise circle with the left hand coming up next to the left ear and the right hand going down in front of the abdomen *(fig 9)*. Pick up the right foot, step forward, and land it on the heel *(fig 10)*. The eyes follow the right hand coming up in front of the chest with the palm facing in. The left hand joins the right hand on the wrist *(fig 11)*. Push forward with the body weight shifting onto the right foot *(fig 12)*.

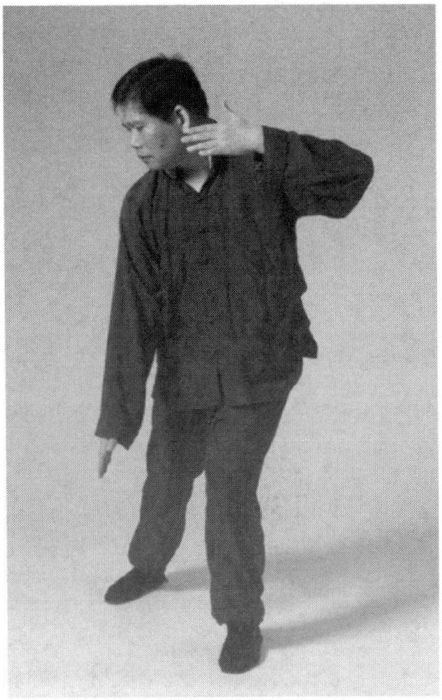

figure 9

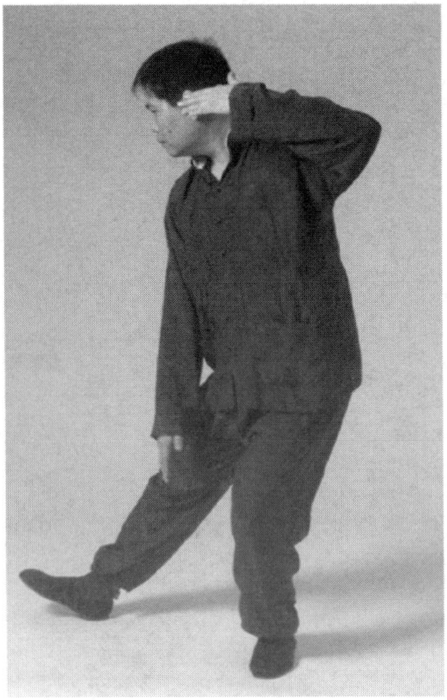

figure 10

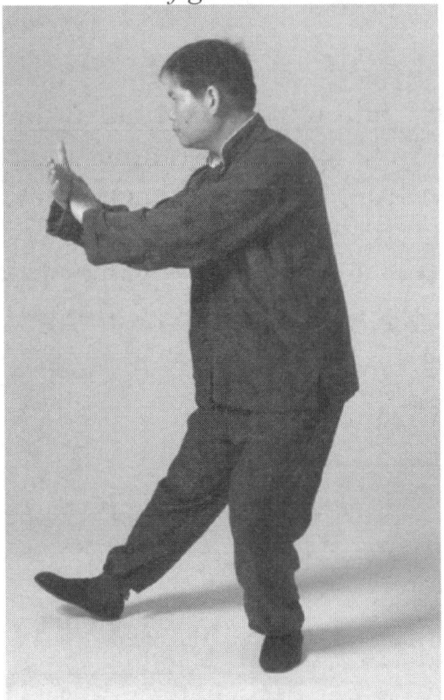

figure 11

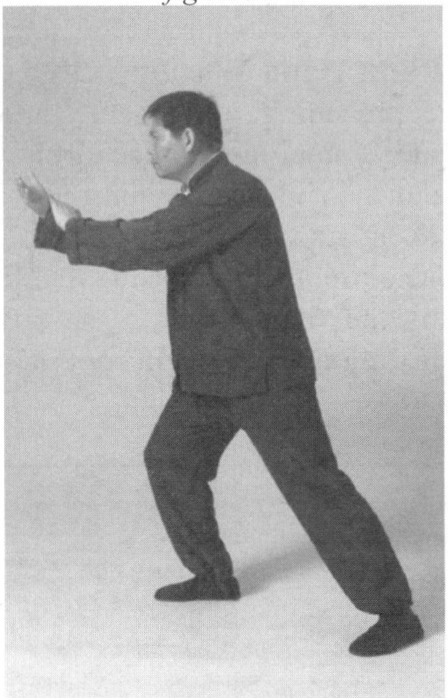

figure 12

Part 3: Roll Back

From the preceding movement, turn the right hand to face down and the left hand to face up *(fig 13)*. Pull the hands back to the hip with the right toes lifting upward *(fig 14)*.

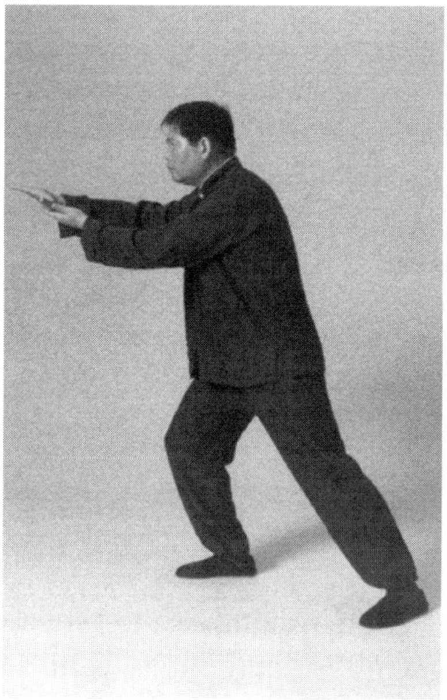

figure 13

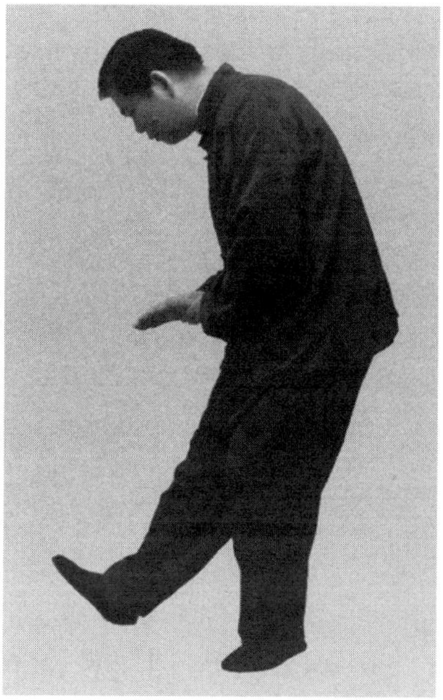

figure 14

Part 4: Press

From the preceding movement, turn the right palm face up and the left palm face down *(fig 15)*. The hands press forward, and the body weight shifts onto the right foot *(fig 16)*.

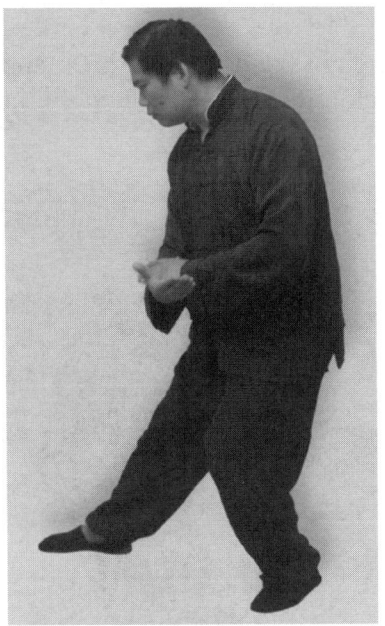

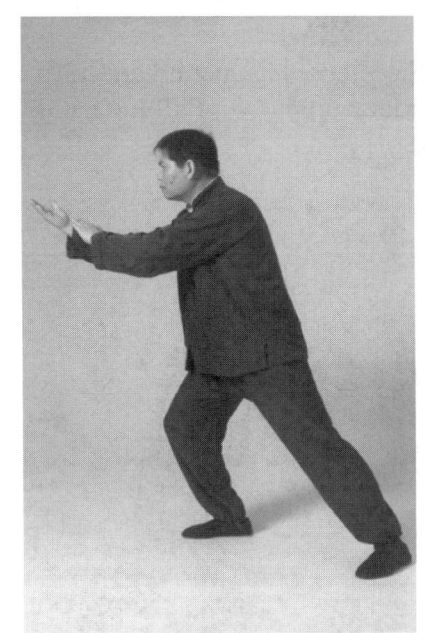

figure 15 *figure 16*

Part 5: Push
From the preceding movement, the hands circle back above the right shoulder with the right toes lifting off the ground *(fig 17)*. Turn the right palm so it faces down. Then push the hands forward with the body's weight shifting onto the right foot *(figs 18 & 19)*.

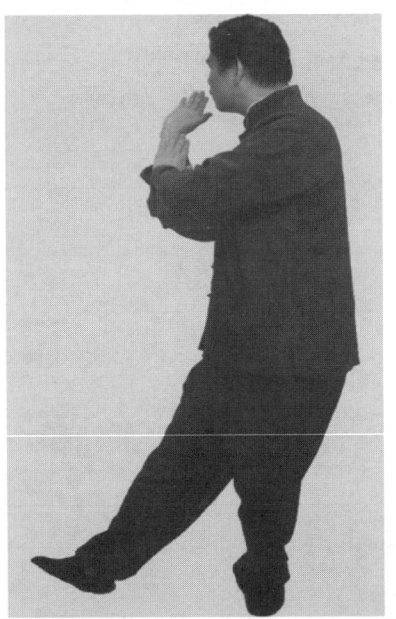

figure 17 *figure 18* *figure 19*

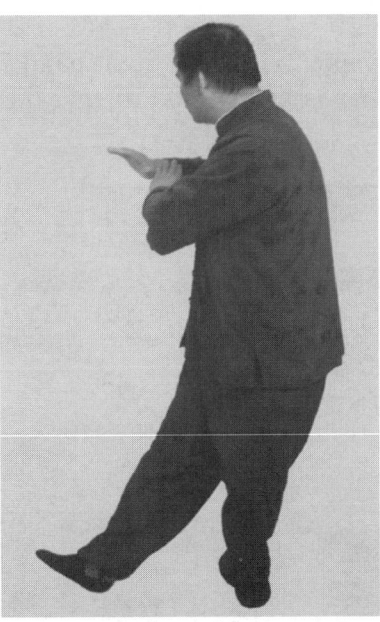

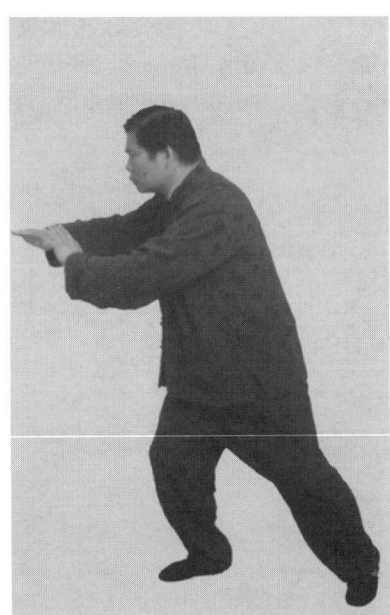

3. Single Whip

From the preceding movement, continue by pushing the hands to the left with the weight shifting onto the left foot and the right toes turning in *(fig 20)*. Circle the hands back to the right with the weight shifting onto the right foot *(fig 21)*. The fingers come together to form a beak; then bend the wrist to form a hook. With the weight on the right foot, pick up the left foot, and step to the left with the toes pointing to the left corner *(fig 22)*. Shift the weight onto the left foot as the eyes follow the left palm across the body to the left *(fig 23)*.

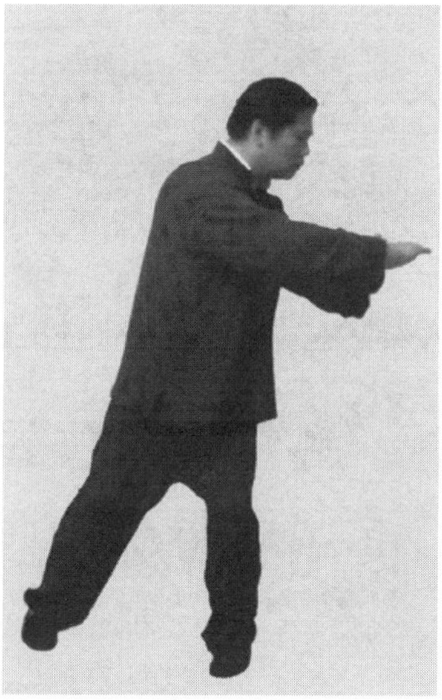

figure 20

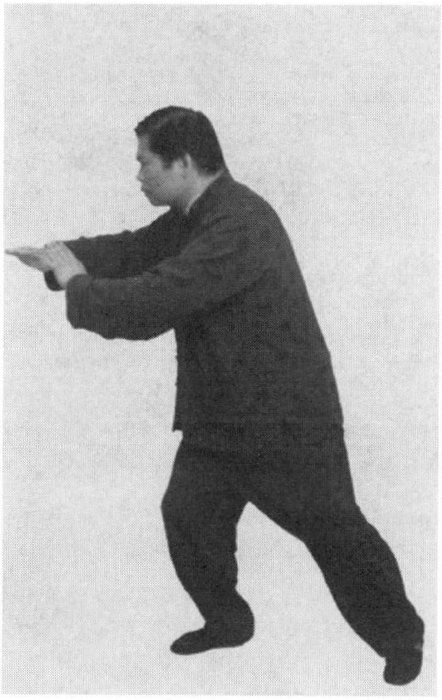

figure 21

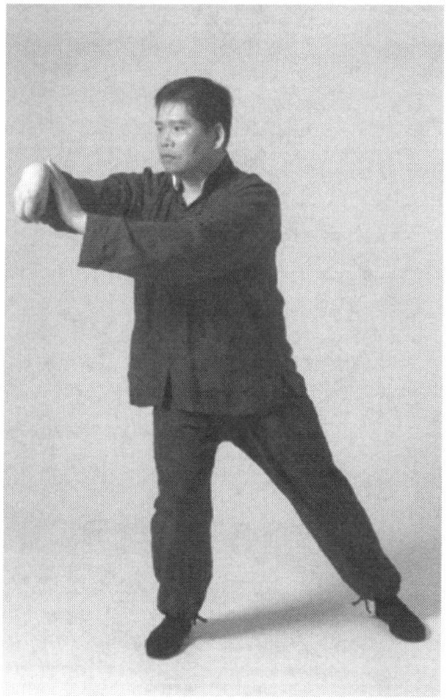

figure 22

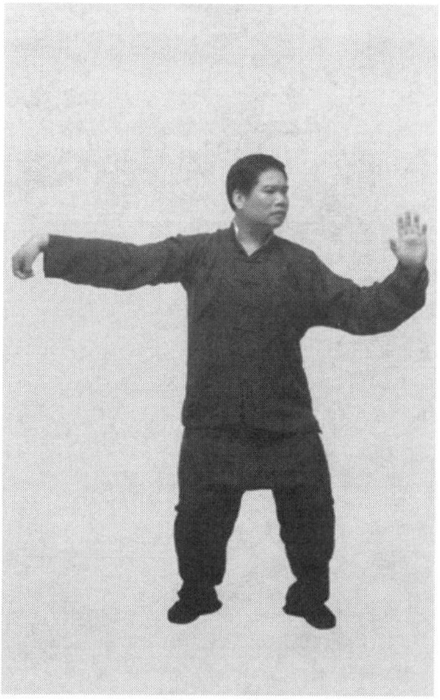

figure 23

4. Play Guitar

From the preceding movement, open the right hand, and swing it forward as the left toes turn out and the left hand comes down to the left hip *(fig 24)*. Pick up the right foot, and step behind the left foot *(fig 25)*. The right hand comes back to the chest, and the left hand thrusts forward *(fig 26)*. With the weight on the right foot, the left foot lifts, then lands on the heel *(fig 27)*.

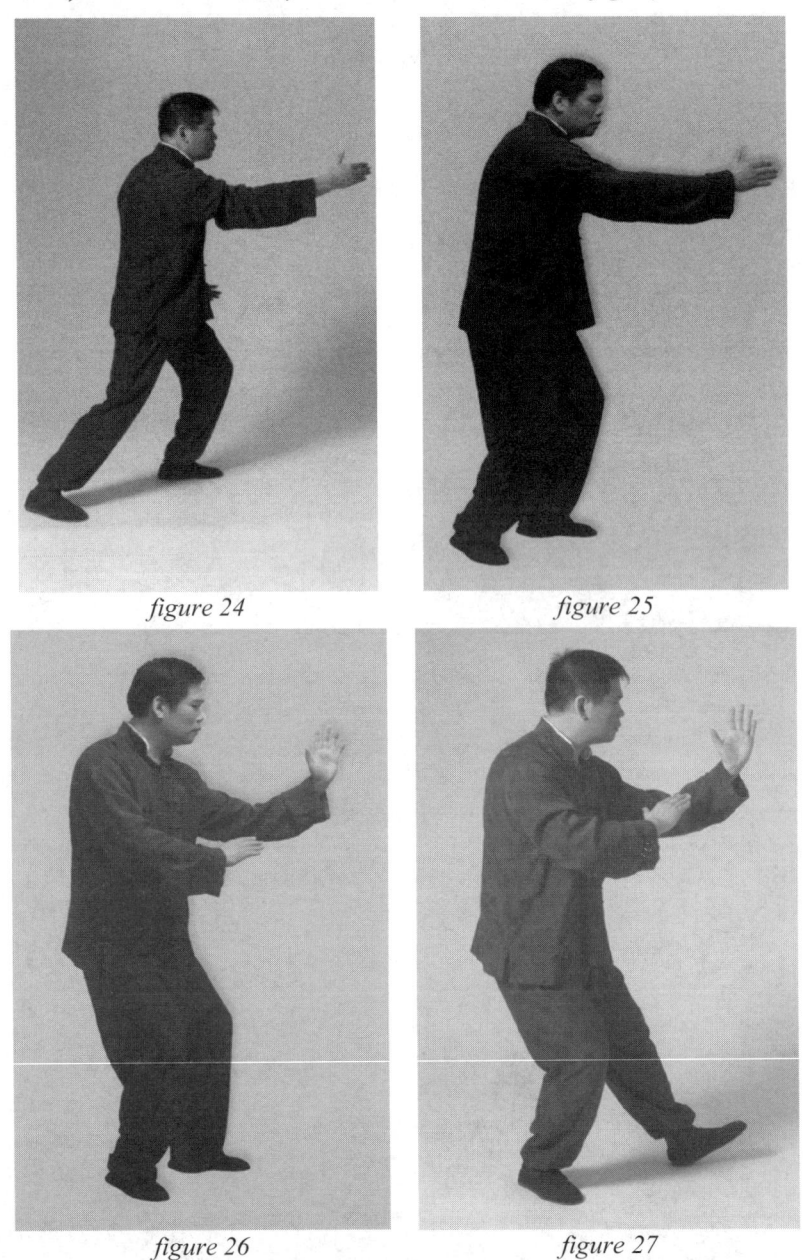

figure 24

figure 25

figure 26

figure 27

5. Step Forward, Parry, Intercept and Punch

From the preceding movement, the two hands come down in front of the chest *(fig 28)*. Thrust the hands forward and upward while shifting the weight forward to stand up on the left foot; the right foot follows, stepping up behind the left foot *(fig 29)*. Shift the weight onto the right foot and lower the body, bringing the hands next to the chest again *(fig 30)*.

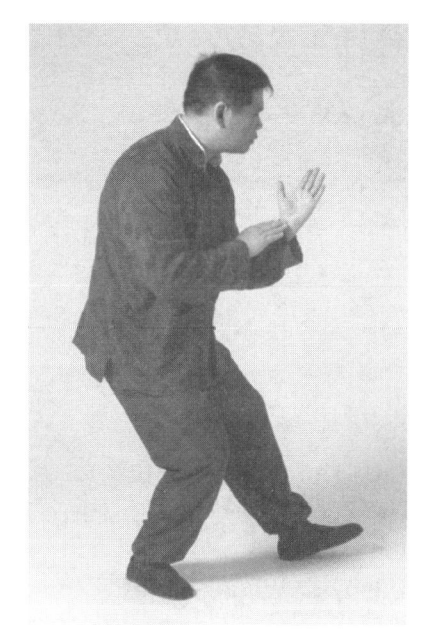

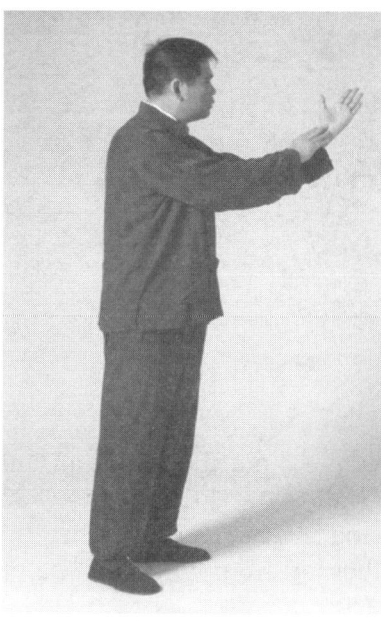

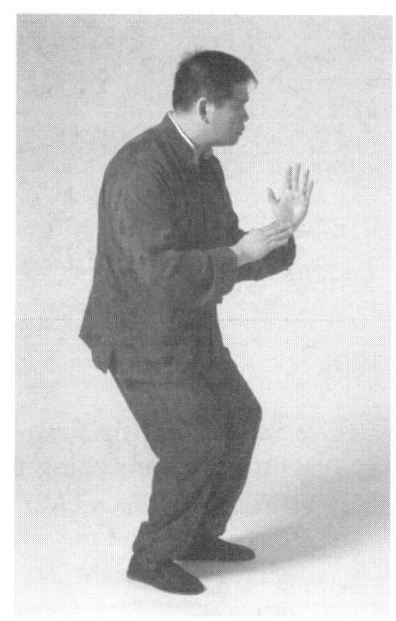

figure 28 *figure 29* *figure 30*

Separate the hands, with the right hand brought back to the right hip then closed into a fist, while the left hand pushes forward. Pick up the left foot, and step forward to the left *(fig 31)*. Shift the weight onto the left foot as the right fist punches forward to join with the left palm *(fig 32)*.

figure 31   *figure 32*

6. Seal Tightly

From the preceding movement, put the left hand under the right wrist. Shift the weight back onto the right foot while open the hands and come back to the chest with the palms facing in *(figs 33 & 34)*. Turn the palms to face out, and shift the weight onto the left foot with the palms pushing forward and downward *(figs 35 & 36)*.

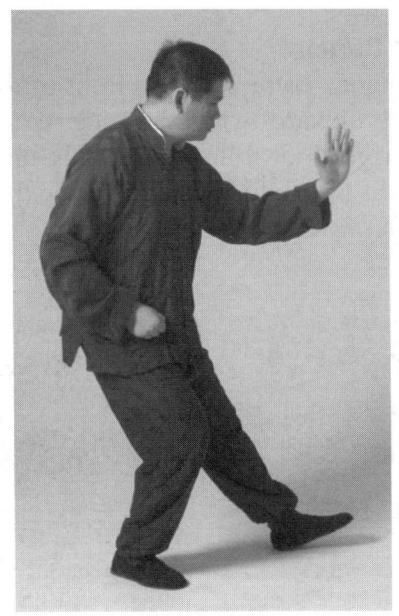

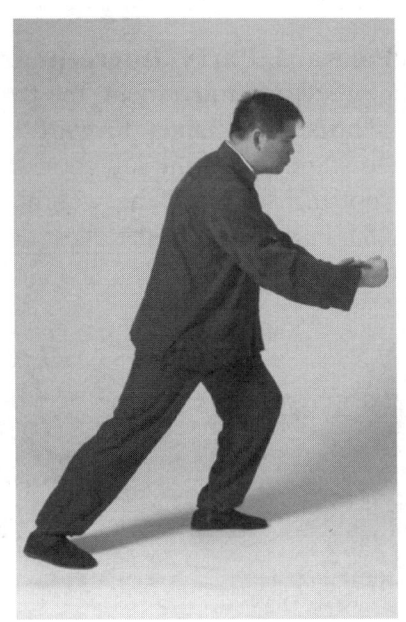

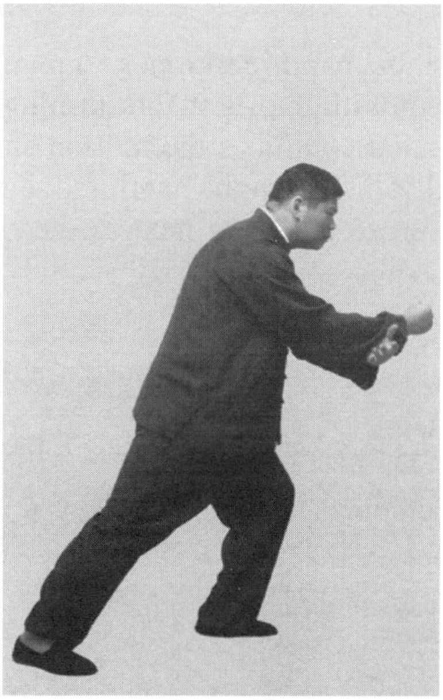

figure 33

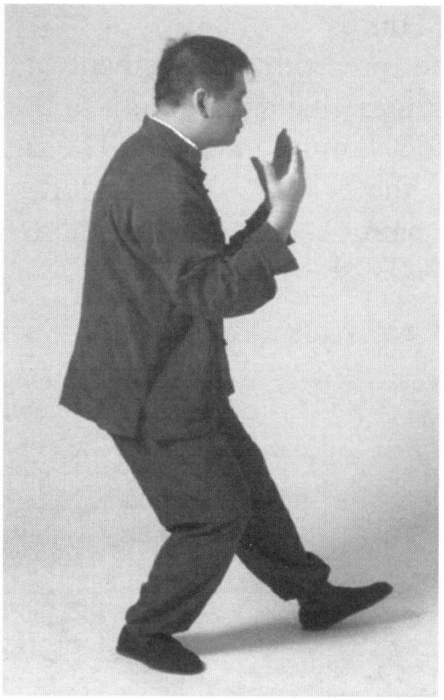

figure 34

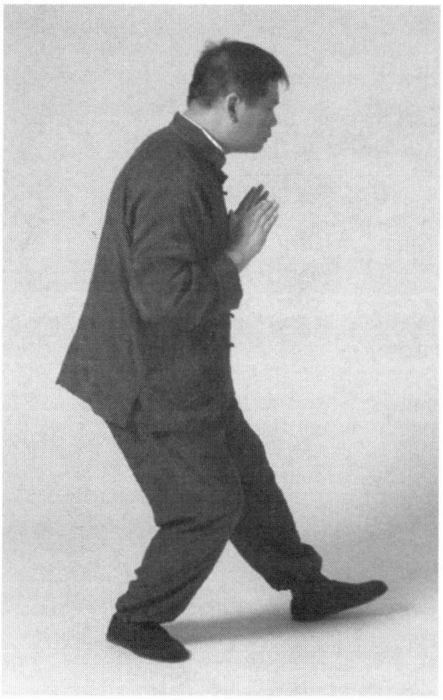

figure 35

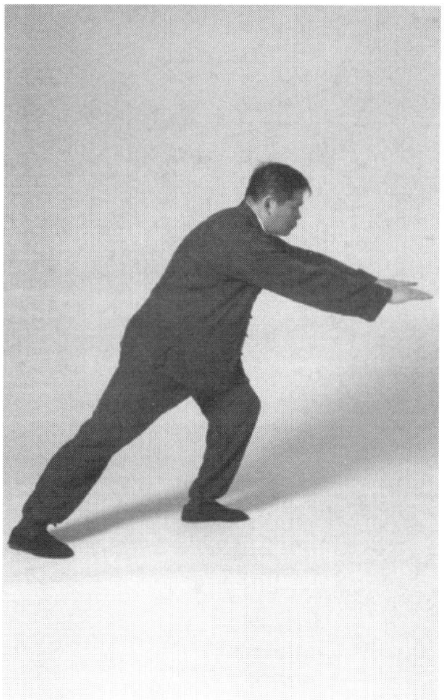

figure 36

7. Cross Hands

From the preceding movement the right hand continues, moving in a downward arc like a pendulum to the right with the right foot turning out and the left foot turning in *(fig 37)*. The right hand continues the motion and comes up above the head *(fig 38)*. The left hand joins the right hand above the head with the palms facing out and the left foot stepping up next to the right foot *(fig 39)*.

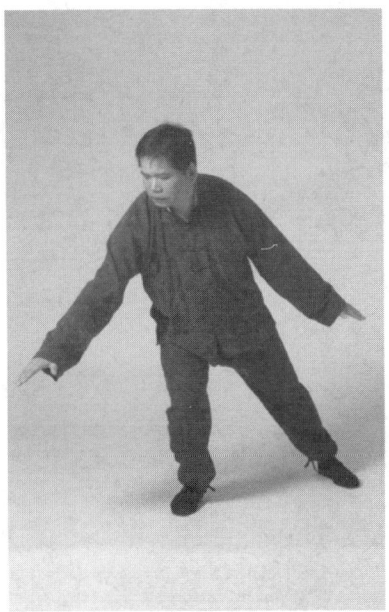

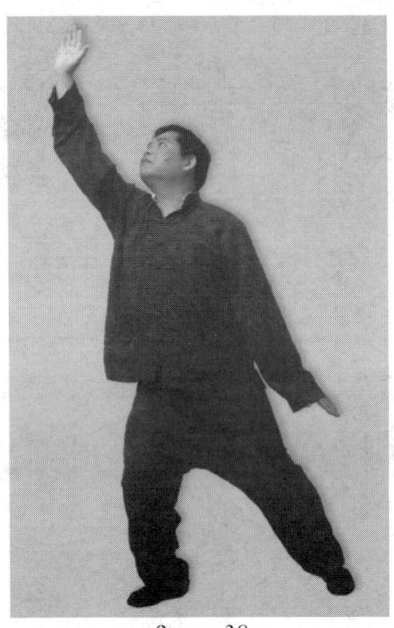

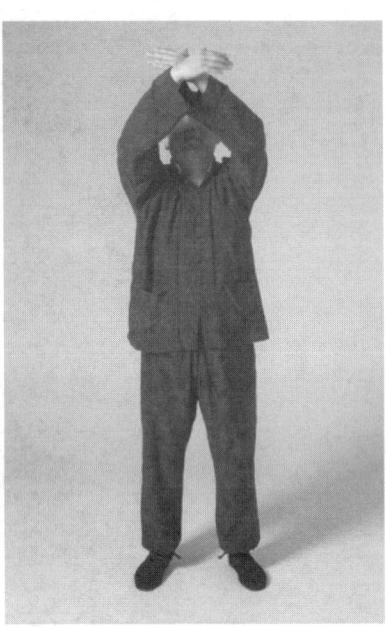

figure 37   *figure 38*   *figure 39*

8. Embrace Tiger Return to Mountain
Part 1: Left Hand Brush Knee
From the preceding movement, shift the weight onto the right foot. The left hand goes down in front of the abdomen, and the right hand arrives next to the right ear with the palm face in *(fig 40)*. Pick up the left foot, and step to the left corner with the heel on the ground *(fig 41)*. Shifting the weight onto the left foot, the left hand goes outside the left knee, and the right hand pushes forward at shoulder level *(fig 42)*.

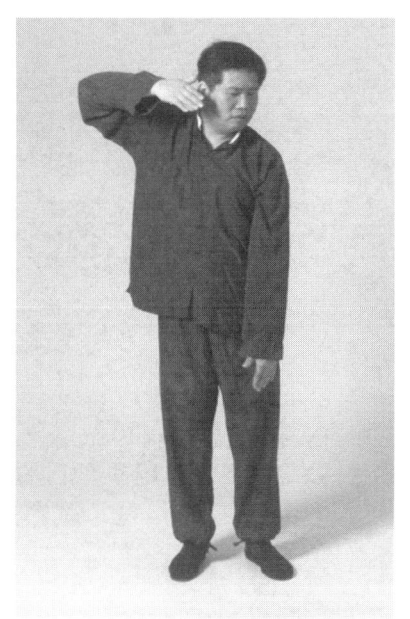

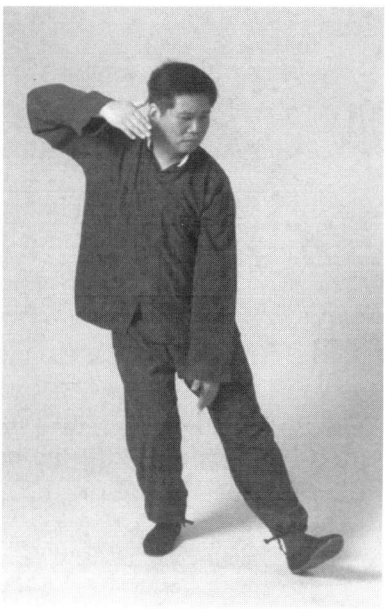

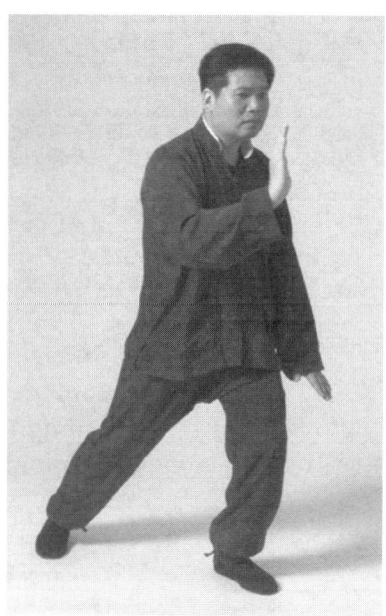

figure 40   *figure 41*   *figure 42*

Part 2: Right Hand Brush Knee
From the preceding movement, shift the weight slightly back onto the right foot while turning the left foot inward and the body to the right. The left hand comes up next to the left ear with the palm face in, and the right hand goes down in front of the abdomen. Shift the weight back onto the left foot *(fig 43)*. Pick up the right foot, and step forward to the corner with the heel on the ground *(fig 44)*. Shifting the weight onto the right foot, the right hand goes outside the right knee, and the left hand pushes forward *(fig 45)*.

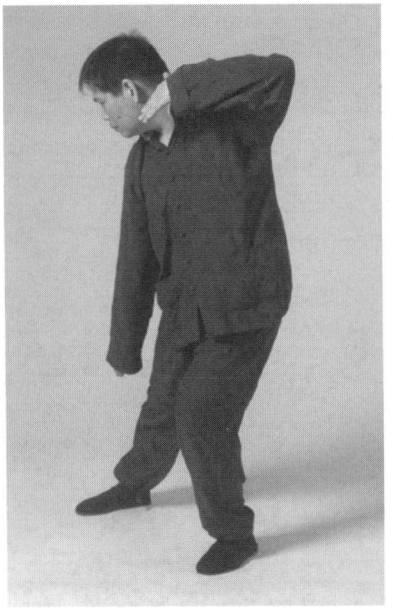

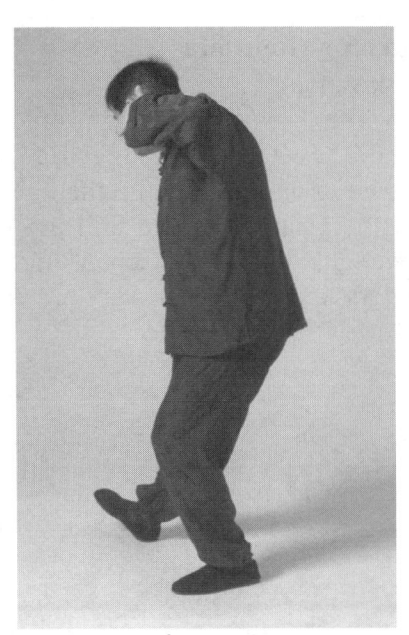

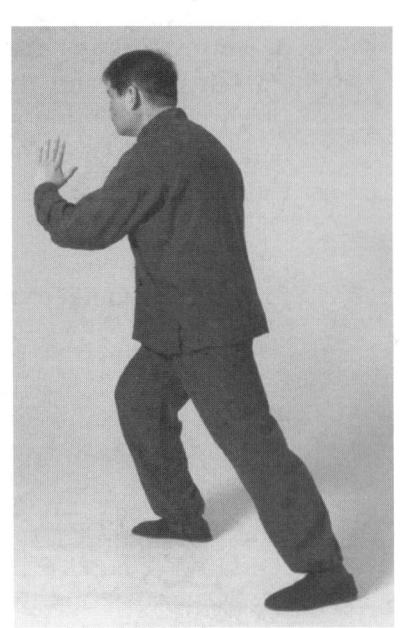

figure 43 *figure 44* *figure 45*

9. Grasp the Sparrow's Tail
Part 1: Roll Back

From the preceding movement, turn the left palm to face up; the right hand then comes up to join the left hand *(fig 46)*. Pull the hands back to the hip in a small clockwise arc with the right toes lifting off the ground *(fig 47)*.

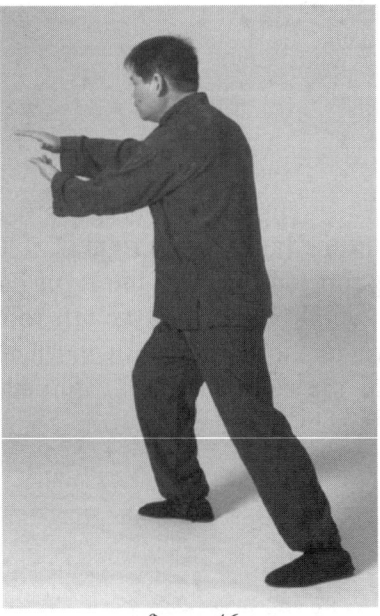

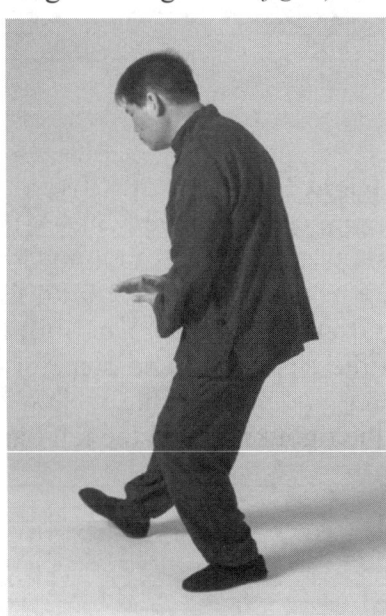

figure 46 *figure 47*

Part 2: Press

From the preceding movement, turn the right palm face up, and place the left palm on top, face down *(fig 48)*. Push the hands forward continuing the small clockwise arc with the weight shifting onto the right foot *(fig 49)*.

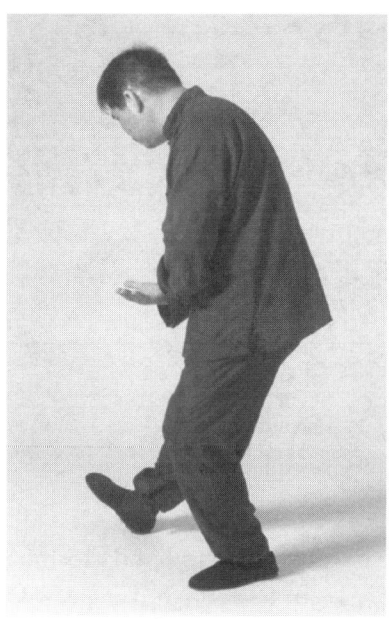

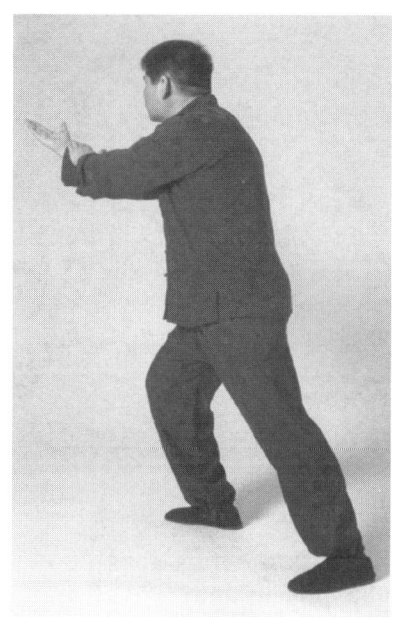

figure 48   *figure 49*

Part 3: Push

From the preceding movement, pull the hands back above the right shoulder with the right toes lifting off the ground *(fig 50)*. Turn the right palm face down as the left hand joins atop the right wrist. Push the hands forward, and shift the weight onto the right foot *(figs 51 & 52)*.

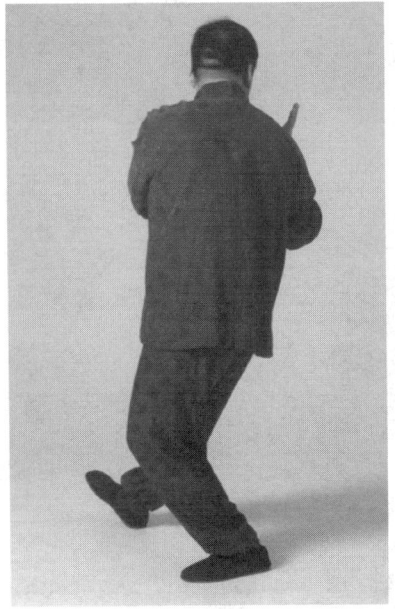

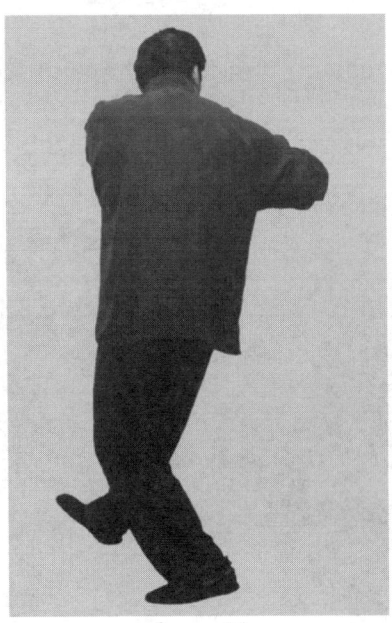

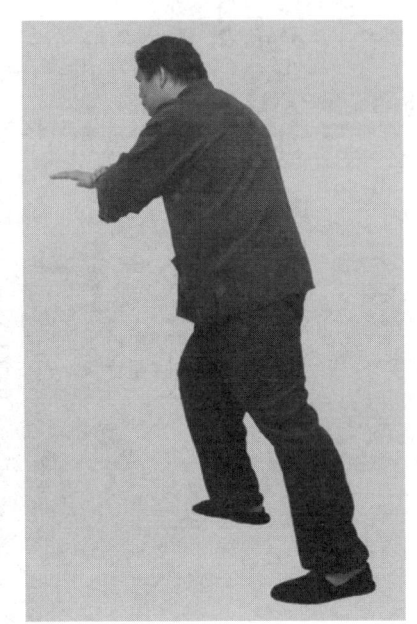

figure 50   *figure 51*   *figure 52*

10. Single Whip

From the preceding movement, continue by pushing the hands to the left with the weight shifting onto the left foot as the right toes turn in *(fig 53)*. Circle the hands back to the right with the weight shifting onto the right foot *(fig 54)*. The right fingers come together to form a beak; bend the wrist to form a hook *(fig 55)*. With the weight on the right foot, pick up the left foot, and step forward to the left. Shift the weight onto the left foot as the eyes follow the left palm across the body to the left *(fig 56)*.

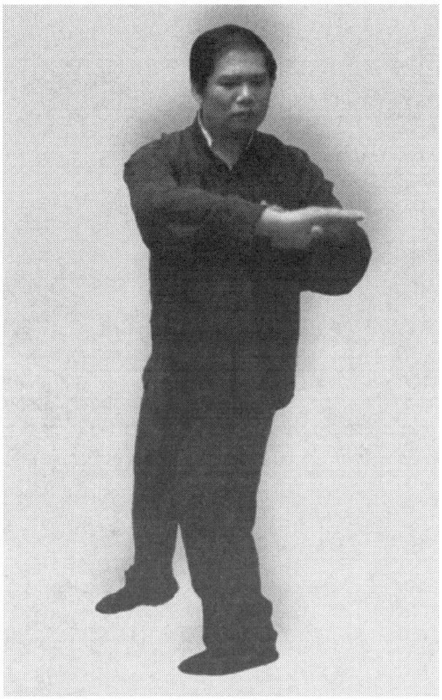

THE 48 MOVEMENT SMALL FRAME SOLO FORM

figure 53

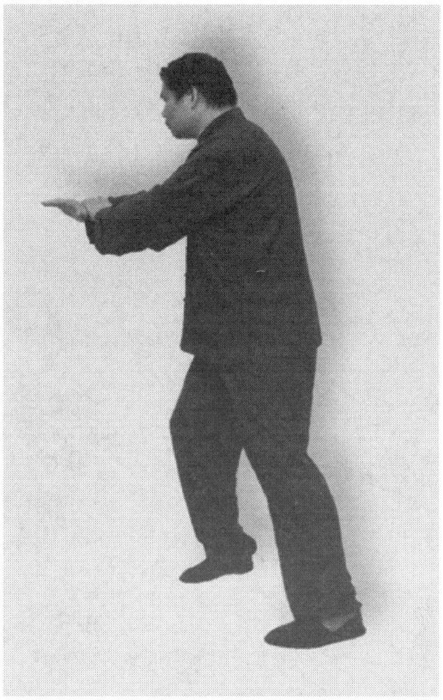

figure 54

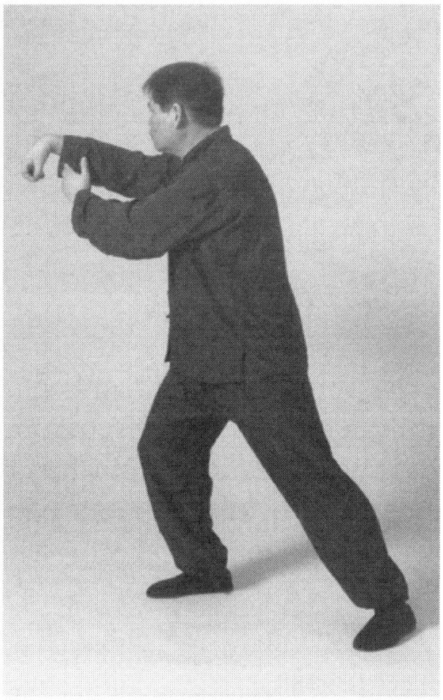

figure 55

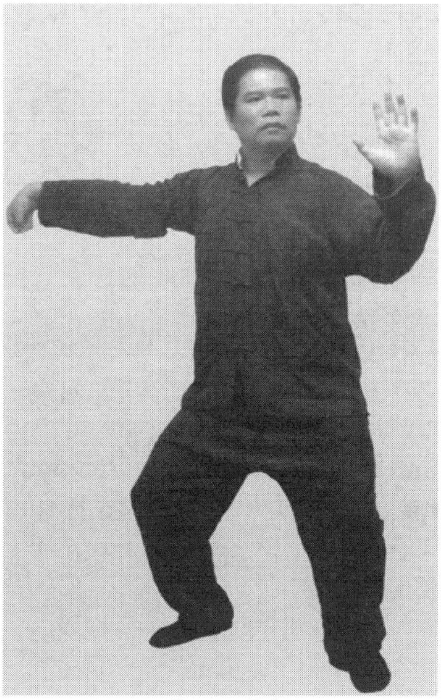

figure 56

11. Fist under Elbow

From the preceding movement, turn the body to the left and the left toes out while the right hand comes in front and the left hand goes in back *(fig 57)*. With the body weight on the left foot, pick up the right foot, and step beside the left foot with the toes pointing to the corner. Then the right hand comes back to

TAI CHI CHUAN – A COMPARATIVE STUDY

the body, and the left hand moves in front of the body *(fig 58)*. Close the right hand into a fist, and shift the body weight onto the right foot while the left hand remains the same. Look forward to the left, and with the body weight on the right foot, place the left foot on its heel, and bring the right fist under the left elbow *(fig 59)*.

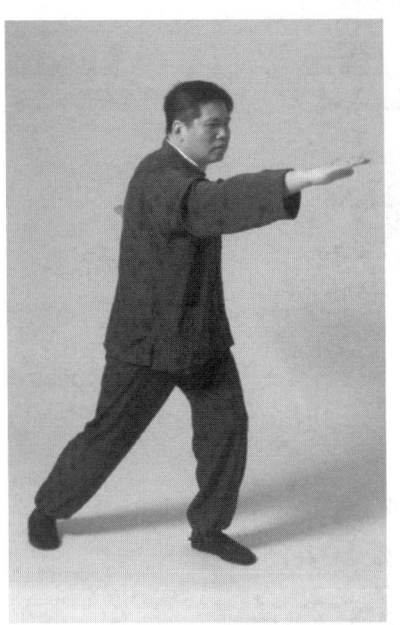

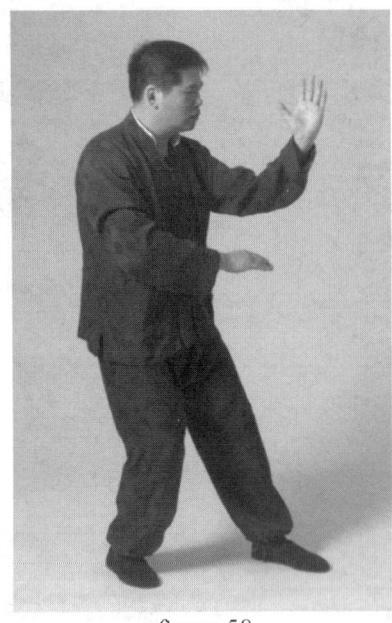

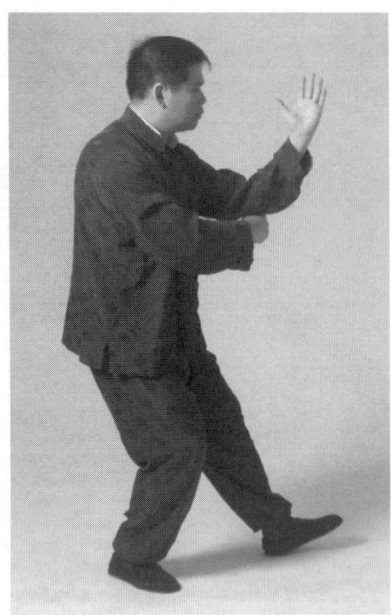

figure 57   figure 58   figure 59

12. Step Backward and Drive Away Monkey (three times)
Part 1: Left Hand Side

From the preceding movement, open the fist, and bring the hands close to the chest with the right hand at the left wrist *(fig 60)*. Shift the weight onto the left foot as the left hand thrusts forward and upward and the right hand remains next to the left wrist *(fig 61)*. Pull the hands back next to the left ear with the left toes lifting off the ground and the body turning to the left *(figs 62 & 63)*.

THE 48 MOVEMENT SMALL FRAME SOLO FORM

figure 60

figure 61

figure 62

figure 63

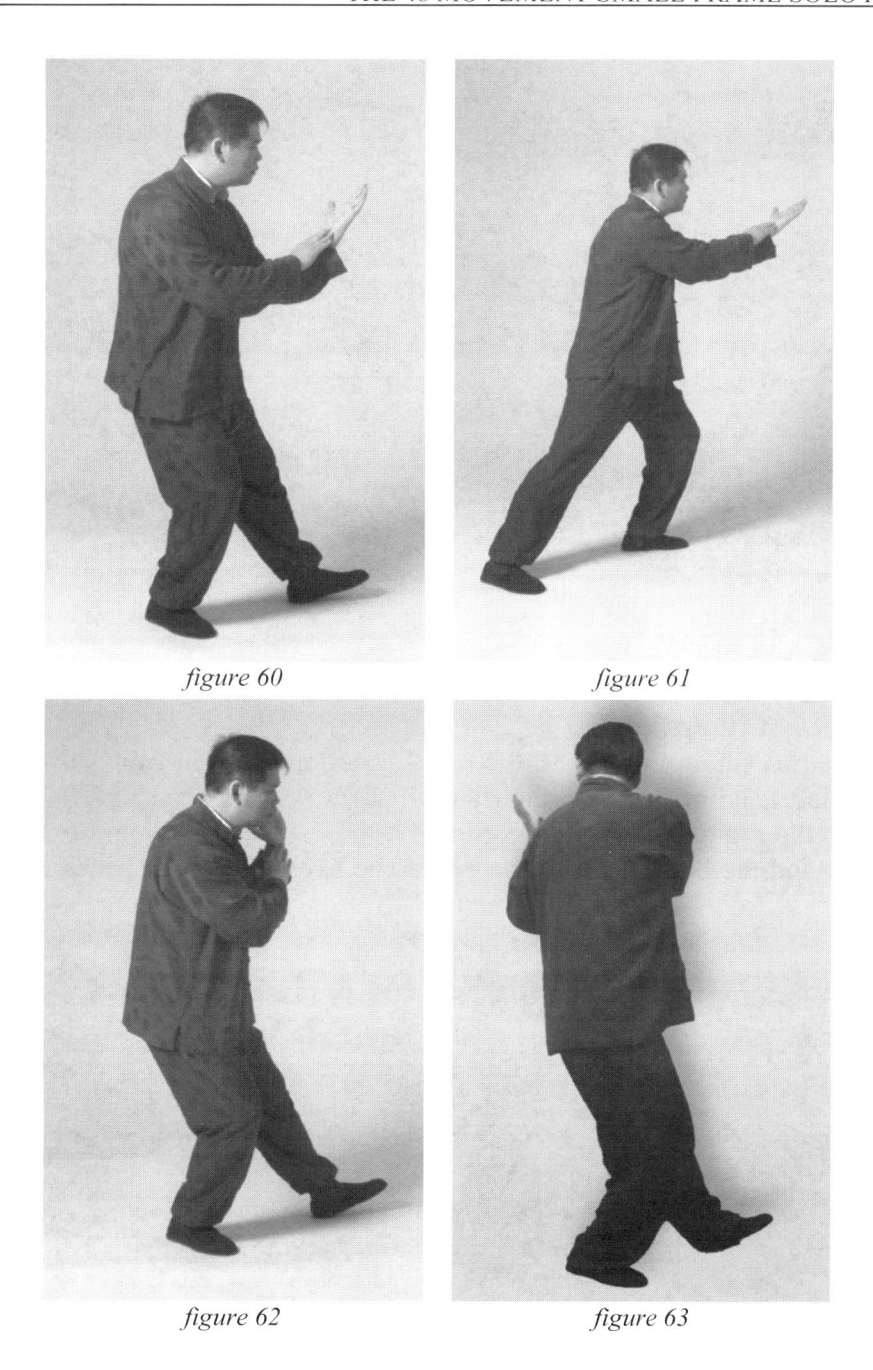

Reposition the body to face forward *(fig 64)*. Pick up the left foot, and step back. The eyes follow the hands with the right hand coming down outside the right knee and the left hand pushing forward from the left shoulder *(figs 65 & 66)*.

TAI CHI CHUAN – A COMPARATIVE STUDY

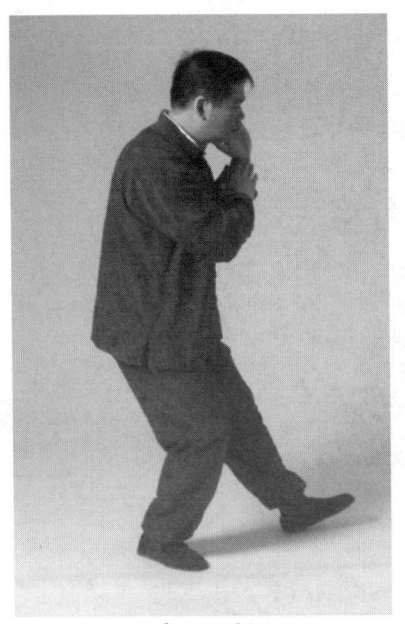

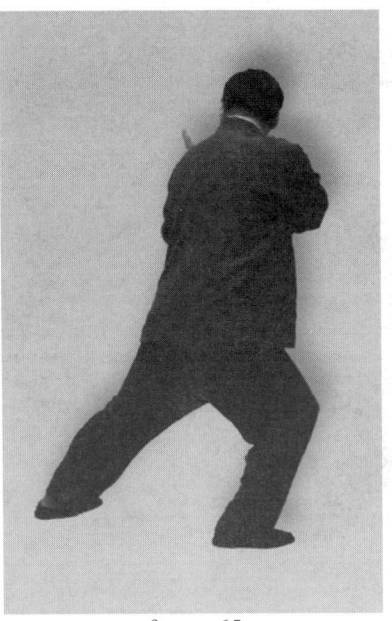

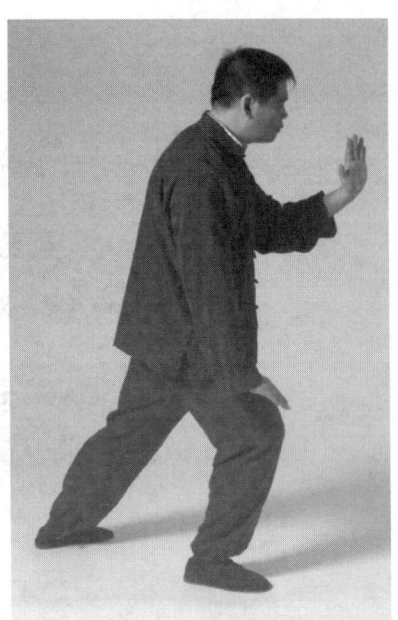

figure 64

figure 65

figure 66

Part 2: Right Hand Side

From the preceding movement, the right hand comes up in front of the body, and the left hand moves onto the right wrist *(fig 67)*. Shift the weight onto the left foot; the right toes lift off the ground as the hands are brought to the right shoulder and the body turns to the right. The eyes follow the hands *(figs 68 & 69)*.

figure 67

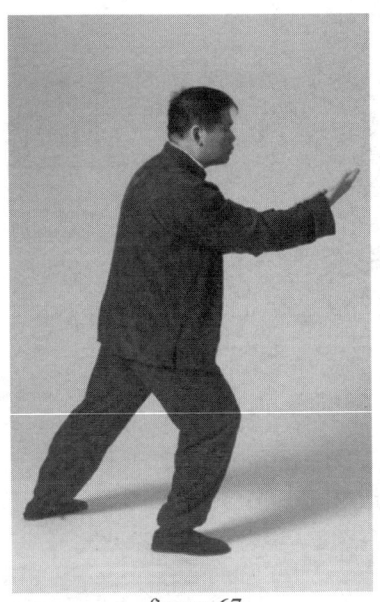

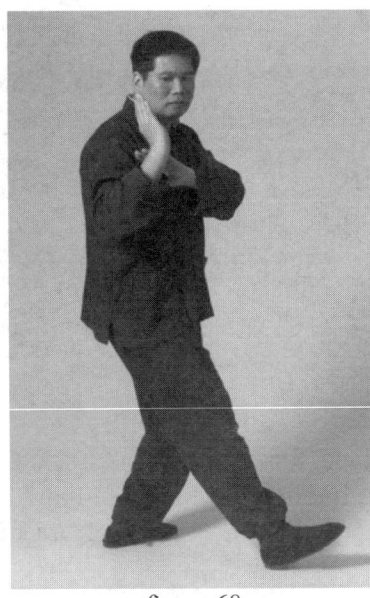

figure 68

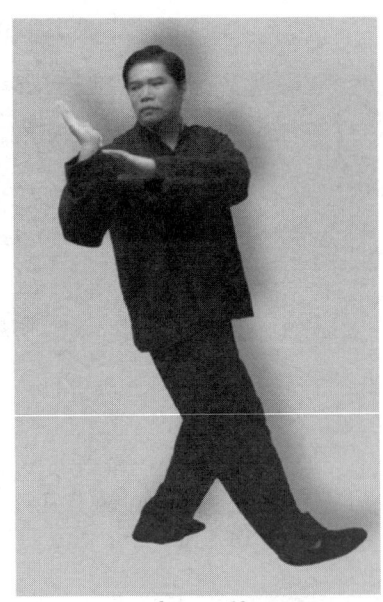

figure 69

Reposition the body to face forward *(fig 70)*. Pick up the right foot, and step back. The left hand goes down outside the left knee, and the right hand pushes forward from the right shoulder *(figs 71 & 72)*.

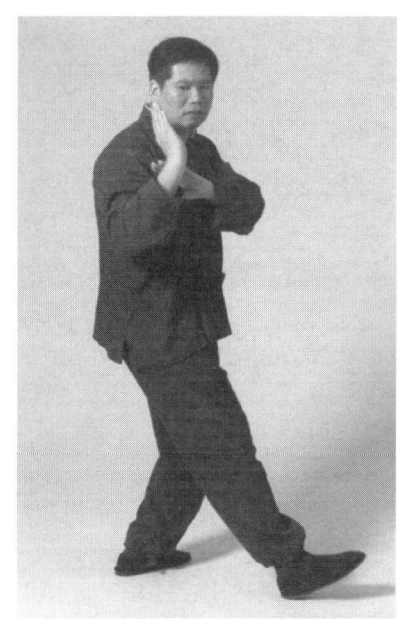

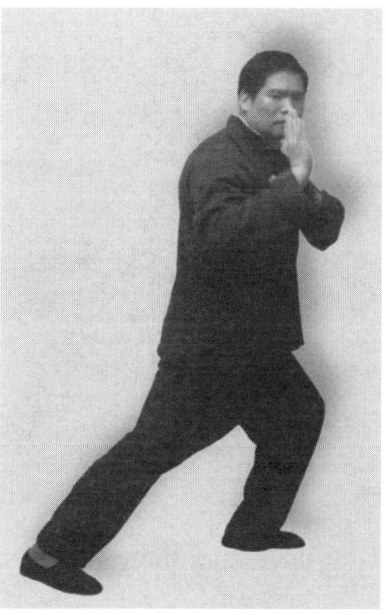

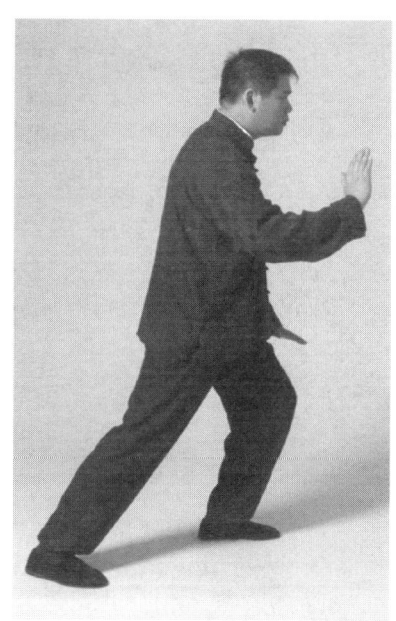

figure 70 *figure 71* *figure 72*

Part 3: Left Hand Side

From the preceding movement, the left hand comes up in front of the chest and is met by the right fingers at the wrist *(fig 73)*. Shift the weight onto the right foot; the left toes lift off the ground as the hands are brought to the left shoulder and the body turns to the left *(fig 74)*. Reposition the body to face forward *(fig 75)*.

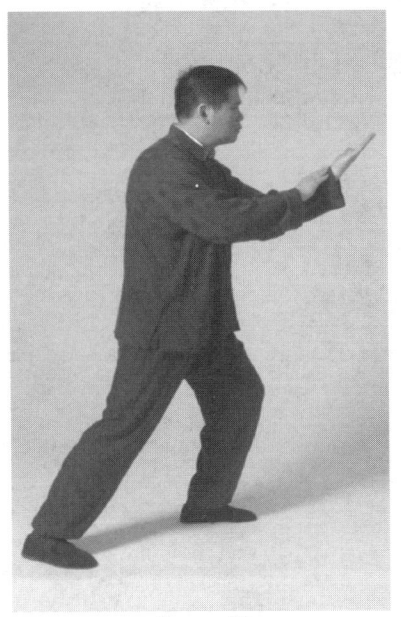

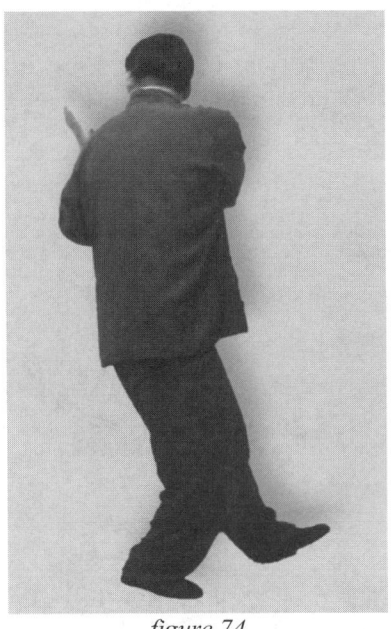

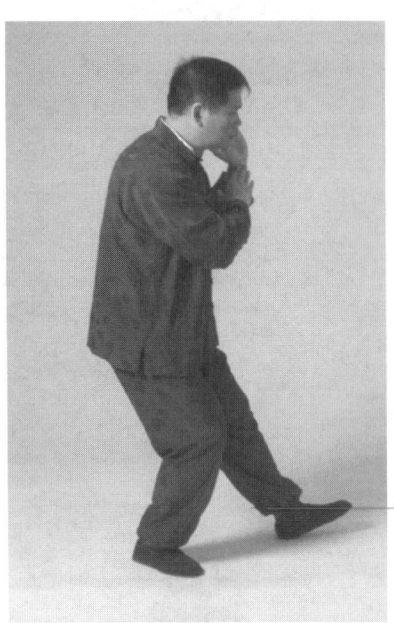

figure 73   *figure 74*   *figure 75*

Pick up the left foot, and step back. The eyes follow the hands, the right hand goes down outside the right knee, and the left hand pushes forward from the left shoulder *(figs 76 & 77)*.

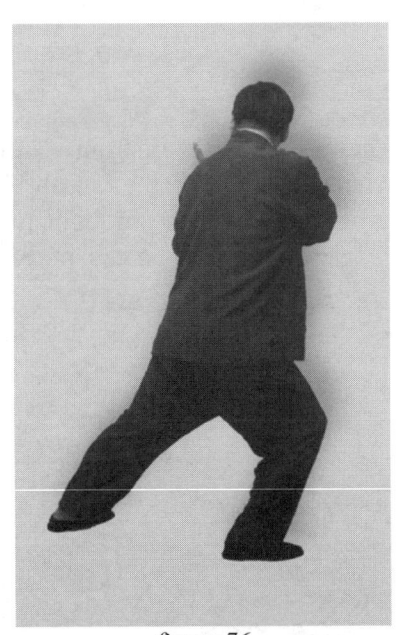

figure 76   *figure 77*

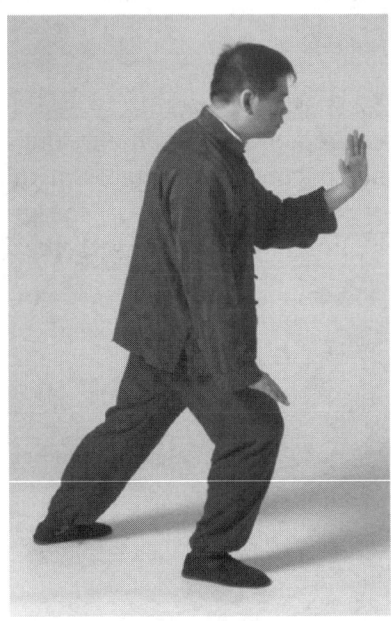

13. Diagonal Flying

From the preceding movement, the right hand comes up to the chest and the left hand goes under the right hand, palm facing up; the eyes look at the left hand *(fig 78, and 79 before the left foot steps)*. Pick up the left foot, and step forward with the toes off the ground *(fig 79)*. Shift the weight onto the left foot while separating the hands with the left hand going up and the right hand going down to the right leg. The eyes are looking at the right hand *(fig 80)*.

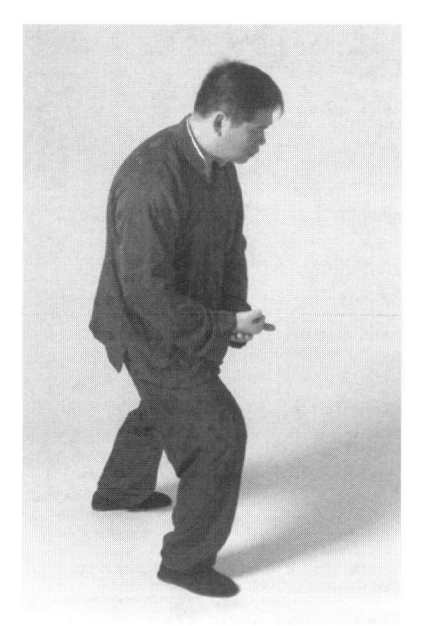

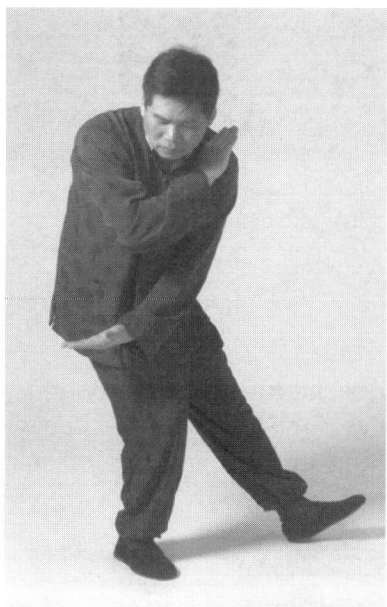

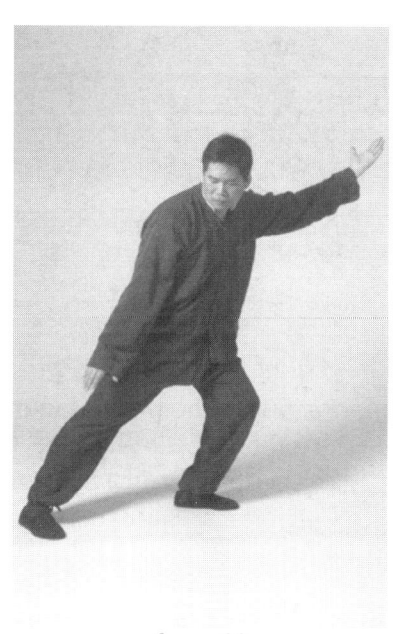

figure 78   *figure 79*   *figure 80*

14. Right Hand Ward Off

From the preceding movement, while adjusting the body to face forward, the right hand comes in front of the abdomen *(fig 81)*. Pick up the right foot, and step forward onto the heel. The eyes follow the right hand as it comes up with the palm face in and the left hand joins it on the wrist *(fig 82)*. Shift the weight onto the right foot, and push the hands forward *(fig 83)*.

TAI CHI CHUAN – A COMPARATIVE STUDY

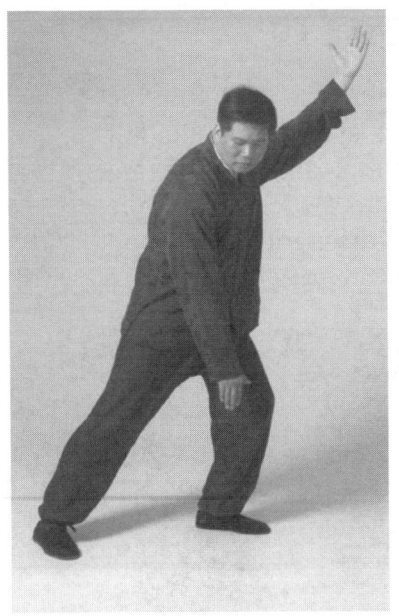

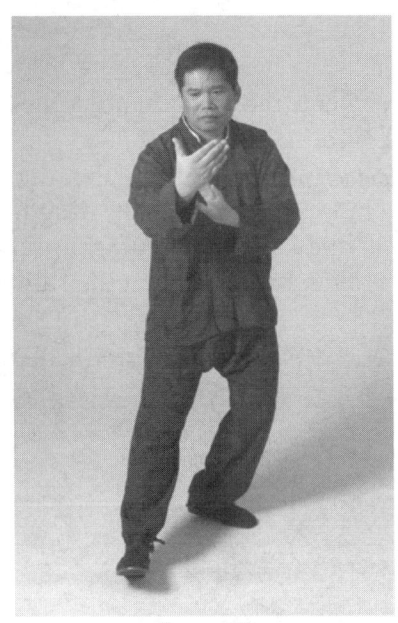

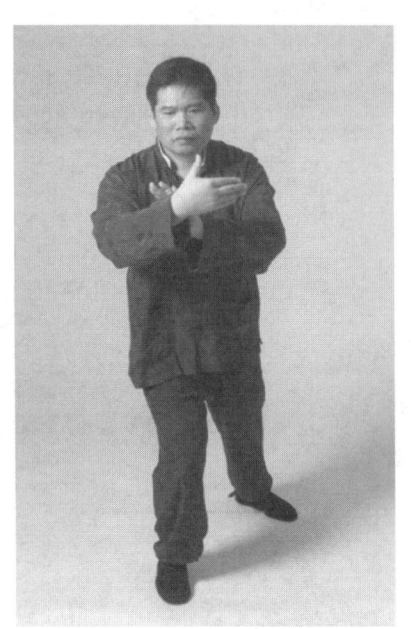

figure 81 *figure 82* *figure 83*

15. Lift Hands

From the preceding movement, turn the right palm to face out *(fig 84)*, and step the left foot up next to the right foot with the knees bent. Separate the hands with the right hand pushing upward and the left hand pushing downward as the legs stand up straight *(fig 85)*.

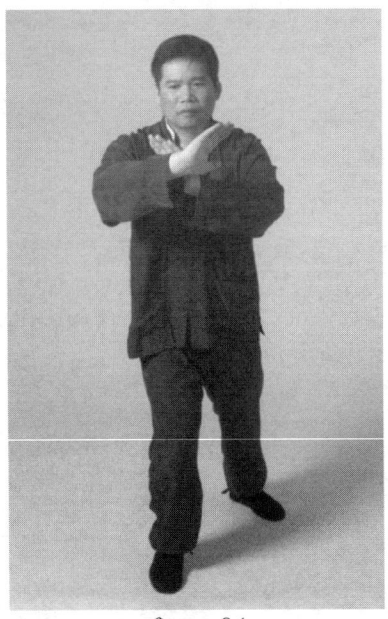

figure 84 *figure 85*

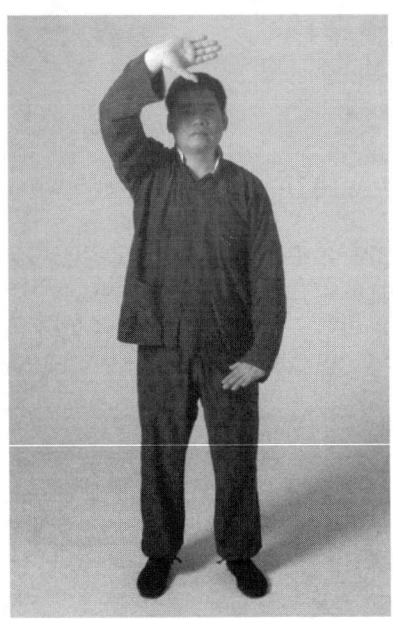

16. White Crane Spread Its Wing

From the preceding movement, the legs remain straight. Bend the body as much as possible to the left *(fig 86)*. The body then comes upright, and at the same time, the left hand comes up next to the right hand above the head *(fig 87)*.

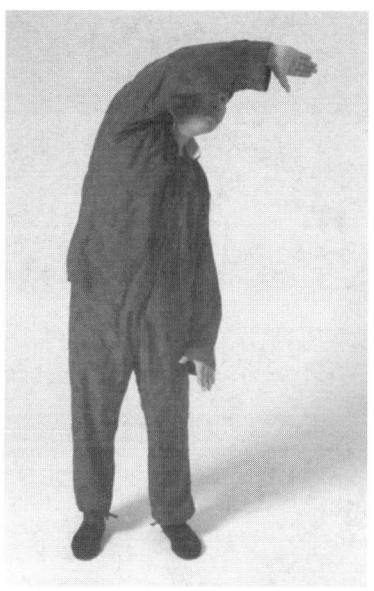

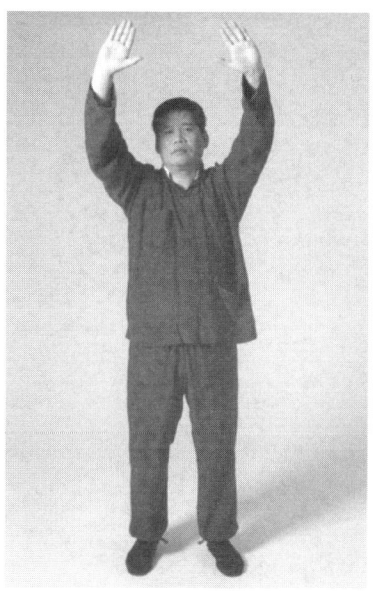

figure 86   *figure 87*

Circling clockwise, both hands reach down to the ground from the right side and come up on the left side with the legs remaining straight *(figs 88 – 91)*.

figure 88

figure 89

figure 90

figure 91

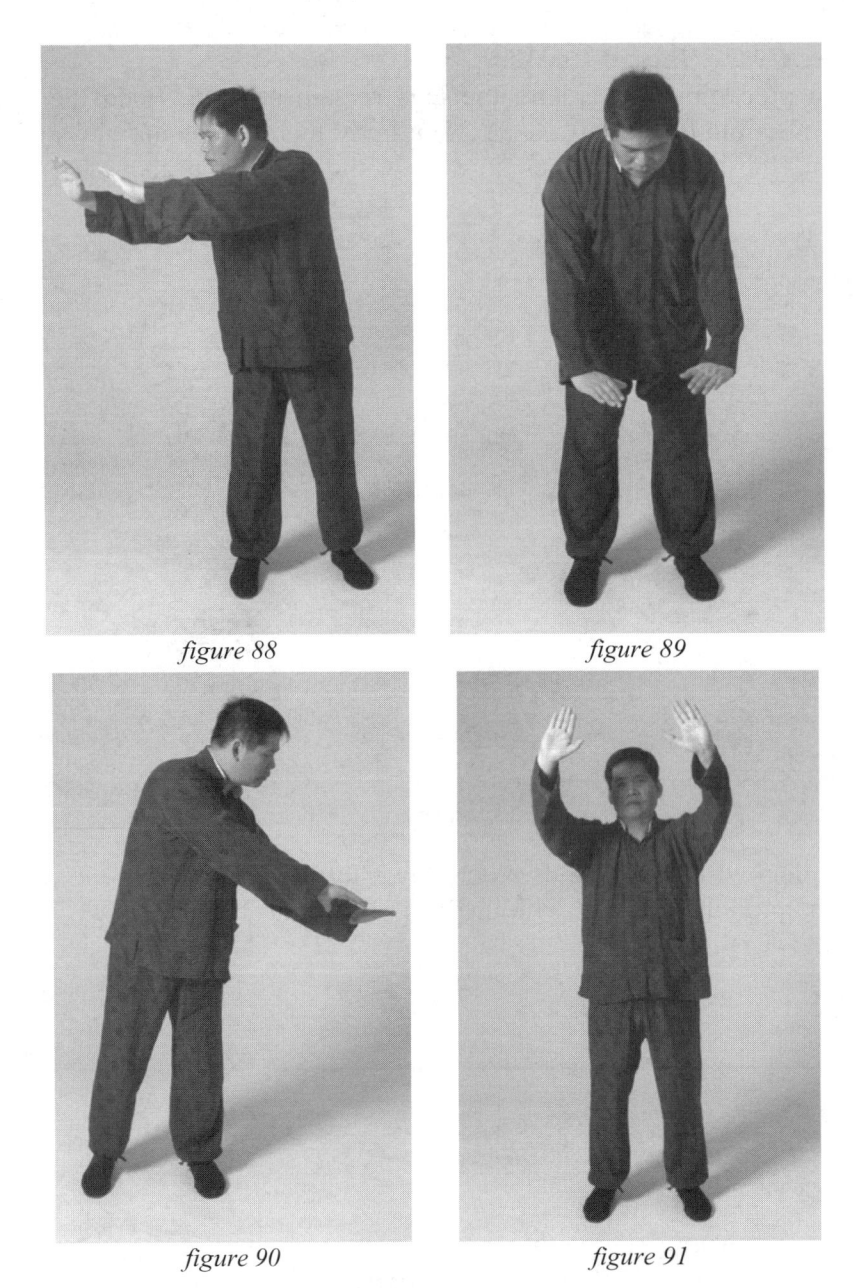

17. Left Brush Knee, Twist Step and Push Right Hand Forward

From the preceding movement, the right hand comes down next to the right ear with the palm face in, and the left hand goes down in front of the abdomen. The legs remain straight, and the eyes look to the left *(fig 92)*. Pick up the left foot, and step forward to the left onto the heel *(fig 93)*. Shift the weight onto the left foot, moving the left hand outside the left knee and pushing the right hand forward from the shoulder *(fig 94)*.

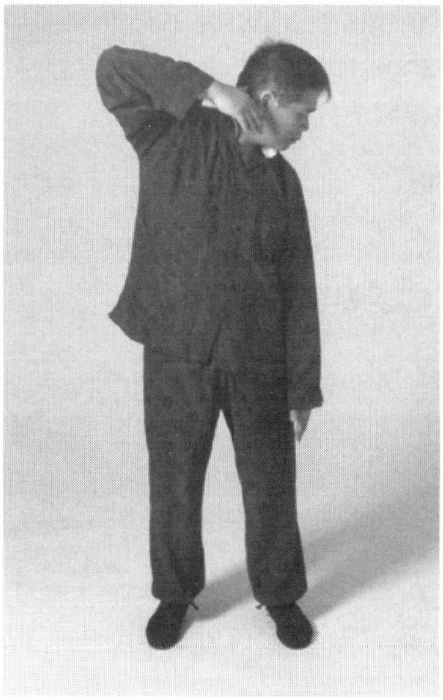

figure 92

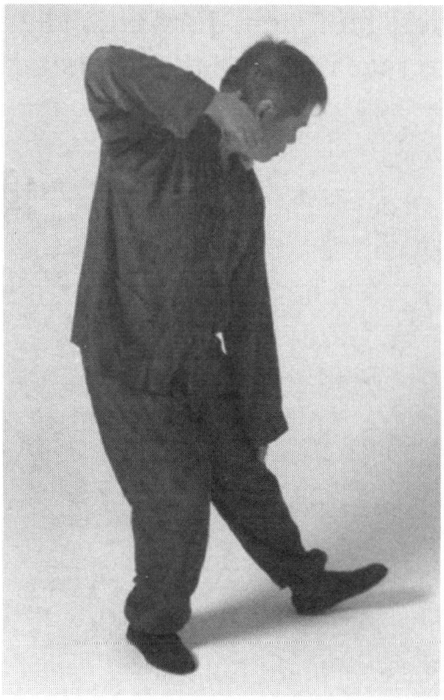

figure 93

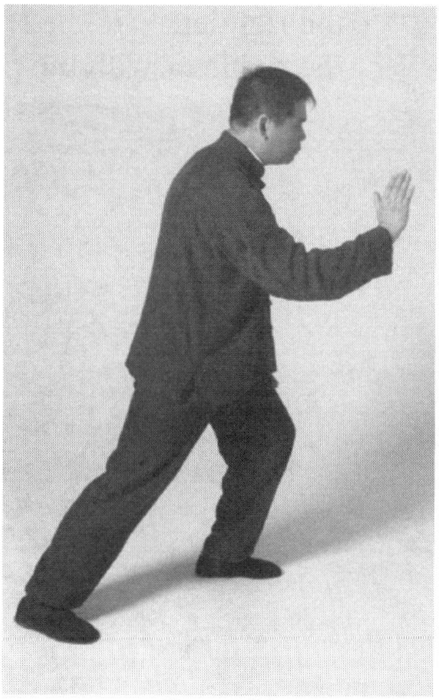

figure 94

18. Pick Up Needle in Sea Bottom

From the preceding movement, the right foot steps up beside the left foot. Squat down with the right hand going down and the left hand coming up in front of the right ear *(fig 95)*.

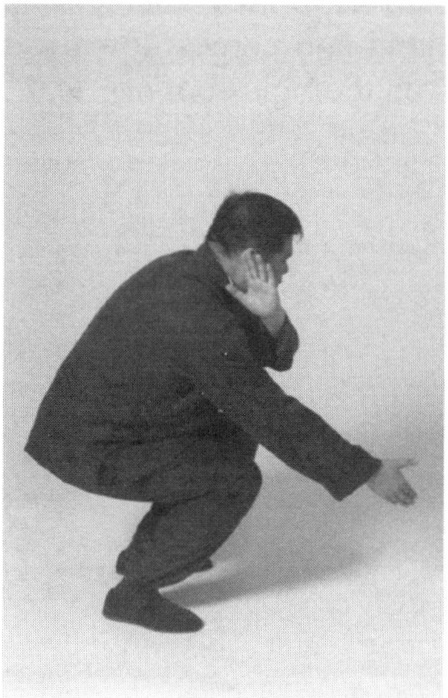

figure 95

19. Fan Back

From the preceding movement, the body rises and the hands position next to the right ear *(fig 96)*. The left foot steps forward. The right hand draws close to the right ear with the palm face out, and the left hand pushes forward *(fig 97)*.

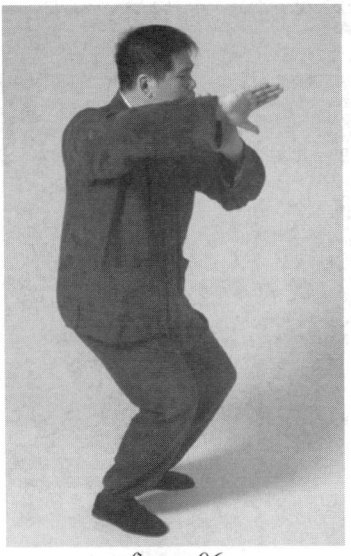

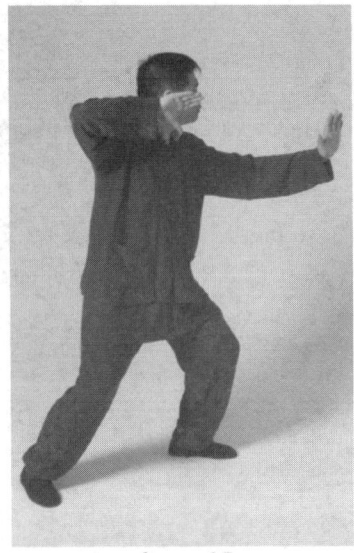

figure 96   figure 97

20. Turn Around and Hit Downward

From the preceding movement, turn the right toes out to turn the body to the right. Shift the weight onto the right foot while the left foot turns inward and the left hand comes up and over to the right *(fig 98)*. The right hand closes into a fist on top of the left hand and comes down to the abdomen as the body lowers and the weight sits on the right foot *(fig 99)*.

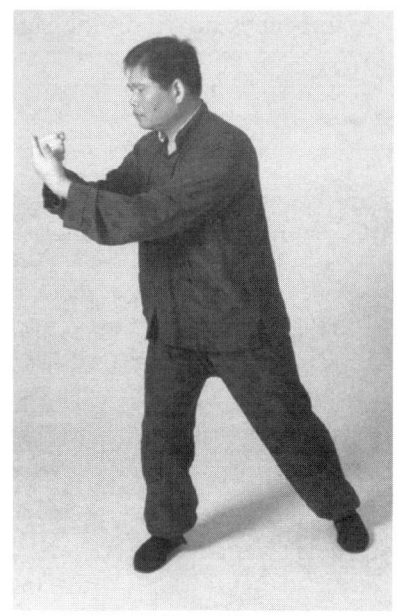

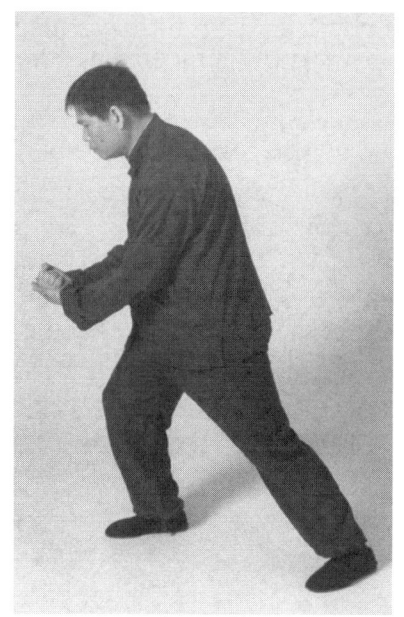

figure 98   *figure 99*

21. Step, Parry and Punch

From the preceding movement, with the weight on the right foot, bring the left fingers to the right inner wrist and extend the hands forward *(fig 100)*. Turn the palms so the left faces up and the right faces down, and bring them back to the body as the weight shifts onto the left foot and the right toes lift *(fig 101)*.

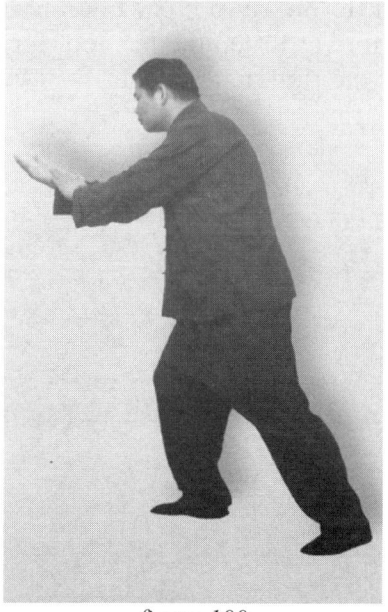

figure 100   *figure 101*

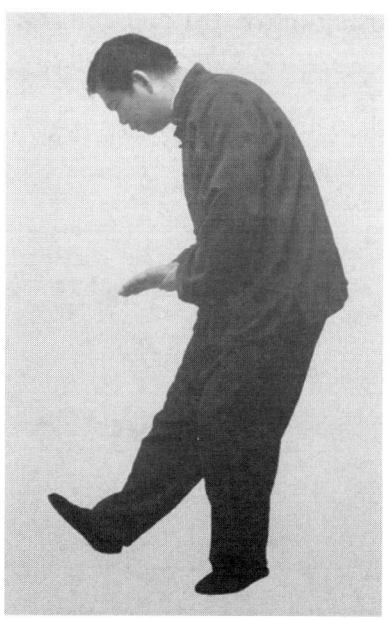

Turn the palms so the right faces up and the left faces down on the right wrist; push forward, shifting the weight onto the right foot *(figs 102 – 104)*.

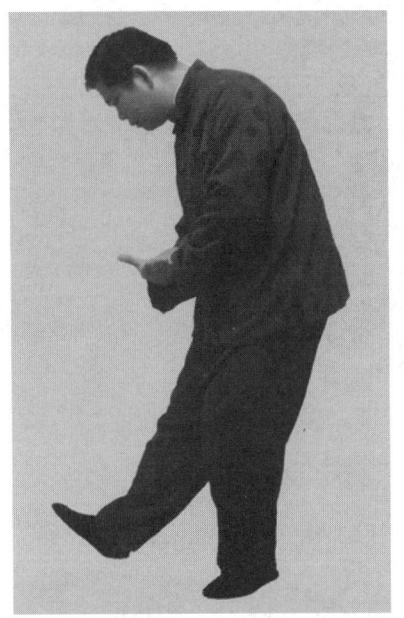

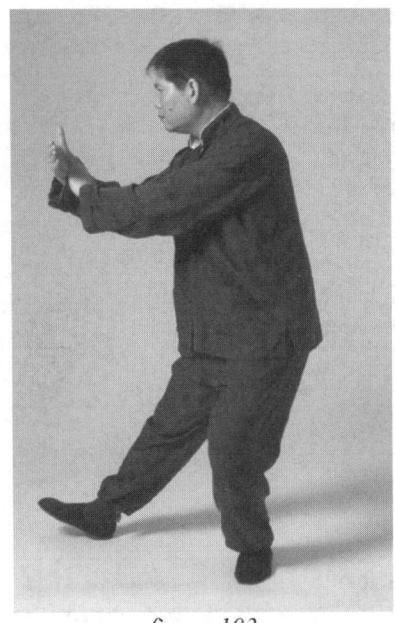

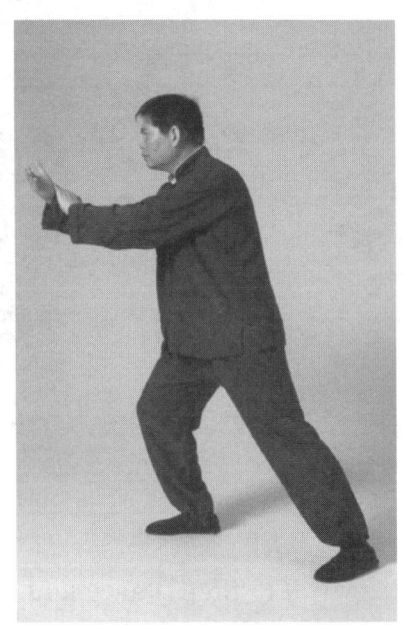

figure 102   *figure 103*   *figure 104*

The body's weight remains on the right foot. Separate the hands with the right hand closing into a fist and coming back to the right hip while the left hand pushes forward. As the left hand pushes forward, step the left foot forward *(fig 105)*. Shift the weight onto the left foot as the right fist punches forward, and is met by the left palm at its wrist *(fig 106)*.

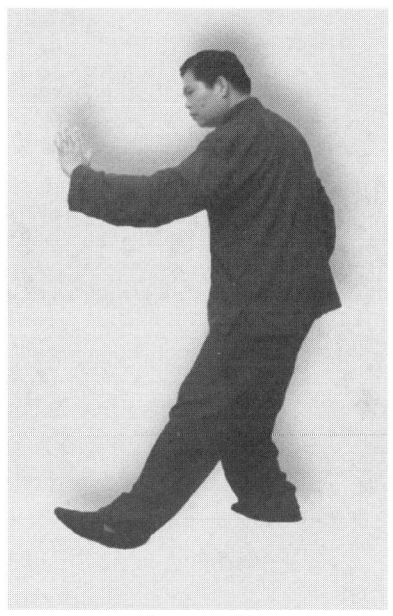

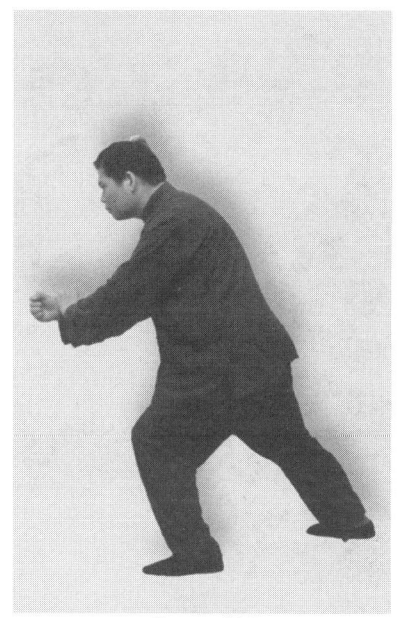

figure 105 *figure 106*

22. Part the Wild Horse's Mane

From the preceding movement, open the right fist, the right hand comes down to the abdomen, and the left hand goes up to the right shoulder *(figs 107)*. Pick up the right foot, and step to the right corner with the heel on the ground *(figs 108)*. Shift the weight onto the right foot while separating the hands with the right hand going up above the shoulder and the left hand going down to the left leg. The eyes are looking at the left hand *(figs 109)*.

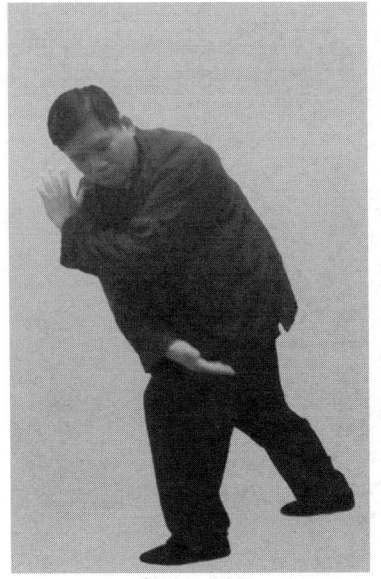

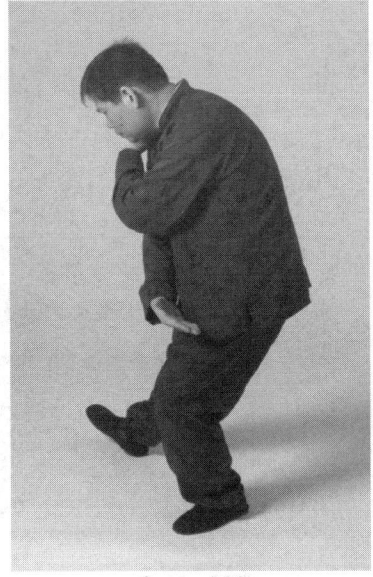

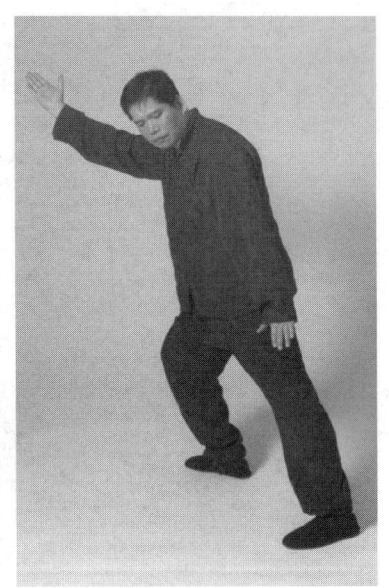

figure 107 *figure 108* *figure 109*

23. Left Warding Off

From the preceding movement, turn the body to the left, bringing the right toes in; the right hand comes down to the left hip, and the left hand comes up to the right shoulder. The body weight shifts onto the left foot *(fig 110)*. The hands remain the same as the weight again shifts onto the right foot *(fig 111)*. The left hand goes down in front of the abdomen, and the right hand comes up in front of the right shoulder; the weight remains on the right foot *(fig 112)*.

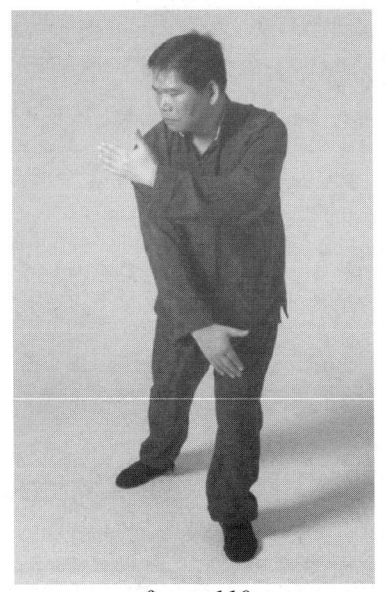

figure 110 *figure 111* *figure 112*

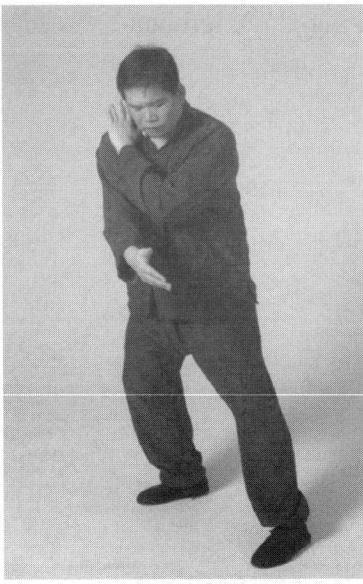

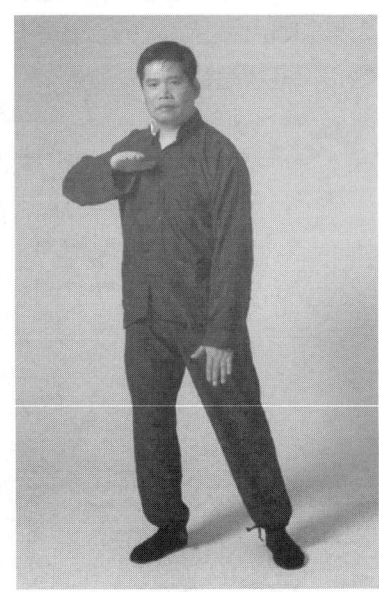

Pick up the left foot, and step forward onto the heel. The eyes follow the left hand as it comes up in front of the face. The right hand joins the left hand on the wrist *(figs 113 & 114)*. Shift the weight onto the left foot as the hands push forward *(fig 115)*.

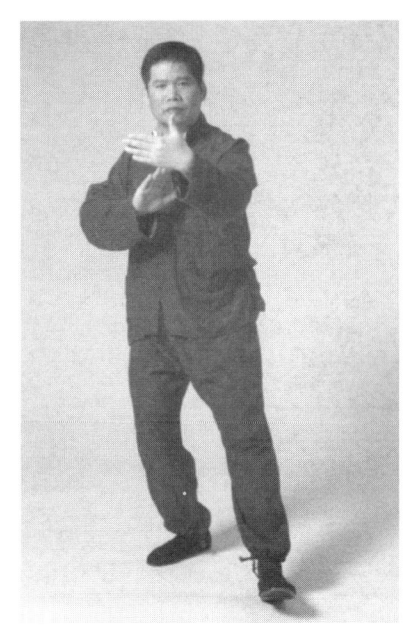

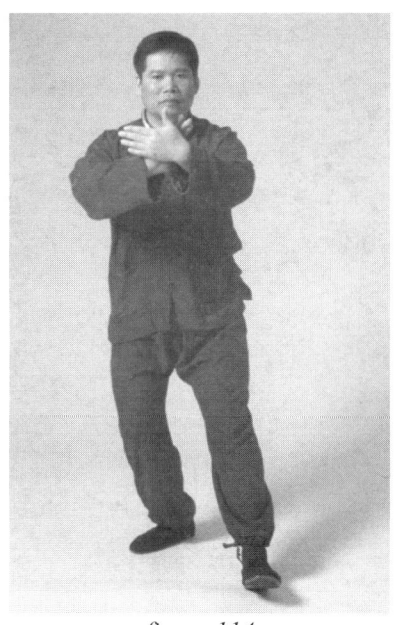

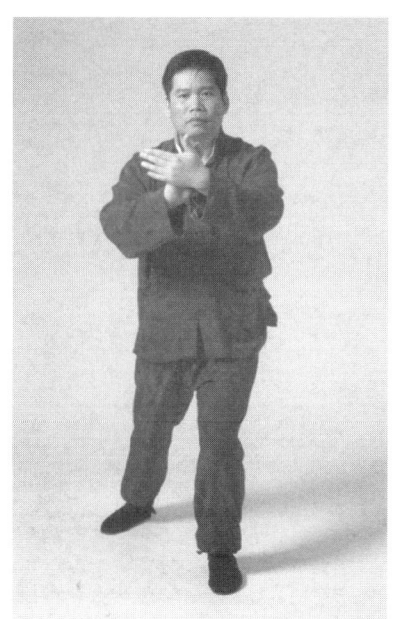

figure 113 *figure 114* *figure 115*

24. Waving Hands Like Clouds (seven times)
Part 1: Left Hand Side

From the preceding movement, the right foot steps up next to the left foot. The right hand then moves to the right side while the left hand arrives near the right shoulder *(fig 116)*. Continuing, the left hand comes up to chin level as the right hand goes down to above the right knee. Pick up the left foot, and step to the left *(figs 117 & 118)*. The hands cross the body to the left, and the weight shifts onto the left foot at the same time *(fig 119)*.

figure 116

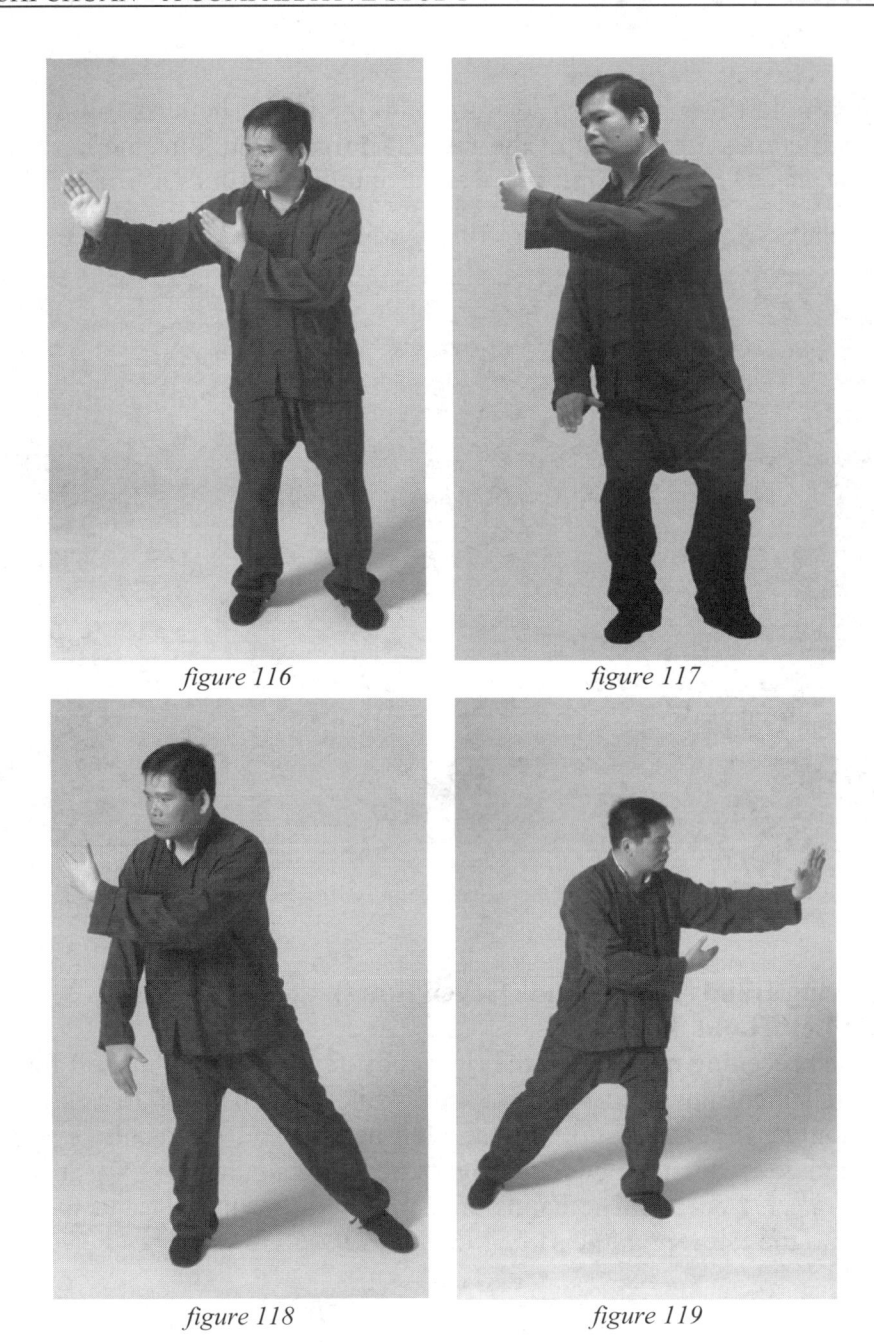

figure 117

figure 118

figure 119

Part 2: Right Hand Side

From the preceding movement, change the position of the hands with the right hand coming up to chin level and the left hand going down above the left knee *(fig 120)*. The right foot steps next to the left foot *(fig 121)*. Shift the weight onto the right foot, and rotate the hands to the right side *(fig 122)*.

figure 120 *figure 121* *figure 122*

Part 3: Left Hand Side

From the preceding movement, change the position of the hands with the left hand coming up to chin level and the right hand going down to above the right knee *(figs 123 & 124)*. Pick up the left foot, and step to the left *(fig 125)*. Shift the weight onto the left foot, and rotate the hands to the left side *(fig 126)*.

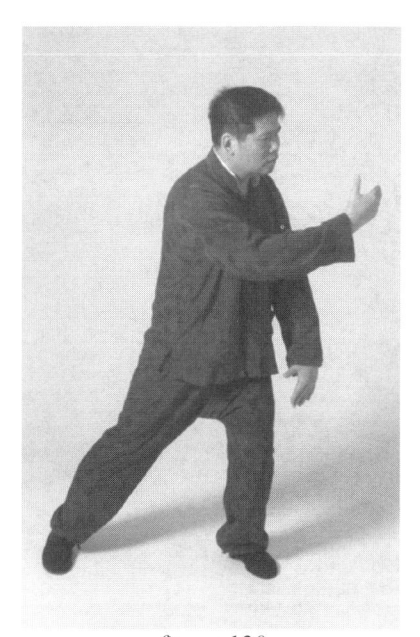

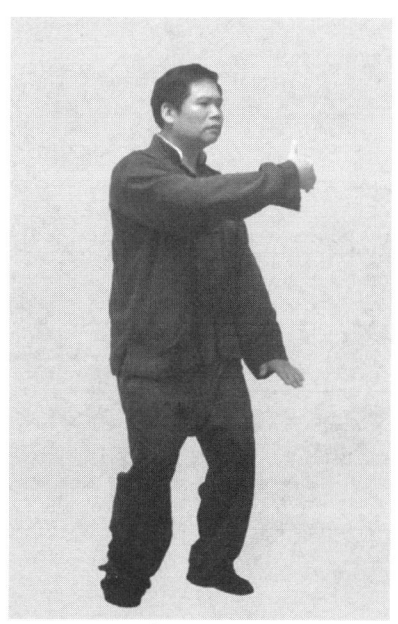

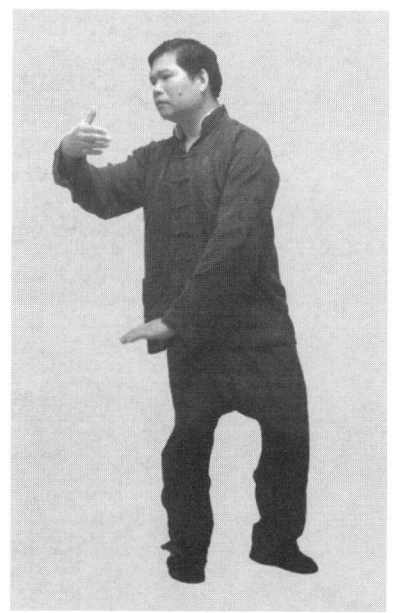

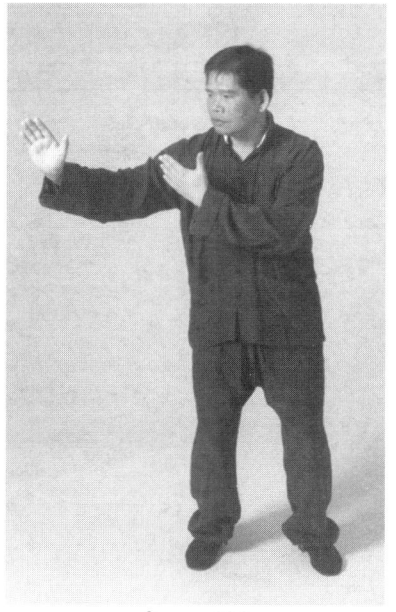

figure 123 *figure 124*

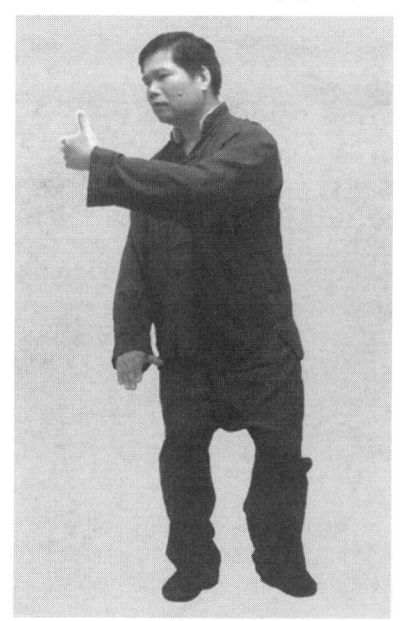

figure 125   *figure 126*

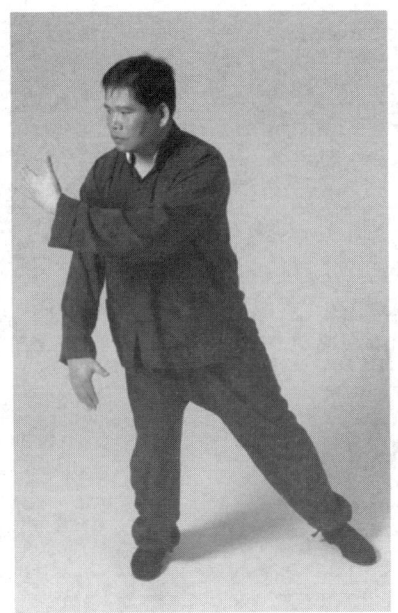

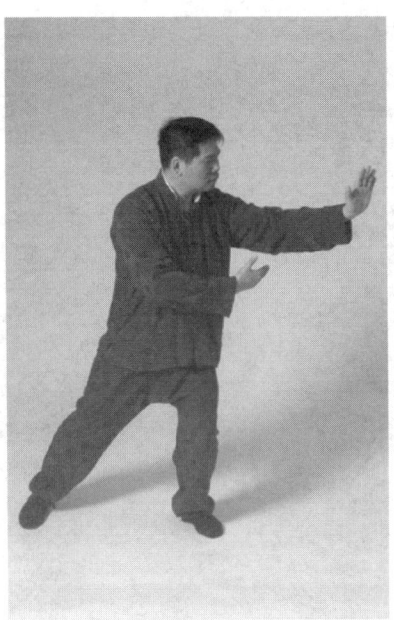

Part 4: Right Hand Side

From the preceding movement, change the position of the hands with the right hand coming up to chin level and the left hand going down to above the left knee *(fig 127)*. Pick up the right foot, and step next to the left foot *(fig 128)*. Shift the weight onto the right foot, and rotate the hands to the right side *(fig 129)*.

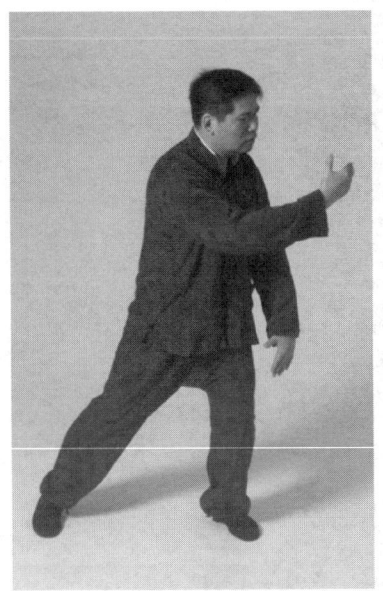

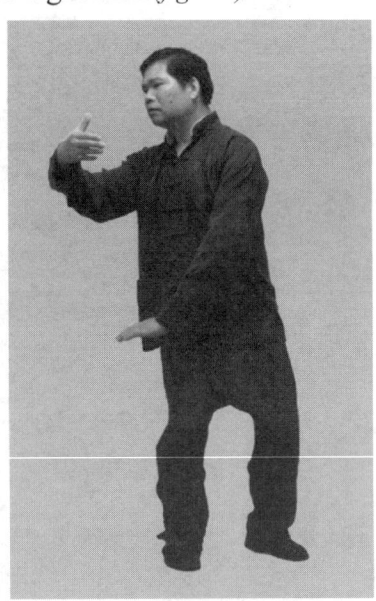

figure 127   *figure 128*   *figure 129*

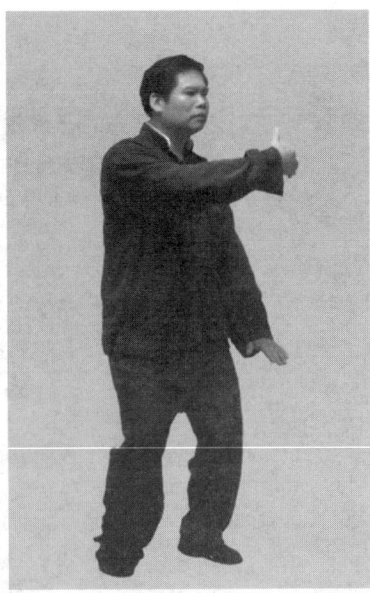

Part 5: Left Hand Side

From the preceding movement, change the position of the hands with the left hand coming up to chin level and the right hand going down to above the right knee *(figs 130 & 131)*. Pick up the left foot, and step to the left *(fig 132)*. Shift the weight onto the left foot, and rotate the hands to the left side *(fig 133)*.

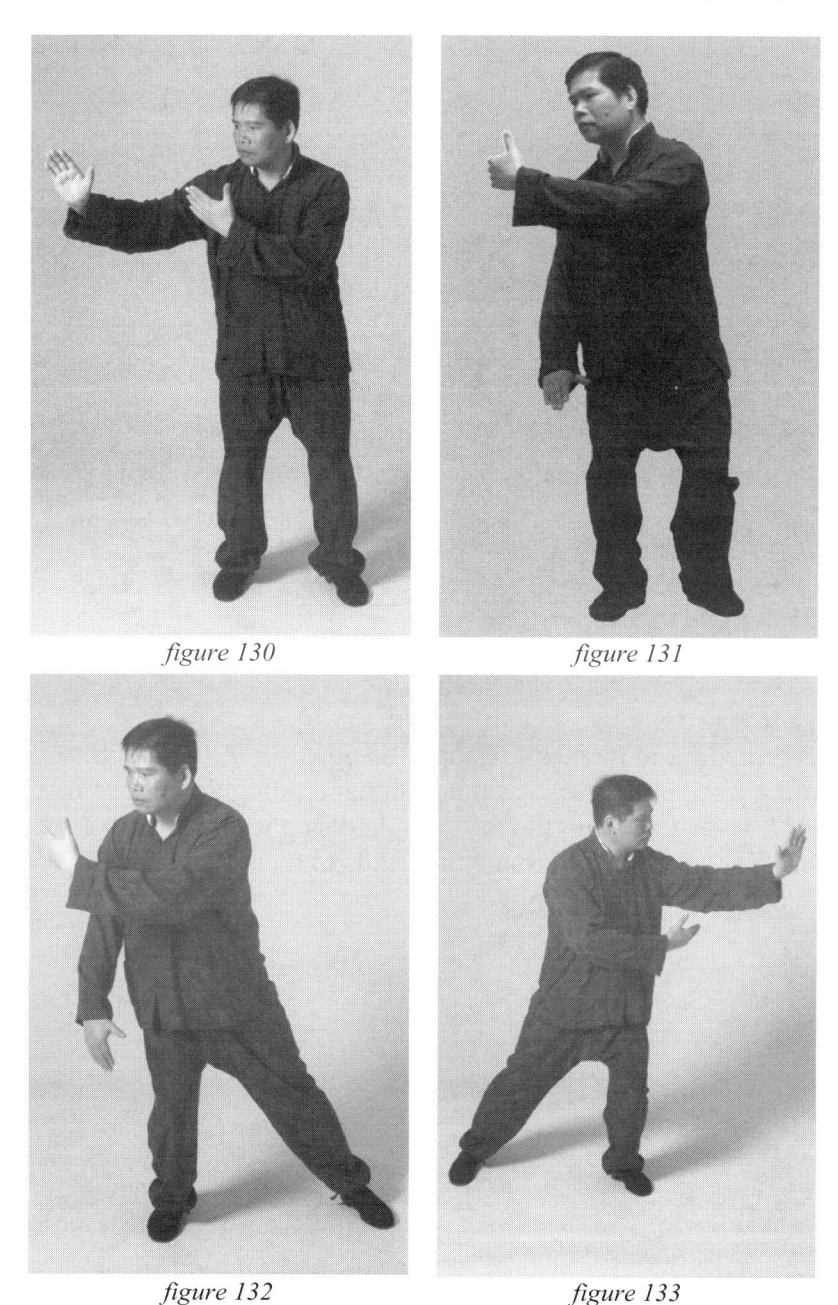

figure 130

figure 131

figure 132

figure 133

Part 6: Right Hand Side

From the preceding movement, change the position of the hands with the right hand coming up to chin level and the left hand going down to above the left knee *(fig 134)*. Pick up the right foot, and step next to the left foot *(fig 135)*. Shift the weight onto the right foot, and rotate the hands to the right side *(fig 136)*.

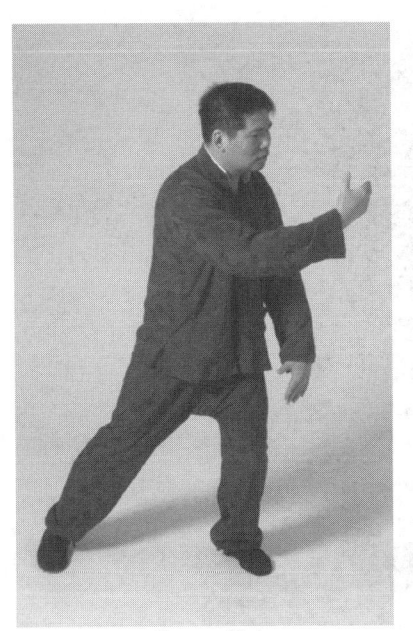

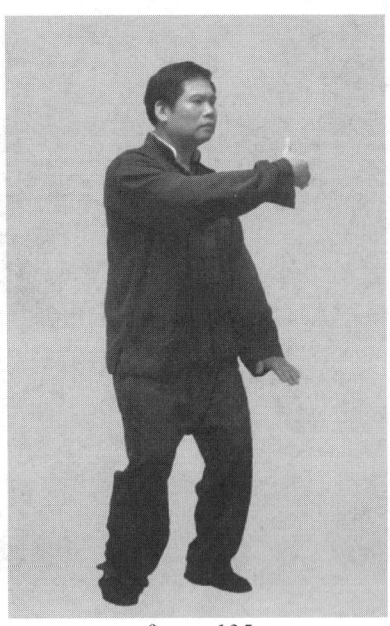

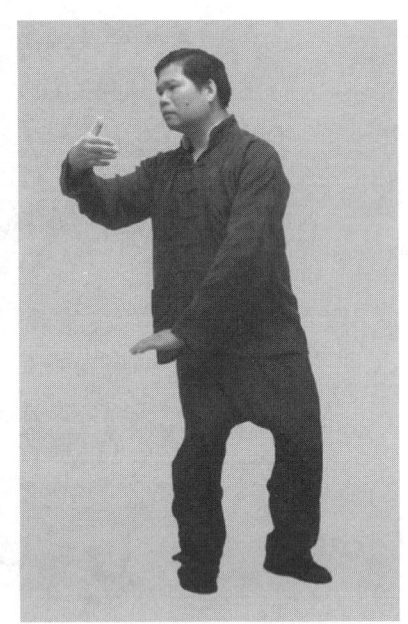

figure 134   *figure 135*   *figure 136*

Part 7: Left Hand Side

From the preceding movement, change the position of the hands with the left hand coming up to chin level and the right hand going down to above the right knee *(figs 137 & 138)*. Pick up the left foot, and step to the left *(fig 139)*. Shift the weight onto the left foot, and rotate the hands to the left side *(fig 140)*.

THE 48 MOVEMENT SMALL FRAME SOLO FORM

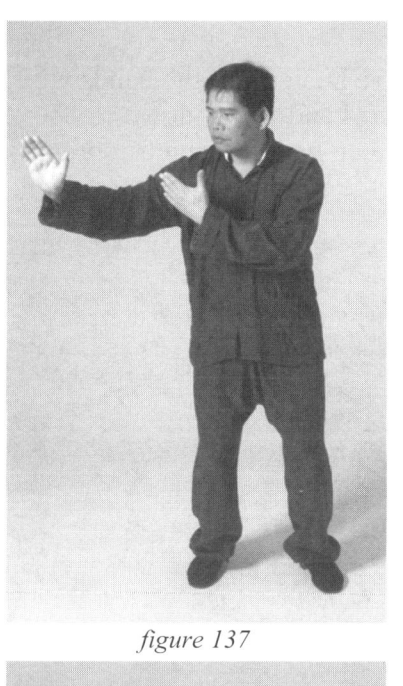

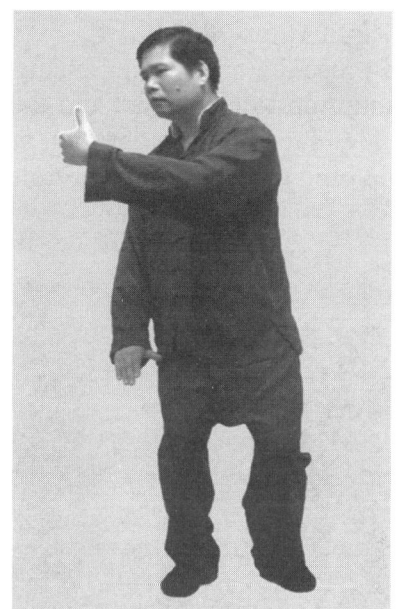

figure 137

figure 138

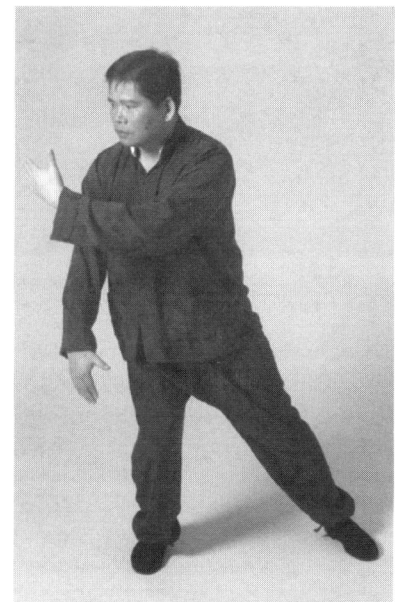

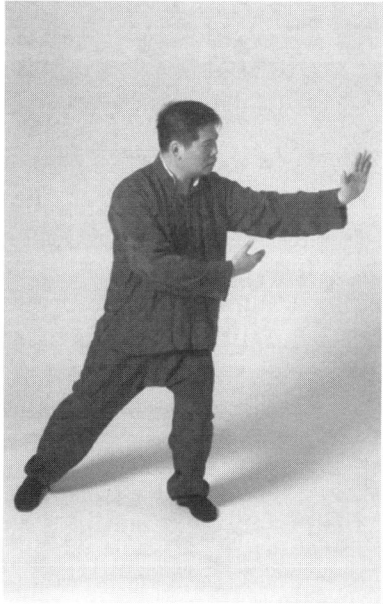

figure 139

figure 140

TAI CHI CHUAN – A COMPARATIVE STUDY

Part 8: Right Hand Side

From the preceding movement, change the position of the hands with the right hand coming up to chin level and the left hand going down to above the left knee *(fig 141)*. Pick up the right foot, and step next to the left foot *(fig 142)*. Shift the weight onto the right foot, and rotate the hands to the right side *(fig 143)*.

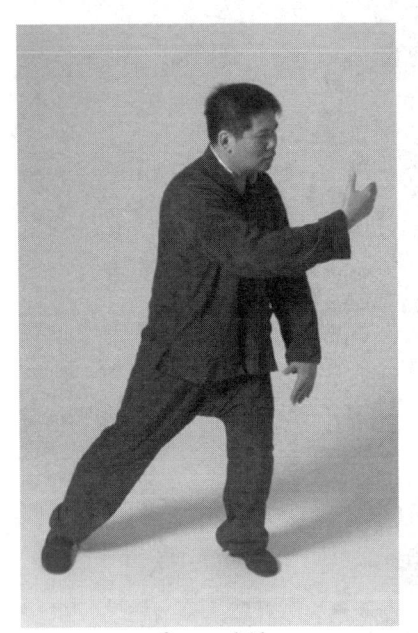

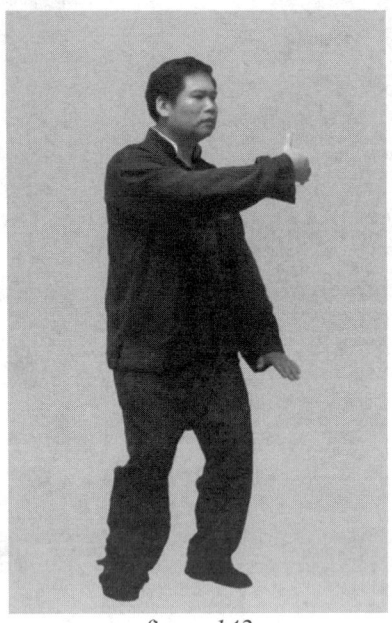

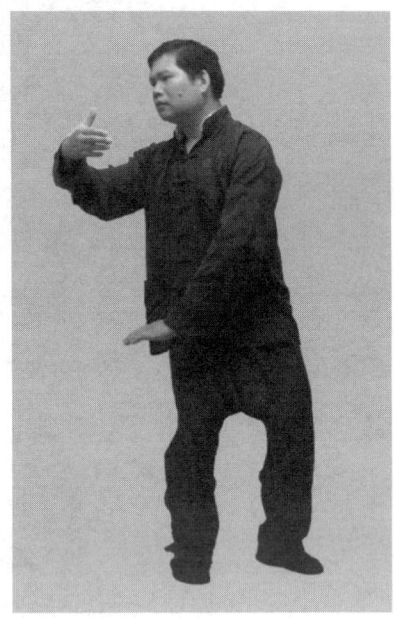

figure 141   *figure 142*   *figure 143*

25. Single Whip

From the preceding movement, bring the right hand's fingers together to form a beak then bend the wrist to form a hook; the left hand comes up next to the right wrist *(fig 144)*. Pick up the left foot, and step to the left with the toes pointing to the corner *(fig 145)*. Shift the weight onto the left foot as the eyes follow the left hand across the body to the left corner. Finally, turn the left palm to face out *(fig 146)*.

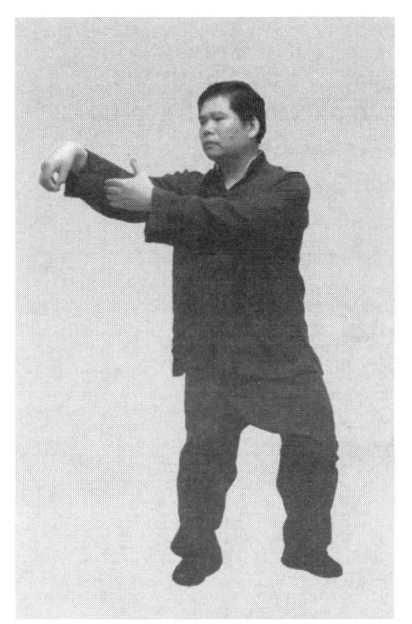

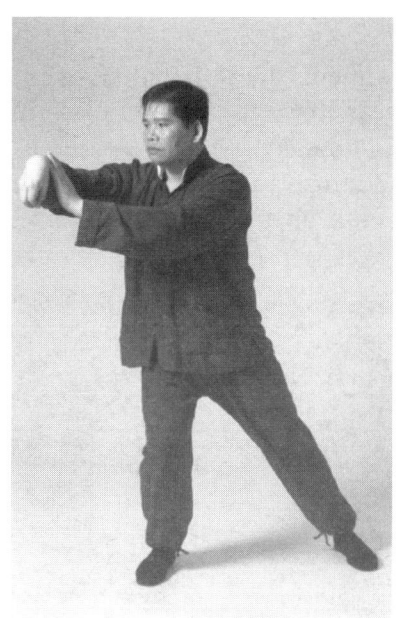

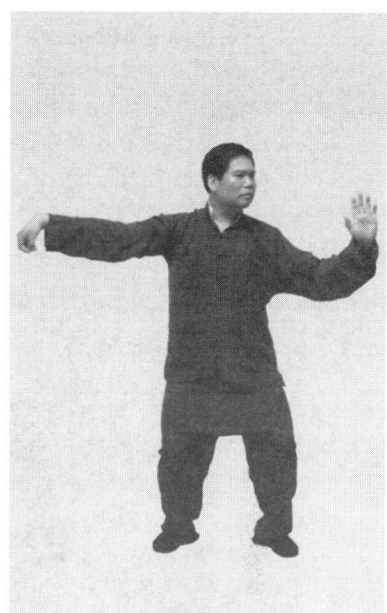

figure 144   *figure 145*   *figure 146*

26. Right High Pat Horse

From the preceding movement, turn the left toes out and the left palm face up while opening the right hook and bringing the right hand toward the right ear *(fig 147)*. The right foot steps beside the left foot as the two hands come together in front of the chest with the right hand above the left hand. The fingers are pointing to the sides *(fig 148)*. Shift the weight to the right foot.

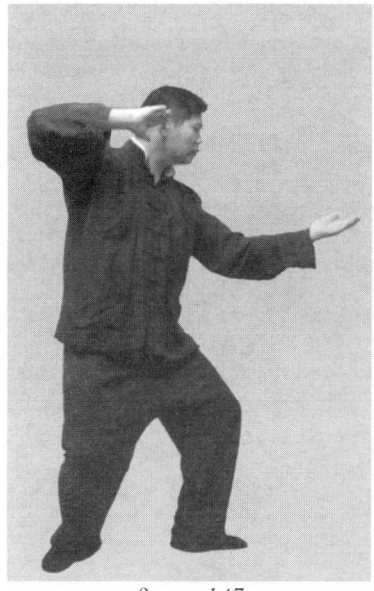

figure 147   *figure 148*

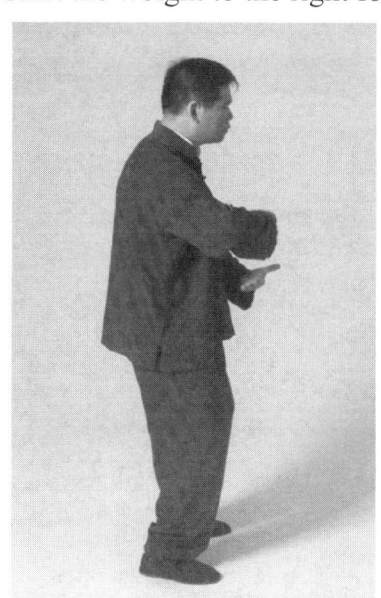

TAI CHI CHUAN – A COMPARATIVE STUDY

27. Right Foot Kicks

From the preceding movement, the left foot steps to the left corner. Shift the weight onto the left foot as the right hand circles clockwise to under the left elbow, and the left hand comes up next to the right ear *(fig 149)*. Separate the hands with the right hand aimed to the right corner and the left hand aimed to the left corner *(fig 150)*. Pick up the right foot, and kick upward to the right corner *(figs 151 & 152)*.

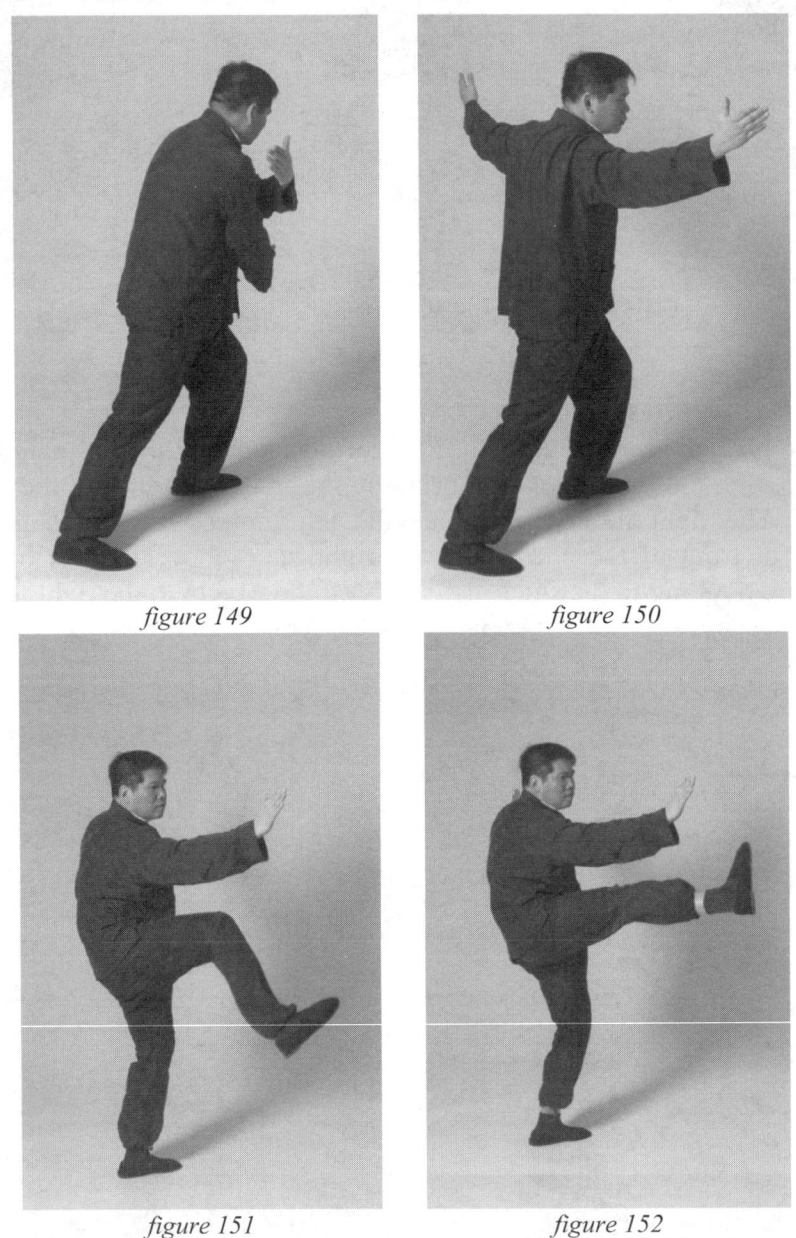

figure 149

figure 150

figure 151

figure 152

28. Left High Pat Horse

From the preceding movement, bring the right foot back, and step down near the left foot; the right hand comes back to the chest with the palm face up while the left hand remains the same *(figs 153 & 154)*. Step the left foot next to the right foot, and bring the left hand down over the right hand *(fig 155)*.

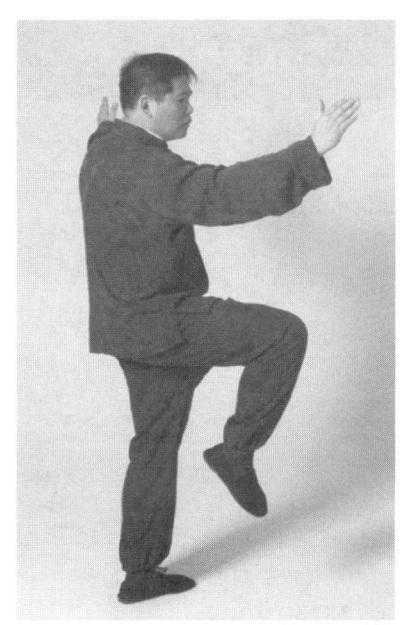

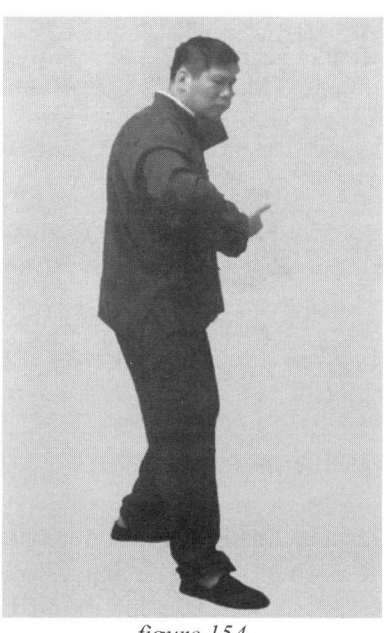

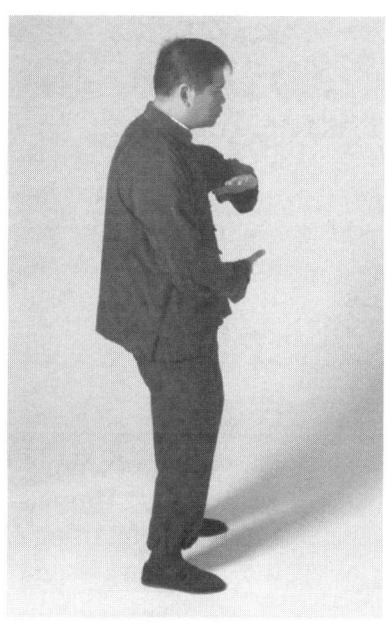

figure 153   *figure 154*   *figure 155*

29. Left Foot Kick

From the preceding movement, step the right foot to the right corner; then shift the weight onto the right foot. Circle the left hand counter-clockwise till it arrives under the right elbow as the right hand comes up to the left ear *(fig 156)*. Separate the hands with the left hand going to the left corner and the right hand going to the right corner *(fig 157)*. Pick up the left foot, and kick upward to the left corner *(fig 158)*.

TAI CHI CHUAN – A COMPARATIVE STUDY

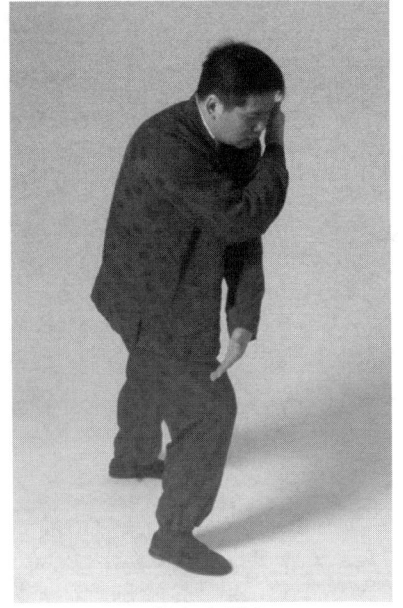

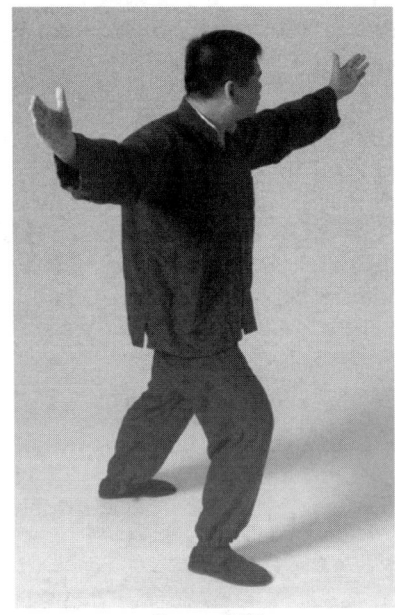

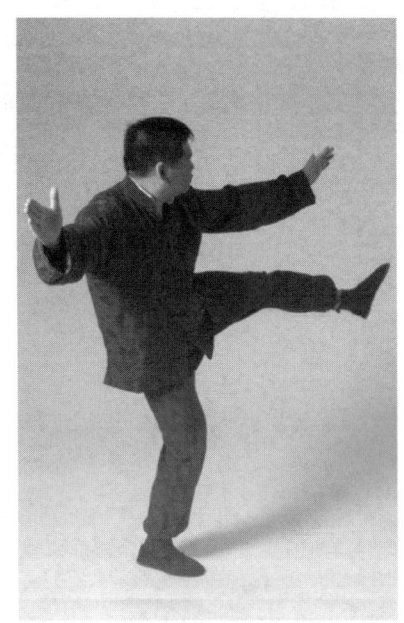

figure 156   *figure 157*   *figure 158*

30. Fair Lady Works on Shuttles (two times)
Part 1: Left Hand Side

From the preceding movement, bring the left foot back; then step down onto the heel towards the left corner. The left hand lowers, and the right hand arrives near the ear *(figs 159 & 160)*. The left hand comes up in front of the chest, and the right hand touches the left wrist *(fig 161)*.

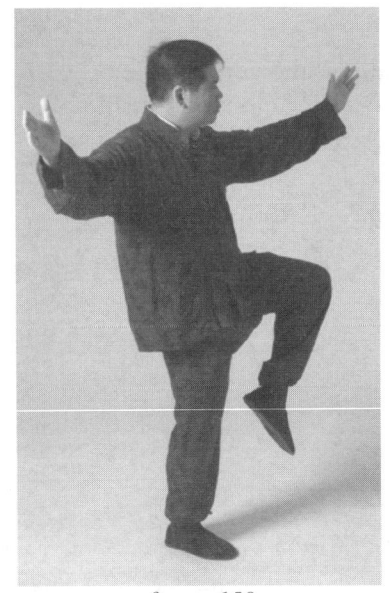

figure 159   *figure 160*   *figure 161*

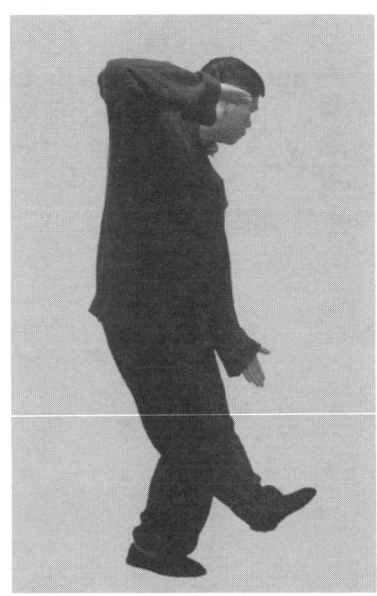

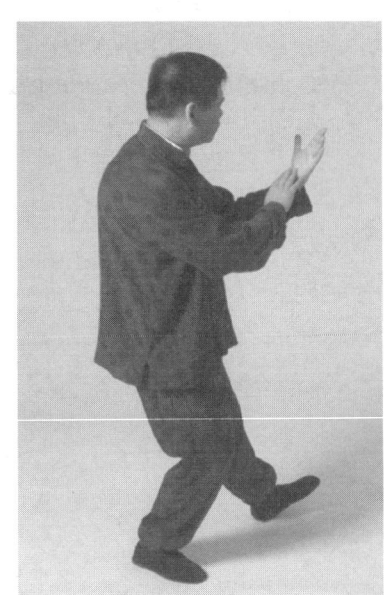

THE 48 MOVEMENT SMALL FRAME SOLO FORM

Shift the weight onto the left foot, and at the same time, push the hands forward *(fig 162)*. Shift the weight back onto the right foot, lifting the left toes up and circling the left palm out and back to face up next to the left ear *(fig 163)*. Shift the weight forward onto the left foot while lifting the left hand above the head and pushing the right hand forward *(fig 164)*.

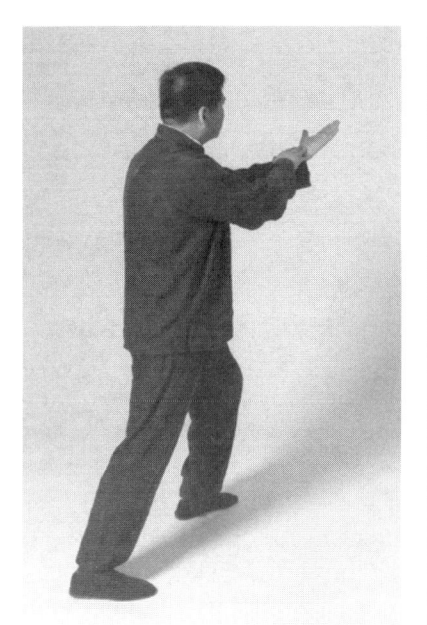

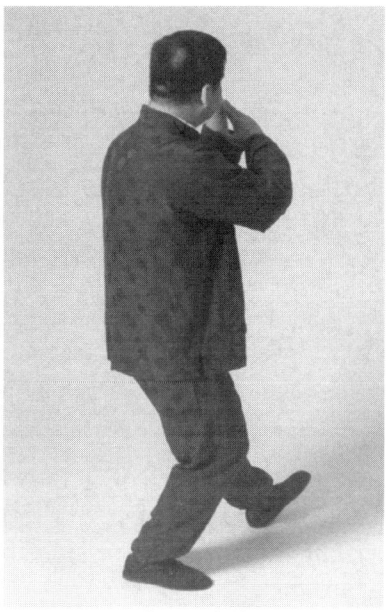

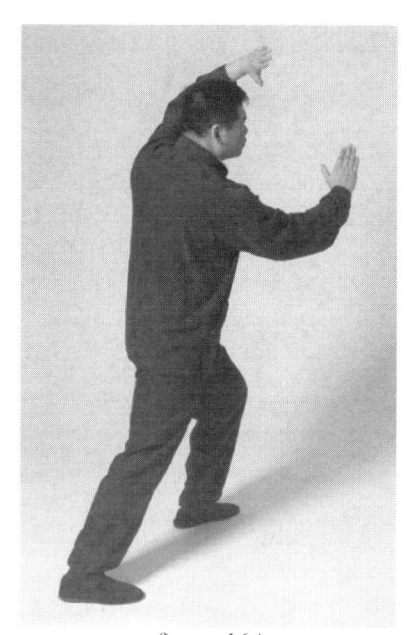

figure 162   *figure 163*   *figure 164*

Part 2: Right Hand Side

From the preceding movement, bring the hands down to the chest with the left hand over the right hand and the palms facing each other. Turn the left foot inward and the body to the right as much as possible *(fig 165)*. Look to the right corner, pick up the right foot, and step to the corner, landing it on the heel as the right hand comes up and the left hand then moves to the right wrist in front of the chest *(fig 166)*. Shift the weight onto the right foot as the hands ward off moving forward together *(fig 167)*.

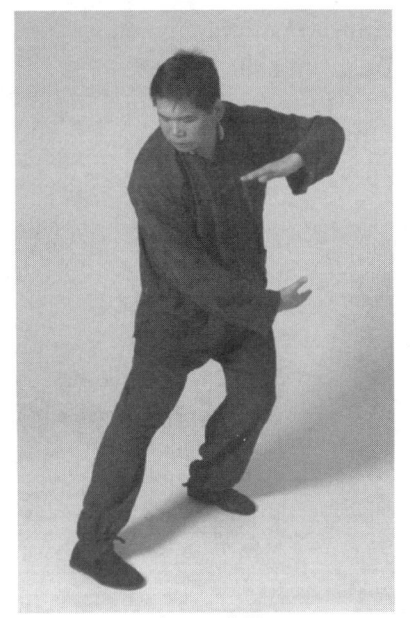

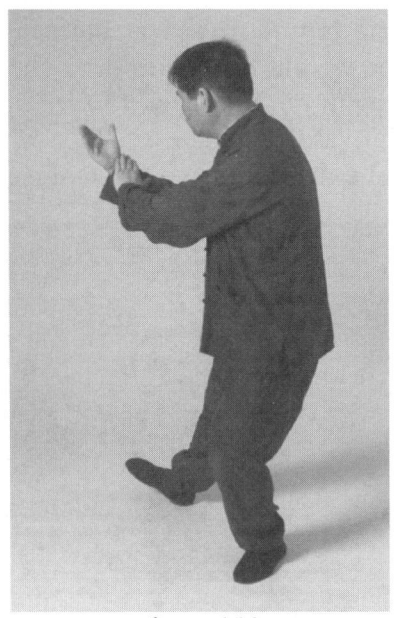

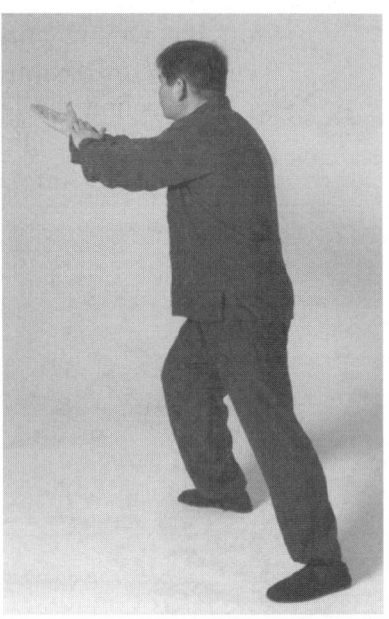

figure 165 *figure 166* *figure 167*

Shift the weight back onto the left foot, lifting the right toes up and circling the right palm out and back to face up near the right ear *(fig 168)*. Shift the weight forward onto the right foot, lifting the right hand above the head and pushing the left hand forward *(fig 169)*.

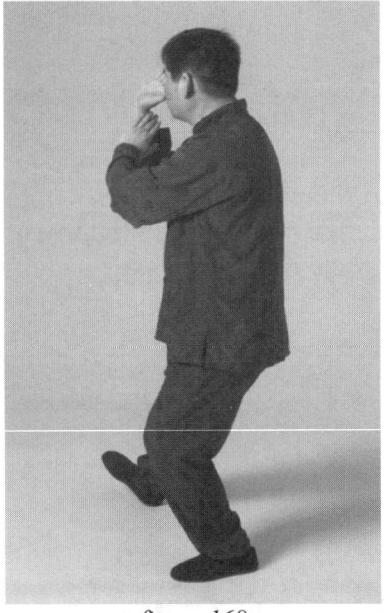

figure 168 *figure 169*

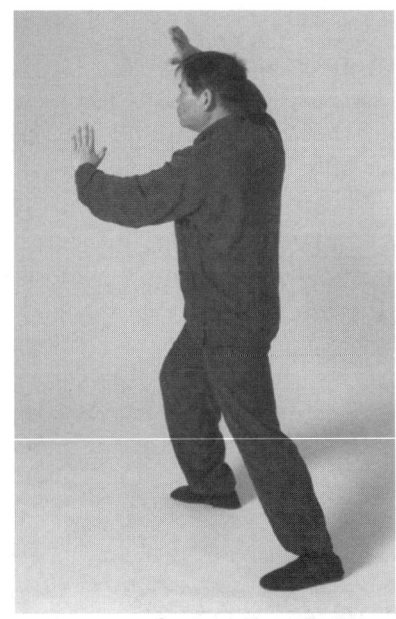

31. Left Warding Off

From the preceding movement, shift the weight onto the left foot, lowering the right hand and bringing the left hand back to the right elbow *(fig 170)*. Turn the body left, bringing the arms along and the right foot inward *(fig 171)*. Shift the weight back onto the right foot as the left hand goes down in front of the abdomen and the right hand comes back in front of the right shoulder with the palm facing down *(figs 172 & 173)*.

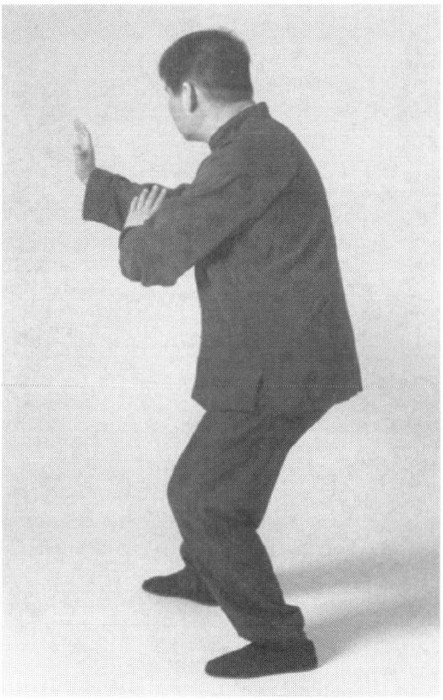

figure 170

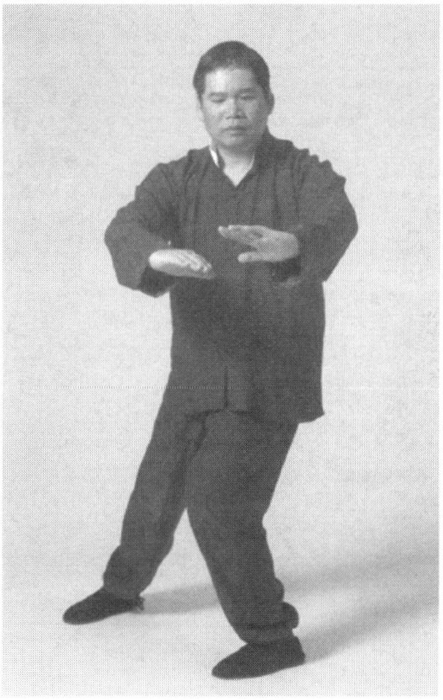

figure 171

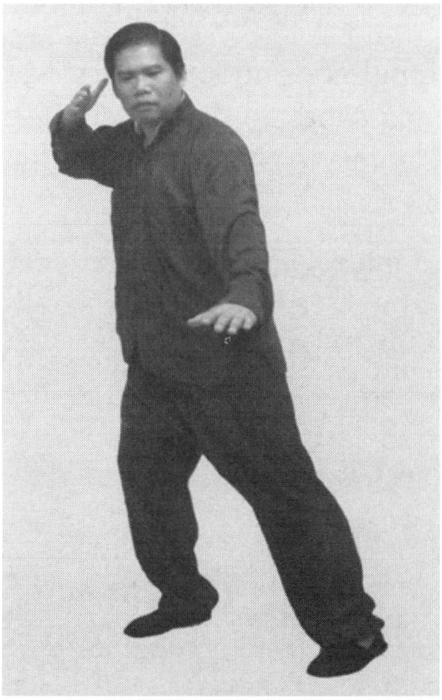

figure 172

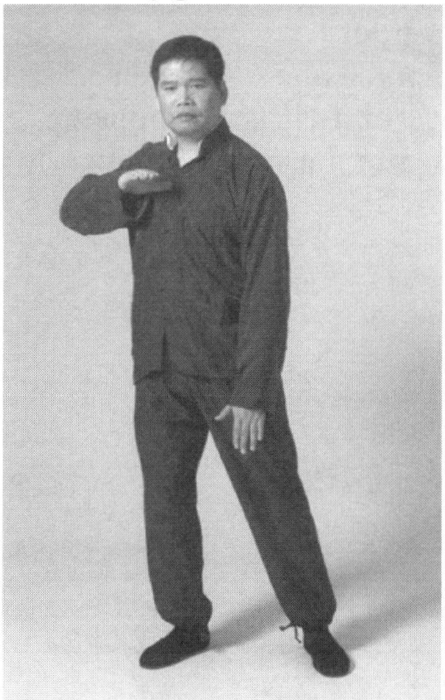

figure 173

Pick up the left foot, and step forward onto the heel. The eyes follow the left hand as it comes up in front of the face. The right hand joins the left hand on the wrist *(figs 174 & 175)*. Shift the weight onto the left foot while pushing the hands forward *(fig 176)*.

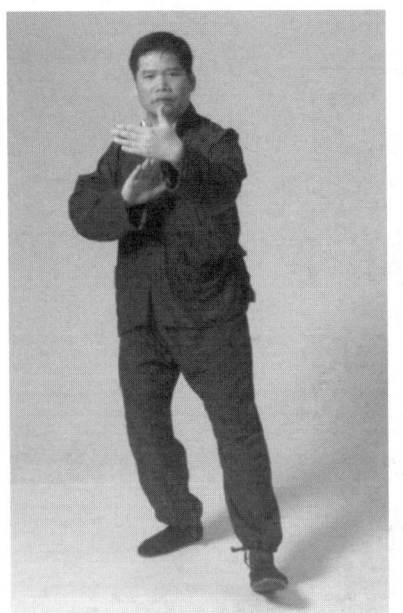

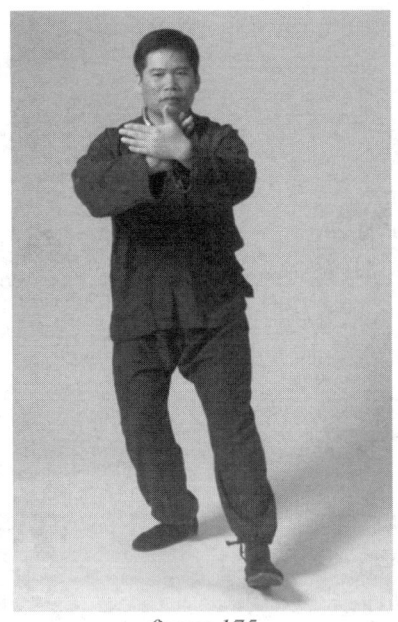

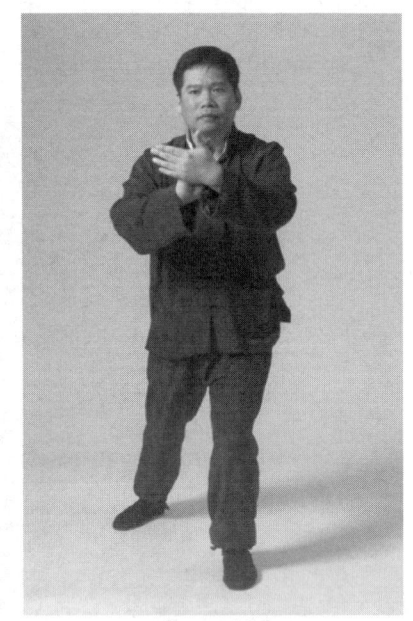

Figure 174 *figure 175* *figure 176*

32. Right Foot Kick

From the preceding movement, the right hand goes under the left wrist and the palms face in. Bring the palms up, and then separate the hands with the right hand going to the right and the left hand going to the left *(figs 177 - 179)*. Pick up the right foot, and kick upward *(fig 180)*.

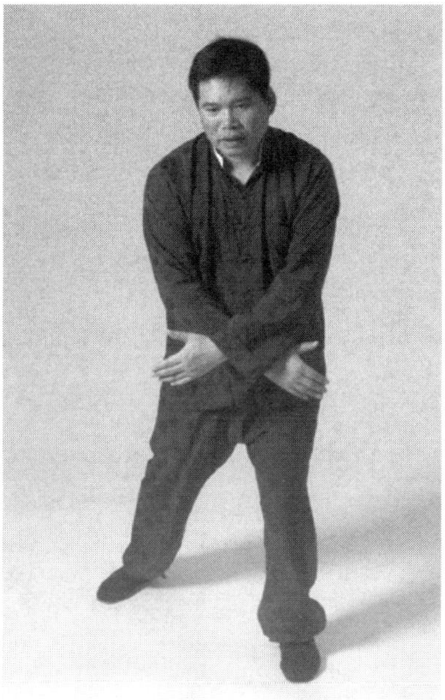

THE 48 MOVEMENT SMALL FRAME SOLO FORM

figure 177

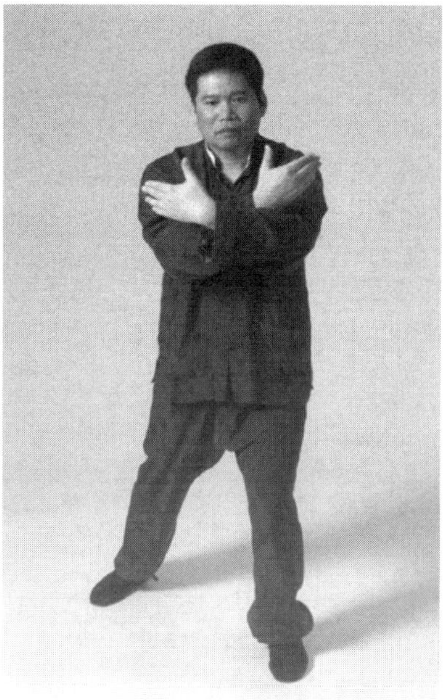

figure 178

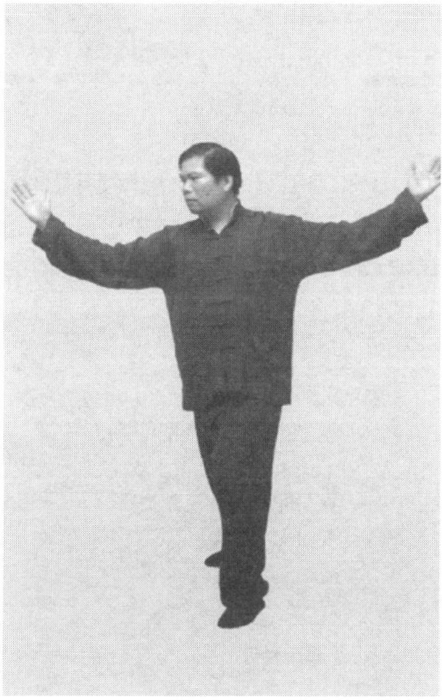

figure 179

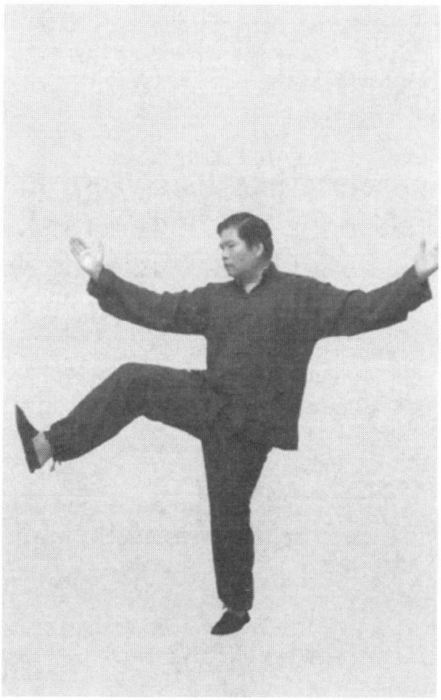

figure 180

33. Left Hit Tiger

From the preceding movement, bring the right foot back *(fig 181)*, and step down behind the left foot with the right hand following down to the right hip, palm facing up, and the left hand coming forward in front of the chest, palm facing in *(fig 182)*. Shift the weight onto the right foot as the left hand continues to the right *(fig 183)*.

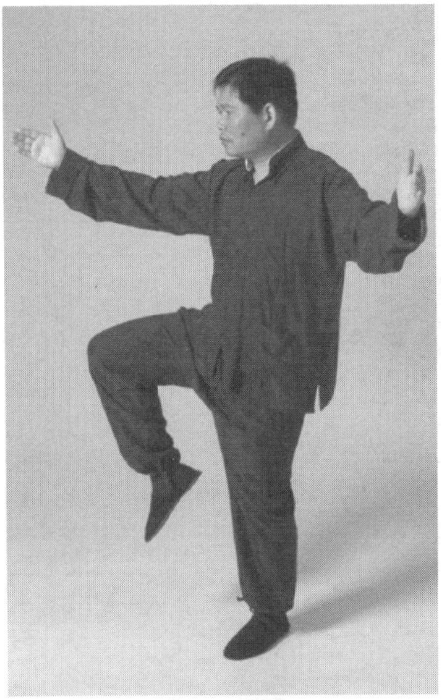

figure 181

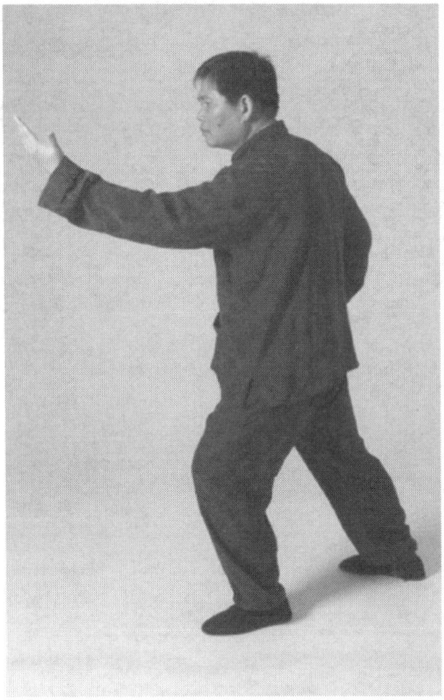

figure 182

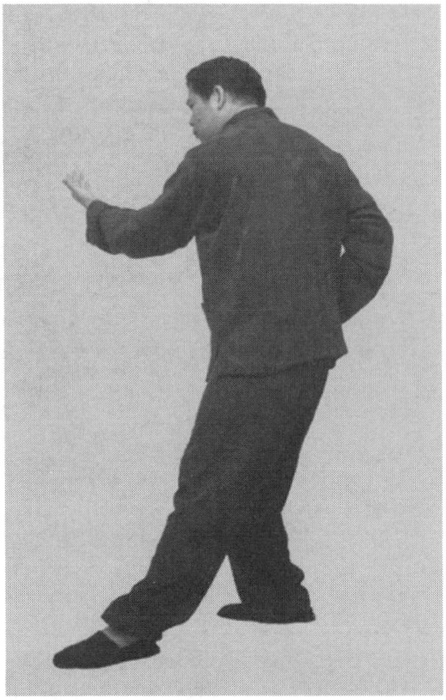

figure 183

Both hands close into fists. Turn the left toes outward, and shift the weight onto the left foot as the body turns left with the fists following. As the weight shifts onto the left foot, circle the left fist up above the head, and bring the right fist before the chest. The right toes turn in *(figs 184 & 185)*.

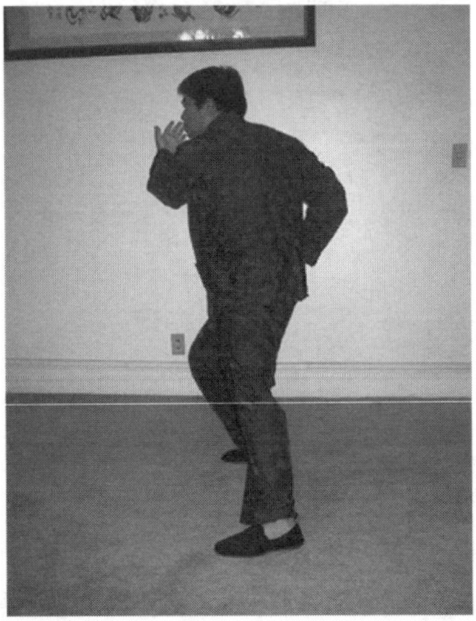

figure 184

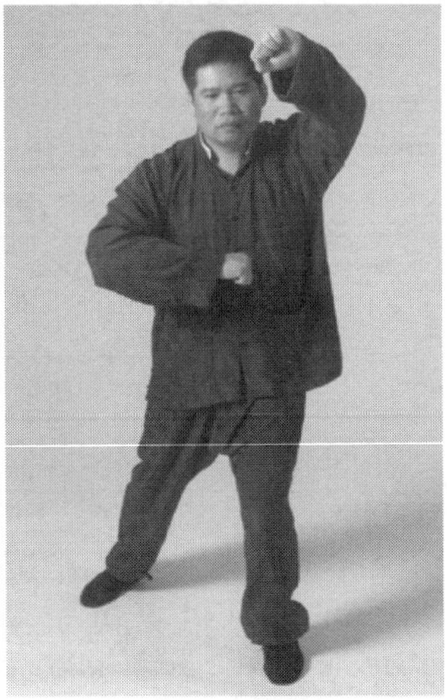

figure 185

34. Hit the Ears with Two Fists

From the preceding movement, while the body turns right and the left toes turn in, turn the arms so the fists face in, and set them in front of the chest *(fig 186)*. Lift the right leg up, and bring the two fists down on top of the right knee as they open into palms *(figs 187 & 188)*.

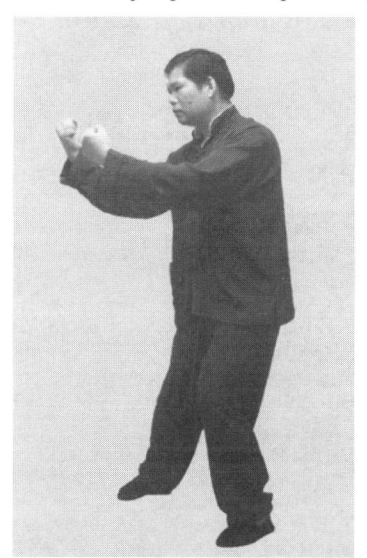

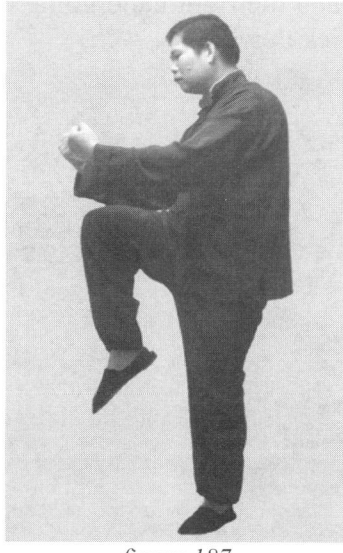

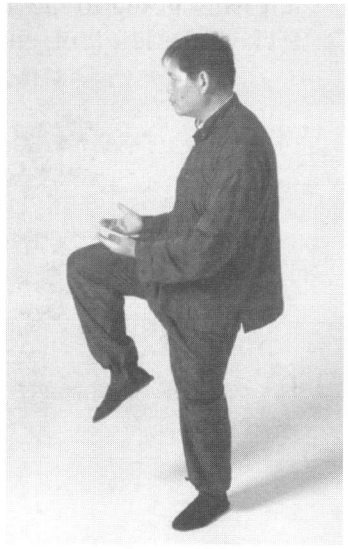

figure 186 *figure 187* *figure 188*

The right foot steps down to the right corner with the heel touching first *(fig 189)*. Shift the weight onto the right foot as the two palms close into fists and come up to face level *(fig 190)*.

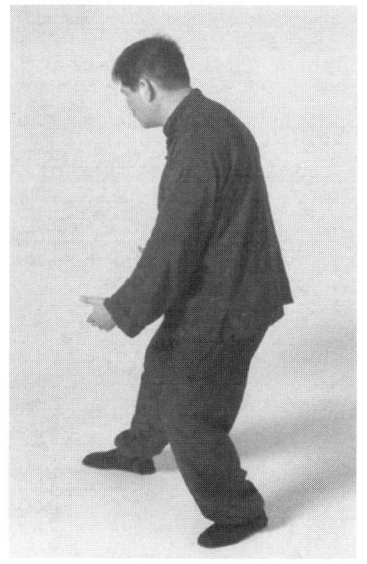

figure 189 *figure 190*

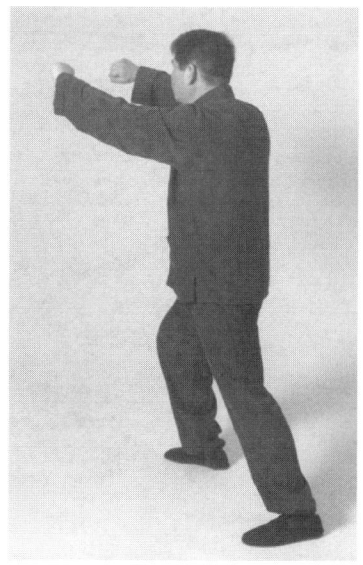

35. Left Foot Kick

From the preceding movement, open the hands, and bring the palms down across the abdomen, the left wrist atop the right and both palms facing in *(fig 191)*. Bring the hands up in front of the face with the palms facing in by turning the wrists. Turn the palms to face out, and separate the hands with the left hand going to the left and the right hand going to the right *(figs 192 & 193)*. Pick up the left foot, and kick upward *(fig 194)*.

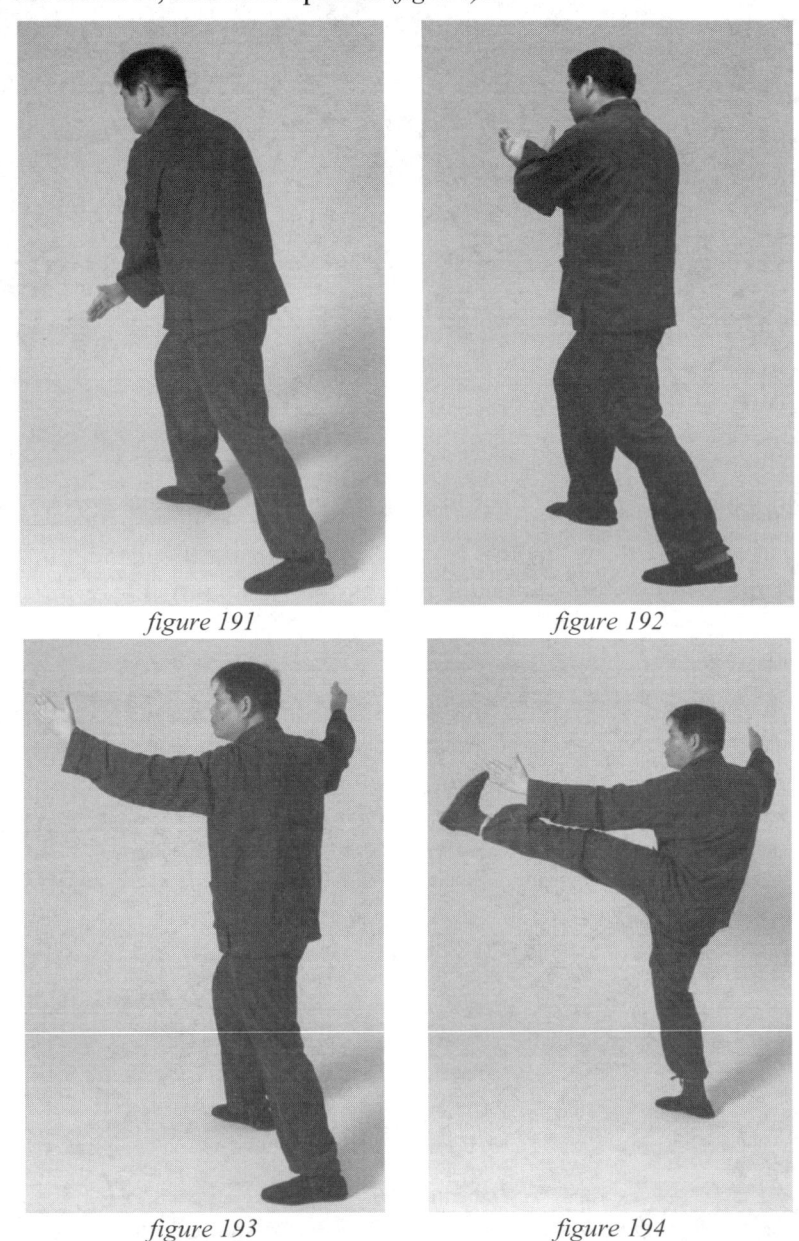

figure 191

figure 192

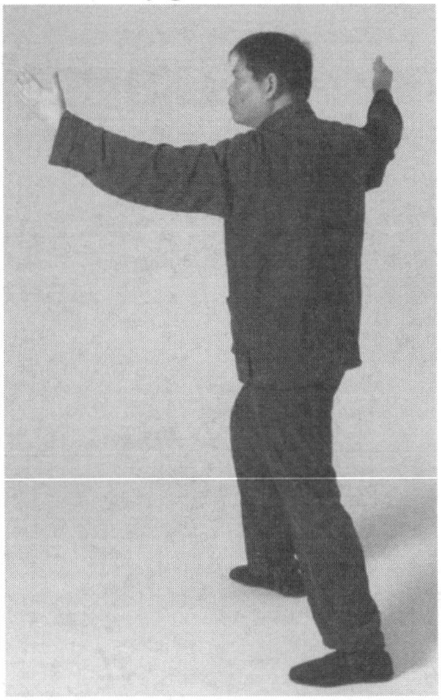

figure 193

figure 194

36. Left Brush Knee, Twist Step and Push Hand (two times)
Part 1: Left Hand Brush Knee

From the preceding movement, bring the left foot back, and step down onto the heel, followed closely by the left hand going down in front of the abdomen and the right hand coming next to the right ear with the palm face in *(figs 195 & 196)*. Shift the weight onto the left foot as the left hand goes outside the left knee and the right hand pushes forward *(fig 197)*.

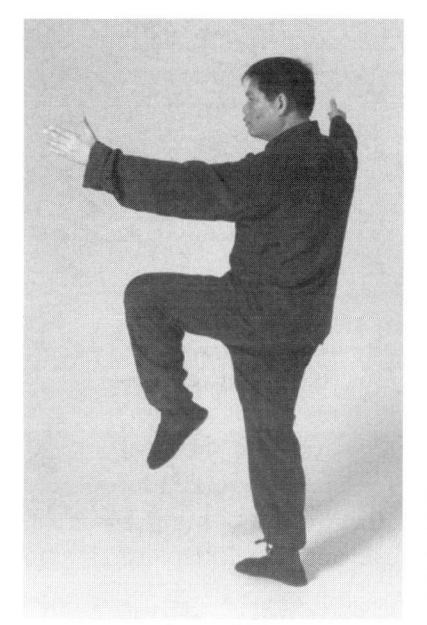

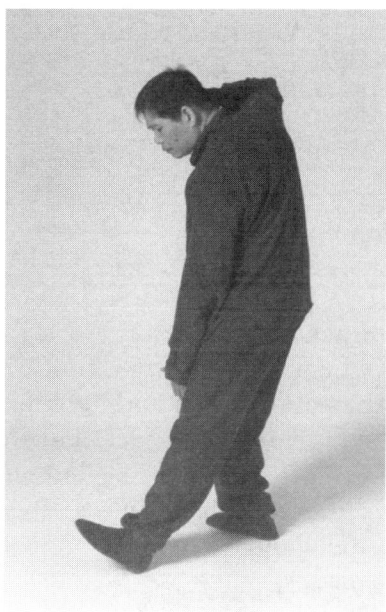

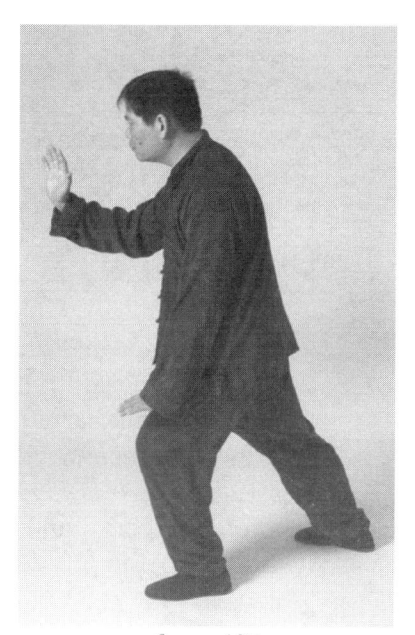

figure 195 *figure 196* *figure 197*

Part 2: Right Hand Brush Knee

From the preceding movement, turn the left foot out. The left hand comes up to the left ear with the palm face in, and the right hand goes in front of the abdomen *(fig 198)*. Pick up the right foot, and step forward onto the heel *(fig 199)*. Shift the weight onto the right foot as the right hand goes outside the right knee and the left hand pushes forward *(fig 200)*.

TAI CHI CHUAN – A COMPARATIVE STUDY

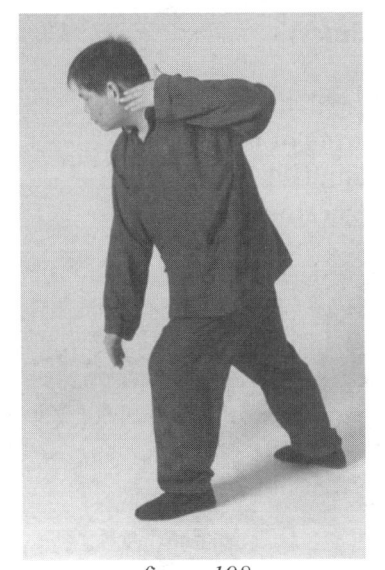

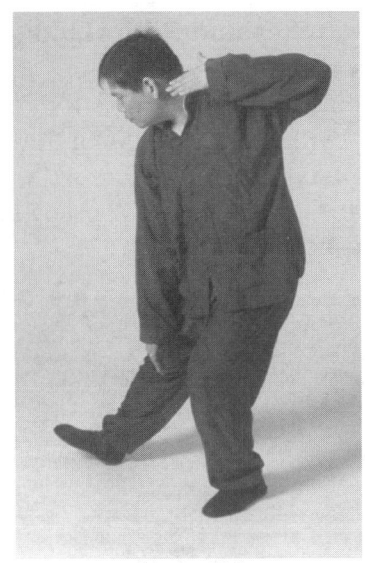

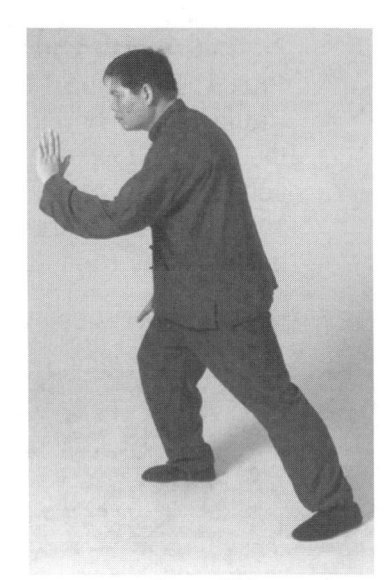

figure 198   *figure 199*   *figure 200*

37. Step Forward and Punch Downward

From the preceding movement, turn the right foot out. The right hand comes up to the right ear with the palm face in and the left hand goes down in front of the abdomen *(fig 201)*. Pick up the left foot, and step forward onto the heel *(fig 202)*. As the weight shifts forward to the left foot, extend the left hand before the chest, and close the right hand into a fist. As the weight continues shifting to the left foot, the right fist punches downward, and the left palm arrives at the right elbow *(fig 203)*.

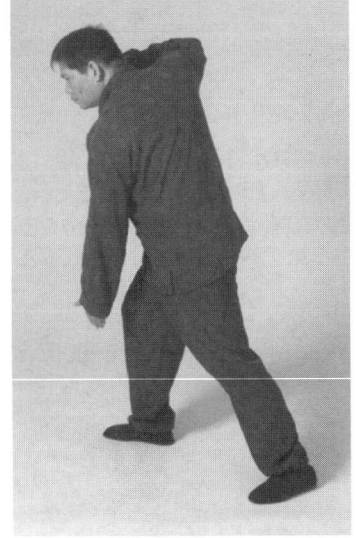

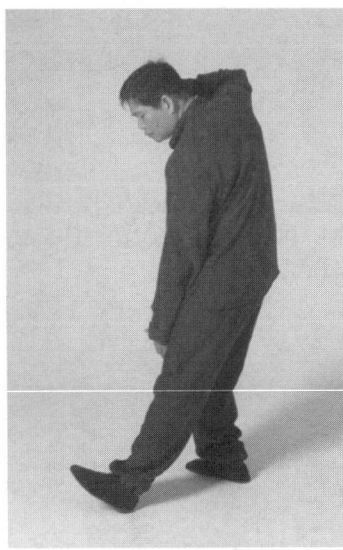

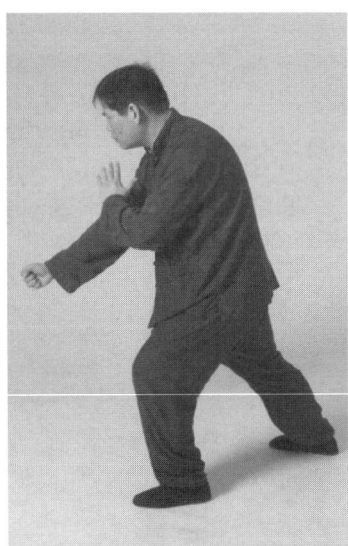

figure 201   *figure 202*   *figure 203*

THE 48 MOVEMENT SMALL FRAME SOLO FORM

38. Step Forward and Grasp Sparrow's Tail
Part 1: Warding Off
From the preceding movement, open the right fist, and bring the right hand up to join with the left hand in front of the abdomen *(fig 204)*. Pick up the right foot, and step forward onto the heel *(fig 205)*. Shift the weight forward, and push the hands forward *(fig 206)*.

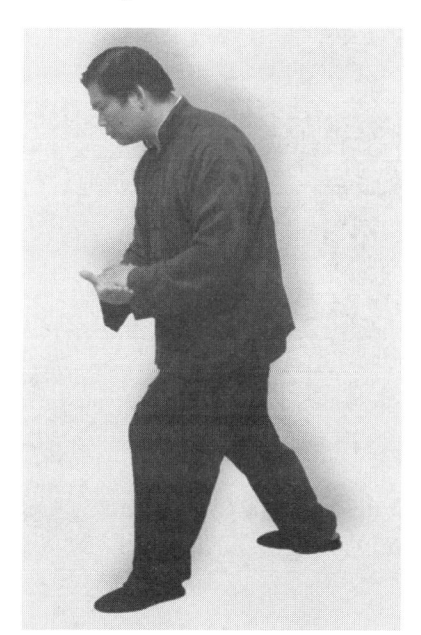

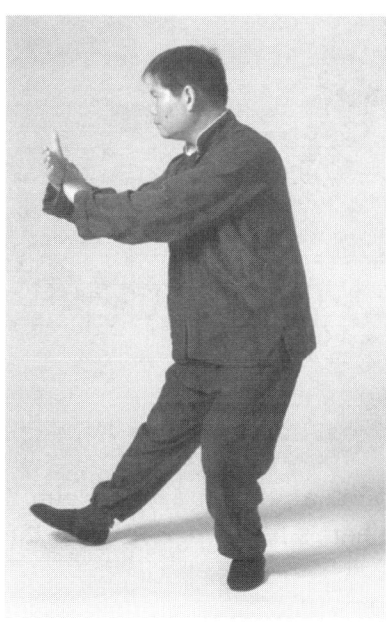

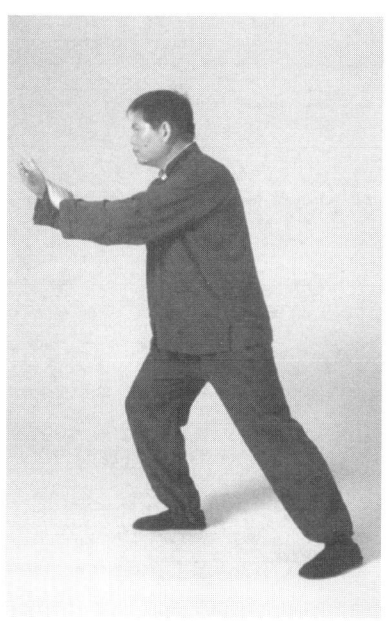

figure 204   *figure 205*   *figure 206*

Part 2: Roll Back
From the preceding movement, turn the right hand to face down and the left hand to face up *(fig 207a)*. Pull the hands back to the hip with the right toes lifting upward *(fig 207b)*.

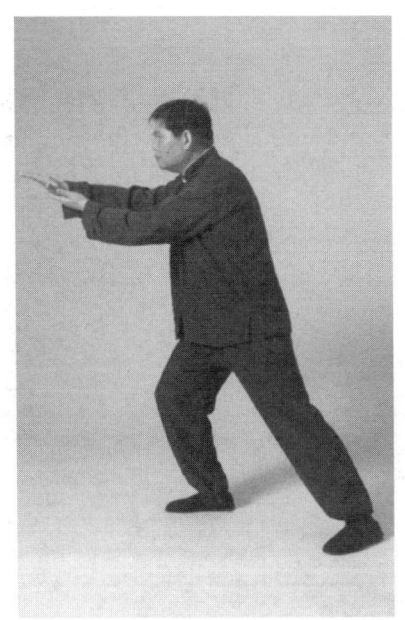

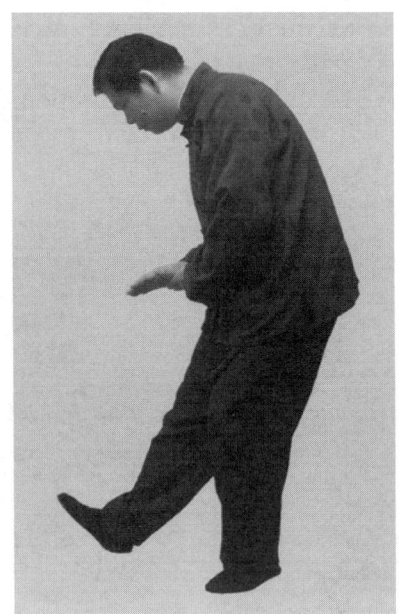

figure 207a *figure 207b*

Part 3: Press
From the preceding movement, turn the right palm face up and the left palm face down *(fig 207c)*. The hands press forward, and the body weight shifts onto the right foot *(fig 207d)*.

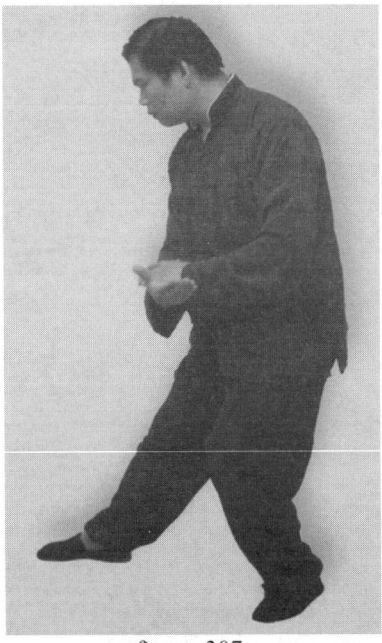

figure 207c *figure 207d*

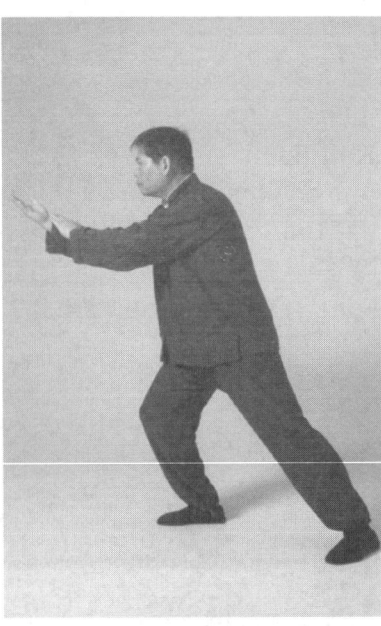

Part 4: Push

From the preceding movement, the hands circle back above the right shoulder with the right toes lifting off the ground *(fig 207e)*. Turn the right palm so it faces down. Then push the hands forward with the body's weight shifting onto the right foot *(figs 207f & 207g)*.

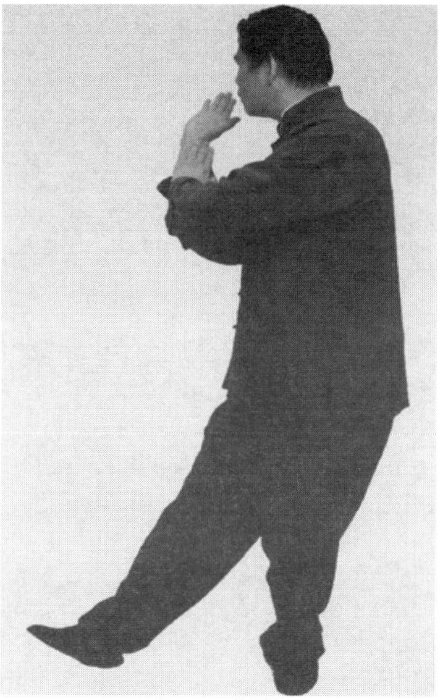

figure 207e

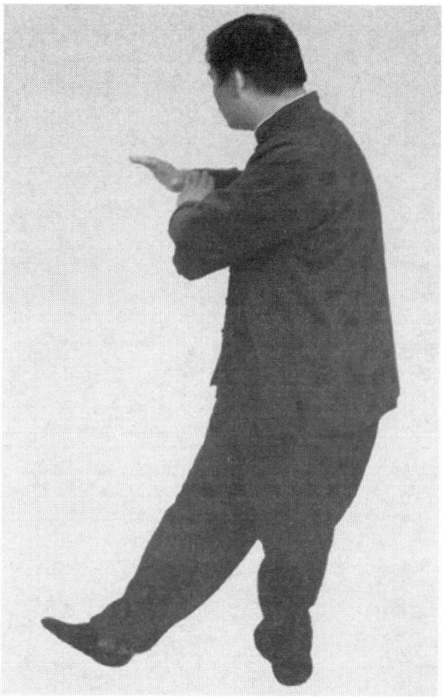

figure 207f

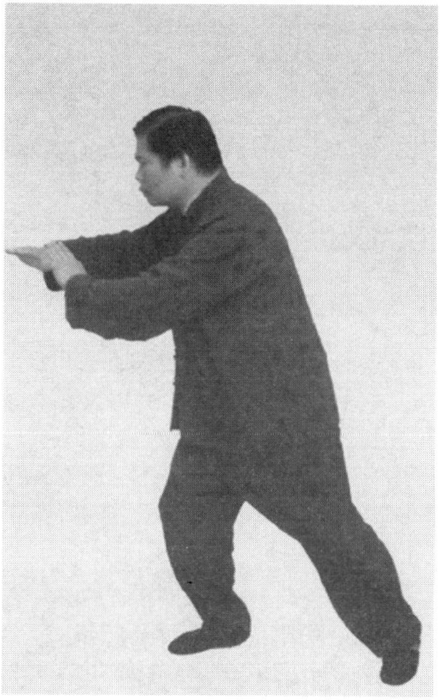

figure 207g

39. Single Whip

From the preceding movement, continue by pushing the hands to the left with the weight shifting onto the left foot and the right toes turning in *(fig 208)*. Circle the hands back to the right with the weight shifting onto the right foot *(fig 209)*. The right fingers come together to form a beak; bend the wrist to form a hook. With the weight on the right foot, pick up the left foot, and step to the left with the toes pointing to the corner *(fig 210)*. Shift the weight onto the left foot as the eyes follow the left palm across the body to the left *(fig 211)*.

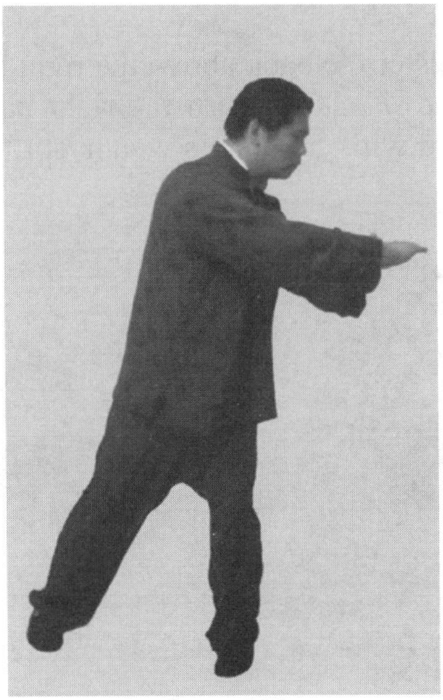

figure 208

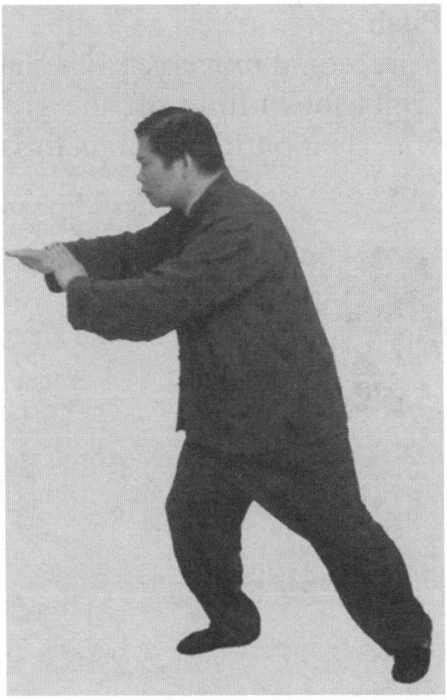

figure 209

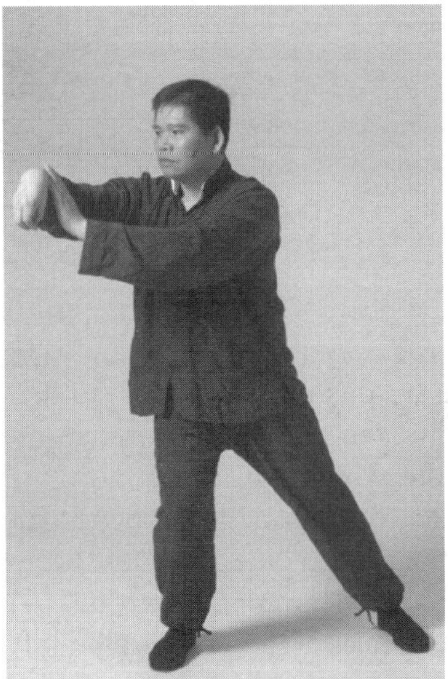

figure 210

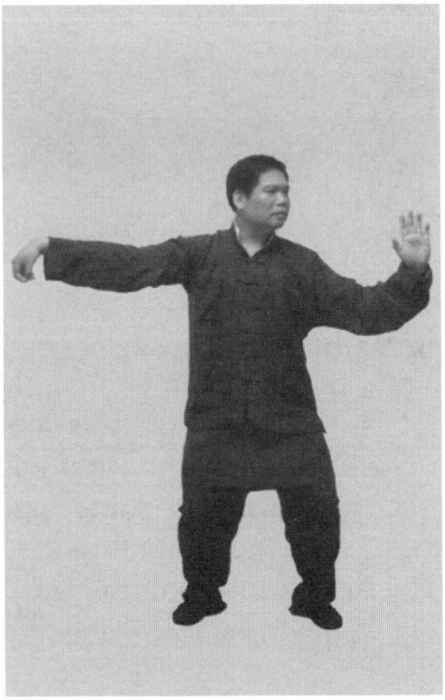

figure 211

40. Lower the Snake Body
From the preceding movement, open the right hand and move it like a pendulum to the left wrist *(fig 212)*. Turn the right foot outward, and bring the hands to the chest *(fig 213)*. Lower the body with the weight on the right foot

and the left toes turning inward. The left hand extends along the left leg *(fig 214)*.

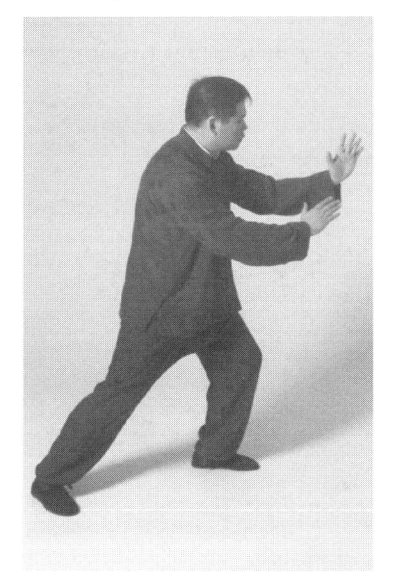

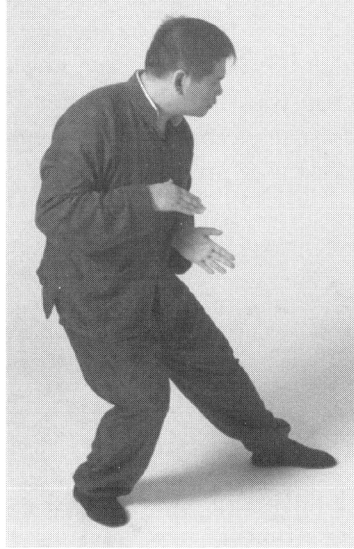

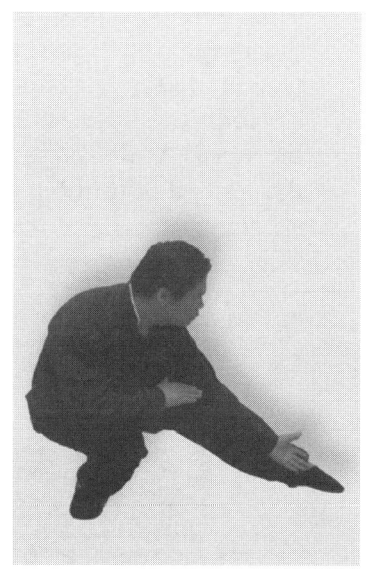

figure 212

figure 213

figure 214

41. Step Forward to Become Seven Star

From the preceding movement, turn the left toes out. Shift the weight onto the left foot, and position the left hand in front of the chest with the fingers pointing up. The right hand arrives on the right hip *(fig 215)*. Pick up the right foot, and step forward onto the toes. Then bring the right hand up to cross outside the left wrist with the palms facing out *(fig 216)*.

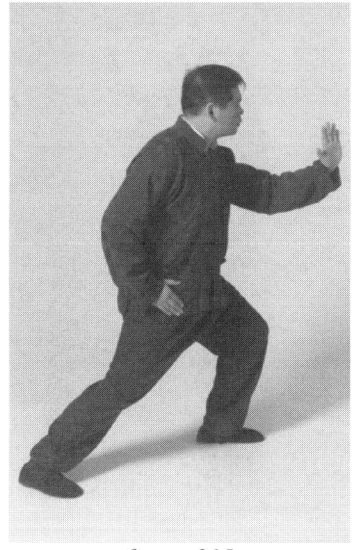

figure 215

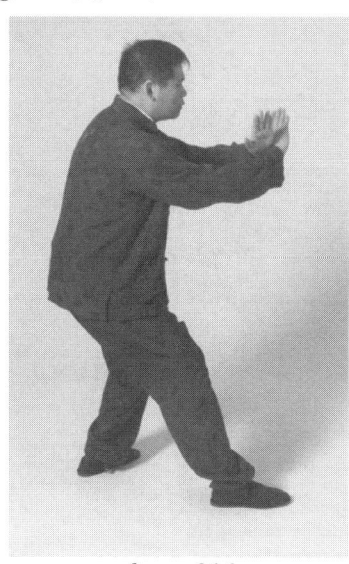

figure 216

42. Retreat to Ride Tiger

From the preceding movement, pick up the right foot, and step back *(fig 217)*. Turn the palms to face down, and bring them back to the chest while shifting the weight onto the right foot *(fig 218)*. Separate the hands with the right palm pushing to the right and the left hand forming a hook and extending to the left. To form the hook, first bring the fingers together like a beak, and then bend the wrist. At the same time that the hands are separating, the left foot lifts off the ground with the toes pointing down. The body still faces forward *(figs 219 & 220)*.

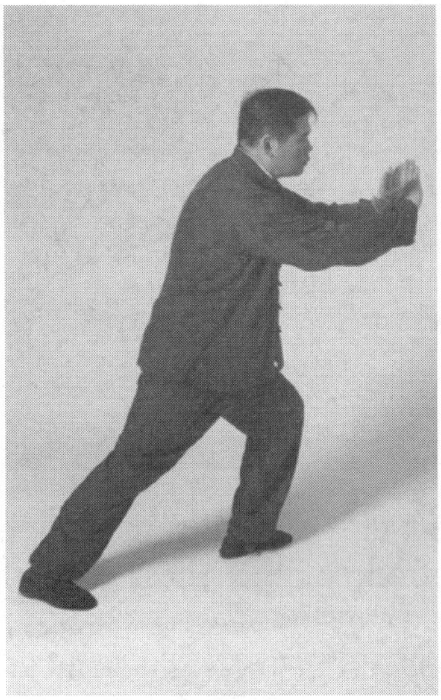

figure 217

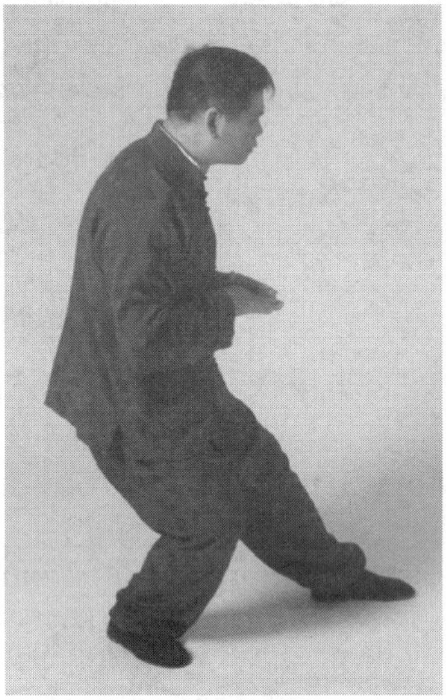

figure 218

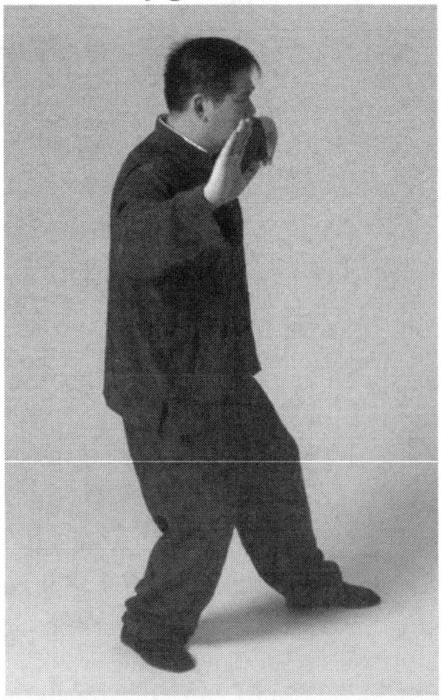

figure 219

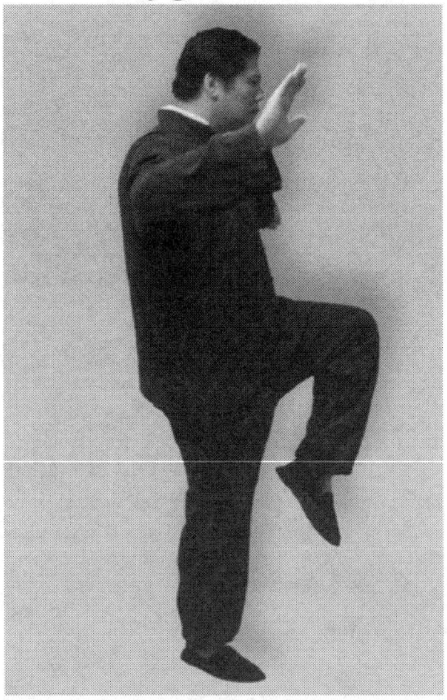

figure 220

43. Turn Around Hit the Face

From the preceding movement, with the left foot still suspended, bring the right hand to the chest *(fig 221)* and the left palm across the body to the right. Pivot on the right toes to the right, turning the body and landing the left foot in front of the right foot. The left hand pushes forward above the right hand *(fig 222)*.

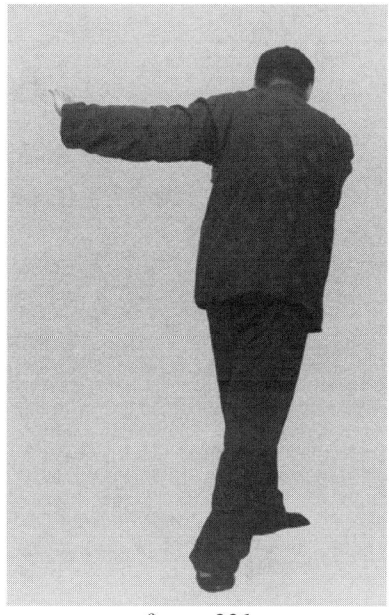

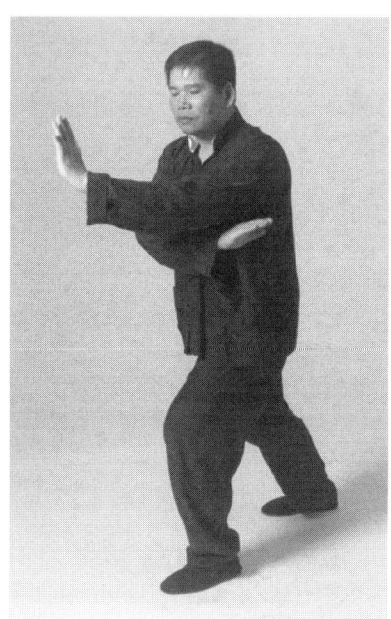

figure 221

figure 222

44. Lotus Kick

From the preceding movement, with the weight on the left foot, turn the left toes inward and the body to the right, moving the hands across the body to the right and turning the right toes out to the right. The right palm arrives facing the right corner, and the left palm faces the right elbow *(figs 223 & 224)*. Pick up the right foot, and do a round kick. As the kick moves from left to right, the hands move across the body from right to left, brushing over the kick *(figs 225 & 226)*.

TAI CHI CHUAN – A COMPARATIVE STUDY

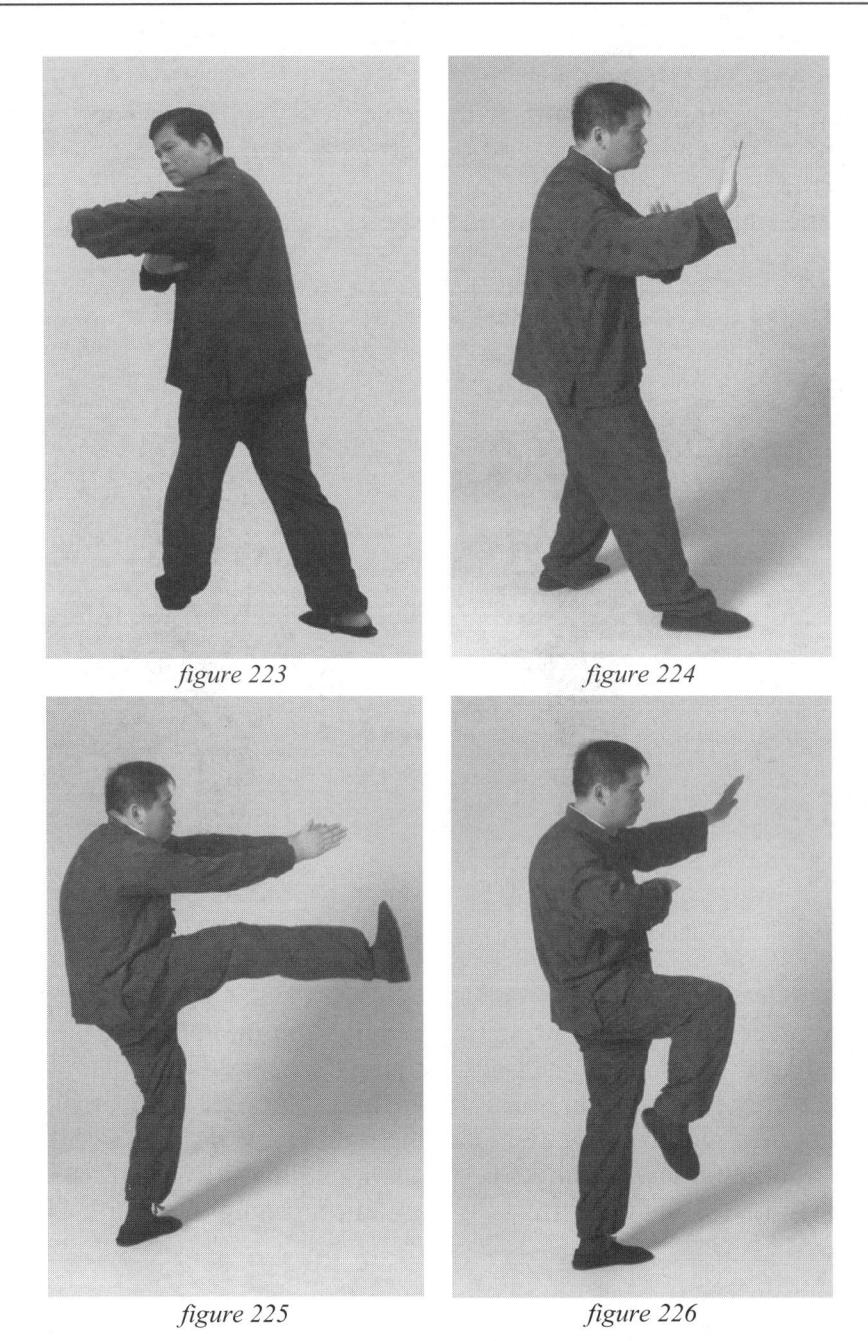

figure 223

figure 224

figure 225

figure 226

45. Shooting Tiger

From the preceding movement, the right foot steps down to the right corner, and the hands come down to the right knee *(fig 227)*. Close the hands into fists; then bring the fists up. Position the right fist near the right ear, and punch the left fist forward to the left corner like a hammer *(figs 228 & 229)*.

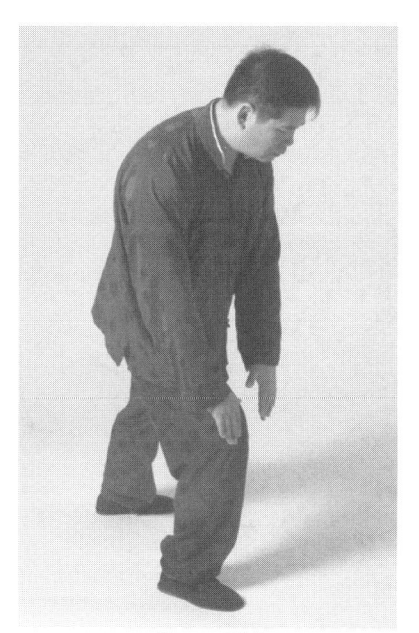

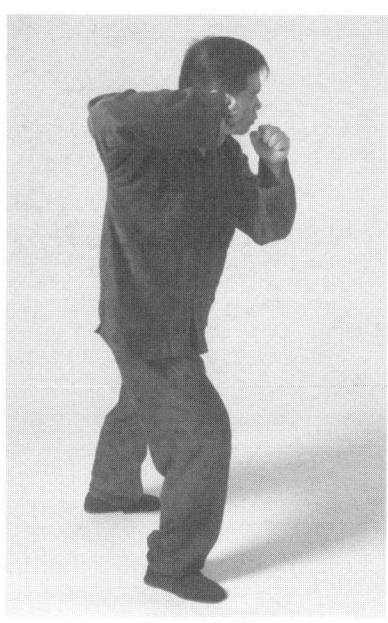

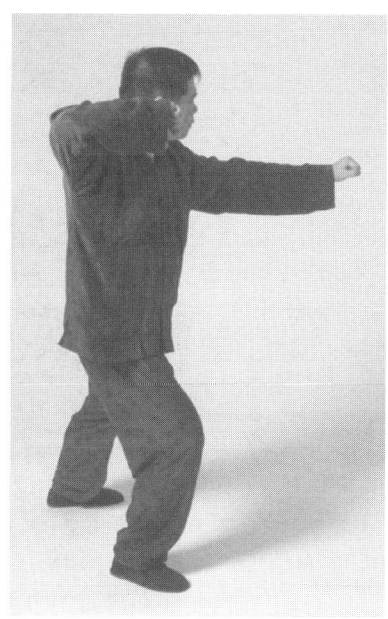

figure 227   *figure 228*   *figure 229*

46. Step Forward, Parry, Intercept and Punch

From the preceding movement, open the left fist, and turn the hand up; then bring it back under the right fist at the abdomen *(figs 230 & 231)*. Pick up the left foot, and step forward onto the heel. Separate the hands by pushing the left palm forward and pulling the right fist back to the right hip *(fig 232)*. Shift the weight onto the left foot, and punch the right fist forward with the left hand coming to the right wrist *(fig 233)*.

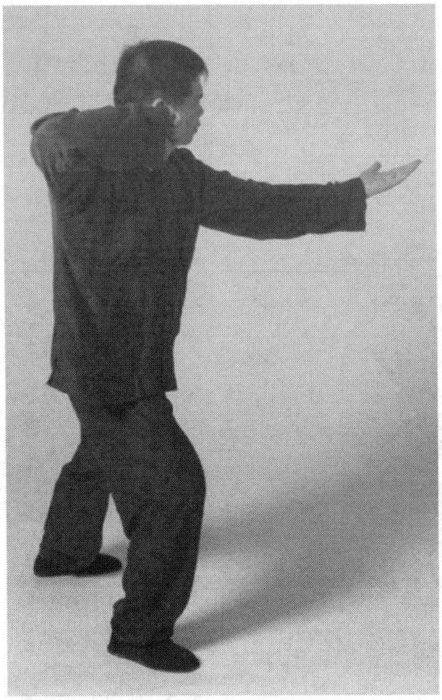

TAI CHI CHUAN – A COMPARATIVE STUDY

figure 230

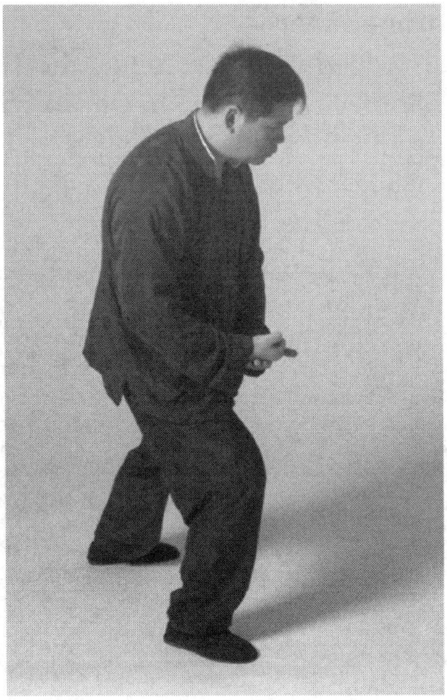

figure 231

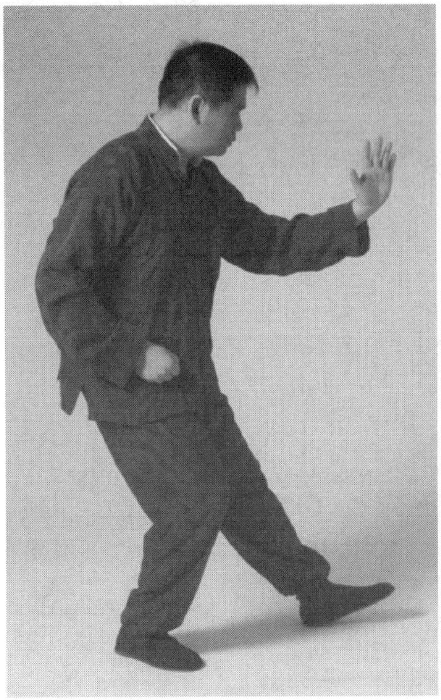

figure 232

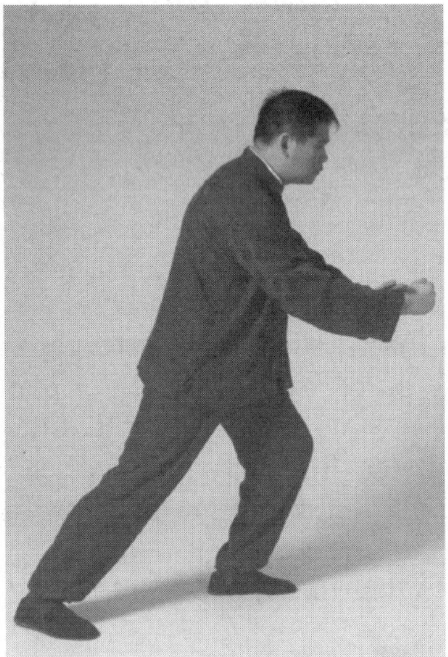

figure 233

47. Seal Tightly

From the preceding movement, put the left hand under the right wrist *(fig 234)*. Open the hands, and bring them back to the chest with the palms facing in as the weight shifts onto the right foot and the left toes lift up *(fig 235)*. Turn the palms to face out. Then push the palms forward and downward while shifting the weight onto the left foot *(figs 236 & 237)*.

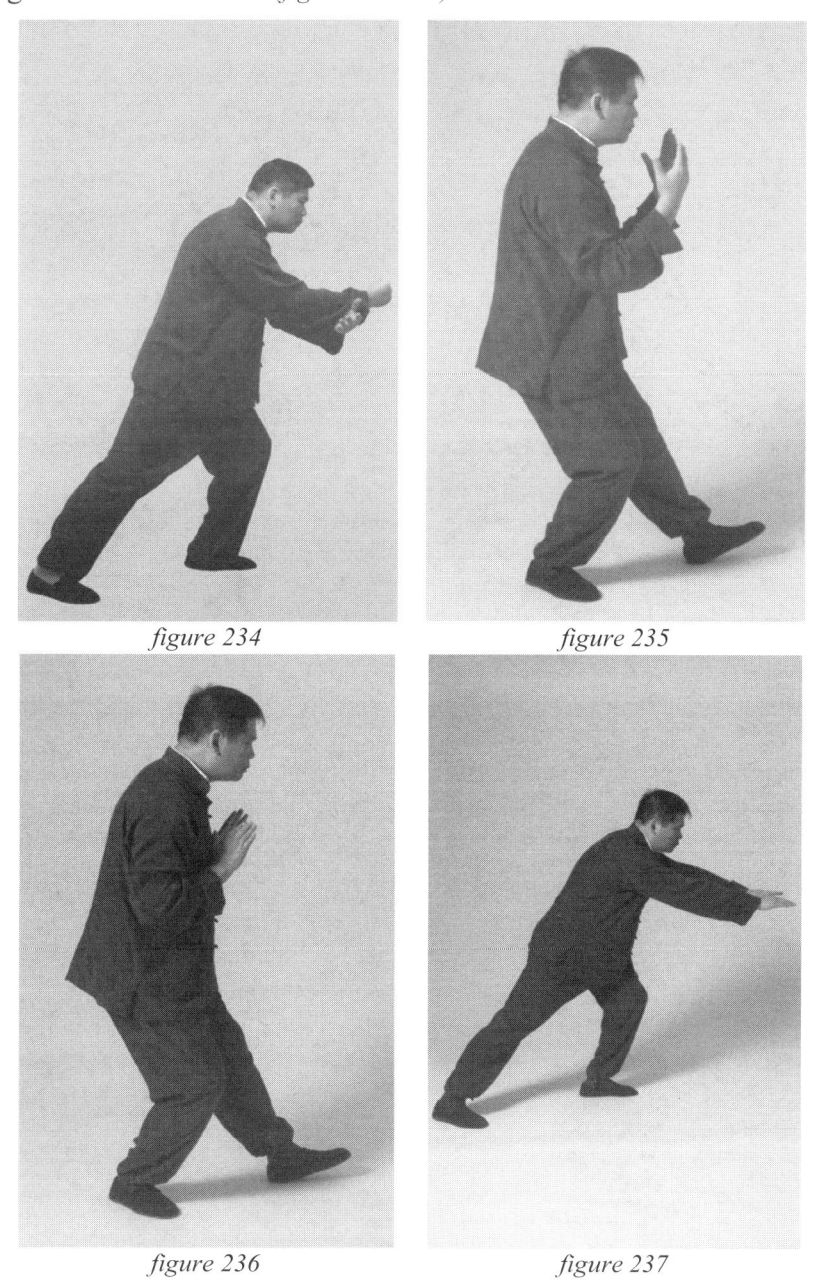

figure 234

figure 235

figure 236

figure 237

48. Closing Tai Chi Chuan

From the preceding movement, the right hand continues, moving in a downward arc like a pendulum to the right with the right foot turning out and the left foot turning in *(fig 238)*. The right hand continues the motion and comes up above the head *(fig 239)*. The left hand follows and joins the right hand above the head with the two palms facing out and the left foot stepping up next to the right foot *(fig 240)*. Lower the hands; then separate them to the sides of the body *(fig 241)*.

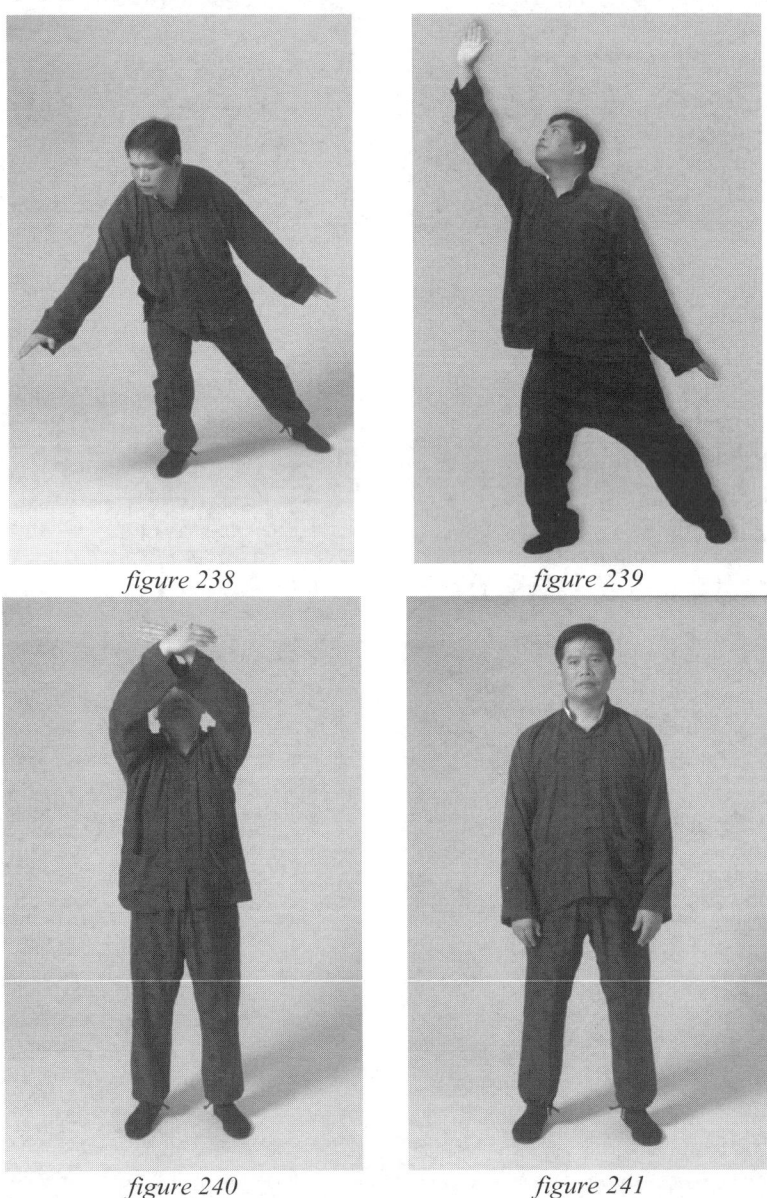

figure 238

figure 239

figure 240

figure 241

Chapter 8
The Three Emphases

After finishing the first seven chapters, a reader may ask, "With so many forms, which should I practice and why?"

Tai Chi Chuan is an internal Chinese martial art. It is different from most of the Chinese martial art systems. And every usage and practice in Tai Chi Chuan differs from our daily life activity. Therefore, one should not compare it with a typical habit or sport. Generally, one can see the differences of Tai Chi Chuan training in three areas:

1. The training emphasizes following principles, not power as with most martial arts.
2. The training emphasizes improving the root, not the function, as many health maintenance exercises do today.
3. The training emphasizes improving the body, unlike most martial arts, which focus on the application of individual techniques.

With these three emphases in mind, one can see that the variations of the solo form are but applying the form to improve the body and *chi*. Different body conditions require different executions of movement, and consequently the results differ. This method is comparable to education; the same knowledge is presented differently to students of different levels. Obviously, the knowledge is presented differently to an elementary pupil than to a high school or college student. Different presentations accommodate varying qualities of a student body and its respective academic levels.

The three forms I introduced in the previous chapters differ in the execution of movements but share a similar philosophy and principle. With these differences in execution come different requirements for the body and its parts. These differences developed into the many styles of Tai Chi Chuan practiced today. In the Large Frame Solo Form, the movements mostly involve the joints and four limbs. While in each movement of the Medium Frame Solo Form, the joints, the four limbs, and the trunk are equally involved. Finally, the movements of the Small Frame Solo Form more greatly involve the trunk than the four limbs. When one is moving the trunk, the internal physiologic organs are more involved. Generally, it is more difficult to move the trunk than the limbs. Therefore, it is better for one to begin with the Large Frame Solo Form and work his or her way to the Small Frame Solo Form. Yang Cheng Fu said, "Begin with larger movement. Later, work with compact movement." For the remainder of this chapter, I would like to further elaborate the three emphases so practitioners will have a clearer understanding of their significance.

1. The training emphasizes principle, not power.
Here, principle refers to the Tai Chi philosophy. Zheng San Feng created Tai Chi Chuan based on Taoist philosophy and Lao Tzu's teaching. Therefore, to study Tai Chi Chuan correctly, one should understand the philosophy of Tai Chi, Yin Yang theory, some of Taoism's canonical works, traditional Chinese medical theory, and *The Internal Classic of the Yellow Emperor*.

In order to better understand Tai Chi Chuan and practice it correctly, one must understand the philosophy of Tai Chi, or Yin Yang theory. The *Tai Chi Chuan Classics* say, "Tai Chi came from Wu Chi, the mother of Yin Yang." Lao Tzu's *Tao Teh Ching* says, "Tai Chi is born from One, One gave birth to two, two gave birth to three, three gave birth to ten thousand things." "Tao" is also known as "Wu Chi" or "Void." "One" refers to "Wu Chi." It is also referred to as "Great Void." This "Great Void" refers to emptiness that is filled with *chi,* or energy. It is the original source of a body's health condition. "Two" refers to the Yin Yang components. The *Tai Chi Chuan Classics* say, "The heaven and earth are one great Tai Chi. The human body is one small Tai Chi." One can see that "two" is manifested in Tai Chi Chuan movements as substantial and insubstantial, hard and soft, fast and slow, opening and closing, round and square, and so on. "Three" refers to three dimensions. One sees this manifested as circular motion or spiral motion in Tai Chi Chuan movements. Therefore, one can see, "Great Void" is the true nature of Tai Chi and its manifestation of relaxation, softness, lightness, and agility.

The requirements of Tai Chi Chuan practices are "apply the mind, not physical power"; "apply the intent to guide the *chi*"; "apply the *chi* to circulate throughout the body." The meaning behind these statements is to have a relaxed, tranquil, and natural body. When the body is natural, tranquil, and relaxed, it is easier for the conscious spirit to appear and function. The concept of "relaxation" in Tai Chi Chuan is the external expression of the yin component. It is equivalent to the concept of "empty and insubstantial" in Taoist philosophy. If the body is relaxed, the *chi* circulates better inside the body. This is as if the body were empty: there is room for more invisible *chi*. The more *chi* the body has, the greater its strength and the better its material composition. The mind and body relaxation requirements are indirectly guided by one's conscious spirit to function better in the processes of mobilizing the body's *chi,* circulating the blood, and clearing the body's meridian channels to cultivate the original *chi*. "Tranquility" is associated with the quality of calmness. Generally, when there is calmness, the conscious spirit appears. This is often expressed as "apply the tranquility to nurture the spirit." The substance called *chi* does not occupy any space, nor does it have mass or shape. It is an intangible substance. In order to improve this substance, one should work with something that shares the feature of intangibility, such as a principle.

2. The training emphasizes the root, not the function.
What is the root of Tai Chi Chuan? It is the original substance that fuels every living thing. As the Taoist literature states, "You can say a thousand words to explain it. It is but clear the mind, enhance the root to cultivate the original *chi*, and strengthen the body condition. This produces a result better than your opponent's." The "root" of Tai Chi Chuan is *chi* cultivation. When the Tai Chi Chuan training emphasizes the root, one is placing emphasis on improving the body condition by increasing the *chi* inside the body. However, when the Tai Chi Chuan training emphasizes the "function," one is placing emphasis on the quality and application of each individual technique. Improving the condition of the *chi,* and the awareness and coordination of the whole body, agrees with Tai Chi Chuan's philosophy.

One can see that the training which focuses on the root aims to enhance the foundation as well as the original *chi*. It yields the best result when it follows the philosophy of having the body's inside and outside attributes working together: "When one enhances the root, the tree will have many leaves. When one supplements the spring, it will last longer." When one is strictly practicing and refining each Tai Chi Chuan movement with specific instruction, it is but following the method of "enhance the root, supplement the spring." When enhancing the original *chi* and the kidney *chi* during Tai Chi Chuan practices by incorporating waist rotation into each movement, the condition of the physiologic organs improves and energizes, and one will have quicker reaction time and better coordination. In addition, enhancing the *chi* also benefits the upper body with agility, the mid-section with vitality, and the lower body with stability. These are the important ingredients for a powerful martial art strike.

Practicing Tai Chi Chuan correctly means following the instruction of "regulate the spirit, regulate the breathing, and regulate the body." This instruction is common to Chi Kung disciplines. Chi Kung is a simple exercise to enhance and nurture the root. Therefore, Tai Chi Chuan is also known as a dynamic Chi Kung exercise of the Taoist school. In Tai Chi Chuan, the instruction for the intent is to provide specific *chi* circulation inside the body so that each movement will agree with Tai Chi Chuan's requirements, features, and rules. With a conscientious effort to develop the root, Tai Chi Chuan practices can enhance the *chi* and refine the body.

Through dedication, the quality of Tai Chi Chuan movements is improved. The improved movements are observably better coordinated, and all the movements are initiated from the rotation of the waist. This improvement is the result of incorporating waist rotation into Tai Chi Chuan practices such as the following: dynamic Chi Kung exercise, Tai Chi Chuan Solo Form practices, solo drill exercise, shaking the spear exercise, and dynamic push hand exercise. These all train the martial fundamentals for more power and coordination and enhance the original *chi*. As one can see, Tai Chi Chuan is a complete Chinese martial art system that has a very extensive curriculum.

The *Tai Chi Chuan Classics* have this to say about balance: "When one part of the body moves, all parts of the body follow. When one part is inactive, all parts should be inactive…. When outside and inside are inactive, apply the inactive to neutralize the active." Throughout the entire Tai Chi Chuan Solo Form practices, if one pays attention to all the active and inactive attributes, one will execute each movement in a balanced and comfortable manner.

3. The training emphasizes the body, not an individual technique.

Here, the body refers to the body's movement, the quality of the movement, and its components. If a person's training emphasizes only the application of individual techniques, he or she will forego Tai Chi Chuan's multiple benefits. This is similar to writing Chinese calligraphy. If one only pays attention to each individual stroke, neglecting the character as a whole, the calligraphy is poorly done.

In some aspects, Tai Chi Chuan is like all martial arts. Each movement must be proper and powerful and stepping must be quick. The body, hands, and feet have to move quickly with coordination and power. The eyes have to be sharp. In sum, the body is very light, balanced, and nimble, and the skin is very sensitive so one can easily detect the opponent's movement and power. This requires the body to be in an optimum condition. One observes that Tai Chi Chuan movements are done slowly and powerlessly. This seems counter to all principles of martial art which imply that each movement has to be done quickly and powerfully. However, there is a common saying among Tai Chi Chuan practitioners: to practice the solo form slowly is to work on the martial fundamentals, and to practice the solo form quickly is to work on the martial application. The Tai Chi Chuan Solo Form is done slowly to work on body mechanics so one is able to move quickly when needed.

To demonstrate all the hard and soft attributes in Tai Chi Chuan, externally one should perform the solo form softly, firmly, and with agility. Internally, one should perform the solo form with concentration, clearly defining substantial and insubstantial. In other words, when the body has hard and soft attributes, the body is able to act very quickly; yielding and discharge powers seem to happen at the same time. The body's coordination and balance appear supported from all directions. The muscles' activities and physiologic organs are highly coordinated. If the body has an excess of either hard or soft attributes, it cannot act harmoniously. This is why the *Tai Chi Chuan Classics* prefer 50% from each attribute as the best combination.

The *Tai Chi Chuan Classics* say, "The mind controls the *chi*; let it calm and sink so the *chi* can penetrate inside the bone…. One should concentrate on the spirit, not on *chi*; if the concentration is on the *chi*, it causes stagnation." These quotations indicate that during Tai Chi Chuan practices, what one should follow and concentrate on—in every movement—is based on the intent, not power. Let the intent move first; then the physical movement follows. If one follows this method, the intent will get there first, followed by the *chi*. When the *chi* gets there, the power will follow. When the movement is calm, stable, and has control, it has the potential to yield a lot of power. If one follows this method of practicing Tai Chi Chuan regularly, the *chi* will penetrate into the bones, and a higher level of *chi* circulation will prepare the body for more rigorous activity. In addition to the above, one practicing Tai Chi Chuan should pay attention to stretching the body and joints to improve the chi circulation, body integration, and the elasticity of muscles and tendons. Also, pay attention to the spiral rotation of the waist, upper and lower body coordination, and unifying inside and outside in each movement. After the body is trained, one can see a simple and gentle waving of the hand yielding a lot of power.

Tai Chi Chuan martial skill should be performed based on the opponent's action. Generally speaking, it should be centered on the opponent's action and situation. The *Tai Chi Chuan Classics* say, "When one has attained skill, one engages the opponent instinctually without thinking. When the technique comes, it will come naturally." This is the result of a well-trained body.

Tai Chi Chuan is one of the traditions of Chinese culture. It has a long history and an extensive body of knowledge. It is both old and new. It is elegant and simple. It is a martial art and a performing art. It is the product of ancient Chinese philosophy, traditional Chinese medicine, Chinese martial art, natural living art, and health maintenance exercises. From this, one can see that it is different from conventional sports. During Tai Chi Chuan practices, high emphasis is placed on the intent directing all the movements, sinking the *chi*, a tranquil mind, a relaxed body, and natural breathing. In addition, as with all martial art training, it is necessary to have the coordination of the hands, eyes, body, and stepping. As such, Tai Chi Chuan is a discipline of bodily integration. Regularly practicing Tai Chi Chuan is good for the body's central nervous system, circulatory system, respiratory system, muscular skeletal system, and body metabolism.

Chapter 9
Envoi

After a recent workshop teaching the 43 Movement Large Frame Solo Form in Europe, one of the students came up to me and asked how he should schedule and prioritize his time to practice all the forms he knew. He had told me before that he knew several Tai Chi Chuan solo forms. My reply to this student's question was directly related to his situation.

I have had the good fortune of studying Yang Style Tai Chi Chuan under four generous teachers, which has given me a better understanding of the scope of the Yang Style system. While growing up, I studied with my father, Gin Soon Chu, and his classmate Ip Tai Tak, both disciples of Grandmaster Yeung Sau Chung, the oldest son of Yang Cheng Fu. After China opened its door to welcome visitors, I ventured there to study first with Professor Fang Ning, a disciple of Tsau Li Shu, who was one of Yang Cheng Fu's senior students; later I studied with Liu Xi Wen, a disciple of Zhang Fu Chen, who was, in turn, a disciple of Yang Cheng Fu, Yang Shao Hou, and Xu Yu Sheng.

In previous chapters, I explained why the Classical Yang Family Tai Chi Chuan has several tai chi chuan solo forms. Although there are several, one does not need to practice them all in order to improve one's martial arts skill. As long as one is dedicated and diligent in practice, one's skill will improve with time. From firsthand knowledge, I have come to understand that skill is developed from practice, not from knowing a lot of forms. One day's labor will reap one day's reward.

Although many Tai Chi Chuan practitioners today say that one Tai Chi Chuan solo form is better than another solo form or that one family's style is better than another's, this is not true. Superiority and inferiority happen only in teaching. Each Tai Chi Chuan solo form was created for a specific purpose. Naming styles for a specific family began only in the last few decades. If one has a copy of a Tai Chi Chuan book in Chinese that was published before the 1950s, most likely the book's title is simply *Tai Chi Chuan* without any family name attached to it. My father summarized it best on this subject when he said, "Tai Chi Chuan is one family." He put this in Chinese writing high up on a wall in our school.

About the Author

Vincent Chu, M.Ed., is the sixth generation lineage practitioner of the Classical Yang Family Style of Tai Chi Chuan. He is the second of three sons of Gin Soon Chu. He began learning Tai Chi Chuan from his father when he was very young. At age 16, he began assisting his father at the Gin Soon Tai Chi Chuan Club in Boston, and he has been teaching at the Brookline Adult and Community Education Program since 1984. To further his understanding and knowledge in Classical Yang Style Tai Chi Chuan, he obtained instruction from Masters Ip Tai Tak, Liu Xi Wen, Ou Wen Wei, and Professor Fang Ning. He has conducted many workshops and seminars in Canada and Europe, and he is a frequent contributor to martial arts publications to share his knowledge. He published his first book, *Beginner's Tai Chi Chuan*, in 2000. Video instruction available from Master Chu include *Tai Chi Chuan for Beginners*, *Yang Family Tai Chi Chuan: Large Frame Short Form*, *Center Harmony Qigong*, *Three Circles Exercise*, *Yang Style Tai Chi Chuan: Medium Frame Solo Form*, *Tai Chi Chuan for Beginners: 15 Techniques Small Frame Solo Form*, *Tai Chi Chuan for Beginners: 12 Techniques Large Frame Solo Form*, *Tai Chi Chuan for Beginners: 8 Techniques Medium Frame Solo Form*, *Tai Chi Chuan for Beginners: 14 Techniques Middle Frame Solo Form*, and *Tai Chi Chuan for Beginners: 12 Techniques Returning Tai Chi Chuan*.

Gin Soon Tai Chi Chuan Federation - Curriculum

I. Tai Chi Chuan Fundamentals
    a. Tai Chi Kung
    b. Center Harmony Qigong
    c. Three Circles Exercise
    d. San Feng Yi Jin Jing

II. Tai Chi Chuan for Beginners
    a. 8 Techniques Medium Frame Solo Form
    b. 11 Techniques AJ Tai Chi Chuan
    c. 12 Techniques Large Frame Solo Form
    d. 12 Techniques Returning Tai Chi Chuan
    e. 14 Techniques Middle Frame Solo Form
    f. 15 Techniques Small Frame Solo Form
    g. 22 Techniques Medium Frame Solo Form

III. Comparative Tai Chi Chuan
    a. 41 Techniques Returning Tai Chi Chuan
    b. 42 Techniques Application Solo Form
    c. 42 Techniques Medium Frame Solo Form
    d. 43 Techniques Large Frame Solo Form
    e. 43 Techniques Middle Frame Solo Form
    f. 45 Techniques A.J. Tai Chi Chuan/ Returning Tai Chi Chuan
    g. 48 Techniques Small Frame Solo Form

IV. Traditional Tai Chi Chuan Solo Forms
    a. Middle Frame Solo Form (Medium Circle Form)
    b. Large Frame Solo Form (Large Circle Form)
    c. Middle Frame Solo Form (Middle Circle Form)
    d. Small Frame Solo Form (Small Circle Form)
    e. Crane Form
    f. Tiger Form
    g. Snake Form
    h. Tai Chi Chung Chuan
    i. 108 Techniques Tai Chi Chuan
    j. Pre-arranged Sparring Set (San Sou)
    k. 13 Animals Forms (chicken, monkey, crane, tiger, bear, snake, phoenix, toad, lion, dragon, magpie, horse, and lynx)

V. Push Hand Exercises
    a. Stationary Step Single Join Hands
    b. Stationary Step Double Join Hands
    c. Dynamic Stepping (Stepping on the Flowers)
    d. Dynamic Step Single Join Hands
    e. Dynamic Step Double Join Hands
    f. Great Pulling (Da Lu)
    g. Opening and Closing
    h. Four Corners and Four Directions
    i. Dynamic Push Hands

VI. Weapons
- a. Tai Chi Staff
- b. Tai Chi Knife
- c. Tai Chi Sword
- d. Tai Chi 13 Spears Set

The Gin Soon Tai Chi Chuan Federation

The Gin Soon Tai Chi Club was founded in 1969 with permission from Grandmaster Yeung Sau Chung to propagate the Classical Yang Family Style Tai Chi Chuan in North America. It is the oldest school teaching Tai Chi Chuan in the Greater Boston Area today.

Although there are many schools of Tai Chi Chuan available in the United States, the Gin Soon Tai Chi Club is different from others because its founder, Grandmaster Gin Soon Chu, is a disciple who studied with and was authorized to teach by Grandmaster Yang Sau-Chung, firstborn and heir of the legendary Yang Cheng-Fu. Grandmaster Chu received a deep and well-rounded training, first from Master Lai Hok Soon and then from Grandmaster Yang Sau-Chung, a training that covered all aspects of Classical Yang Family Style Tai Chi Chuan.

The school has attracted many students from around the world with its traditional approach to training characterized by personal individualized attention, emphasis on correct forms, personal development, integration of body, *chi*, and intent, repetition, mutual respect, and hard work.

Over the years, many students have graduated from the school and become instructors themselves. In 1995, the Gin Soon Tai Chi Chuan Federation was established to better serve our members who come from different countries.

We are receptive to teaching workshops and seminars (private or group) at the headquarters or abroad. All of the instruction is given by Grandmaster Gin Soon Chu and his sons, Master Vincent Chu and Master Gordon Chu.

Gin Soon Tai Chi Chuan Federation
33 Harrison Avenue, 2nd floor
Boston, MA 02111
Tel: (617) 542-4442
Website: www.gstaichi.org

Classical Yang Style Tai Chi Chuan Video Series by Vincent Chu

1. Tai Chi Chuan For Beginners (vcd)
   Running Time: 55 Minutes
   Price: $29.95

2. Yang Family Tai Chi Chuan: Large Frame Short Form (vcd)
   Running Time: 52 Minutes
   Price: $39.9

3. Center Harmony Qigong (vhs or vcd)
   Running Time: 45 Minutes
   Price: $29.95

4. Three Circles Exercise (vhs or vcd)
   Running Time: 45 Minutes
   Price: $29.95

5. Yang Style Tai Chi Chuan (two dvd set)
   Running Time: 3 hours 10 minutes
   Price: $99.95

6. Tai Chi Chuan For Beginners: Fifteen Techniques Small Frame Solo Form (dvd)
   Running Time: 57:58 minutes
   Price: $24.95

7. Tai Chi Chuan For Beginners: Twelve Techniques Large Frame Solo Form (dvd)
   Running Time: 74 minutes
   Price: $24.95

8. Tai Chi Chuan For Beginners: Eight Techniques Medium Frame Solo Form (dvd)
   Running Time: 59 minutes
   Price: $19.95

9. Tai Chi Chuan For Beginners: Fourteen Techniques Middle Frame Solo Form (dvd)
   Running Time: 87 minutes
   Price: $24.95

10. Tai Chi Chuan For Beginners: Twelve Techniques Returning Tai Chi Chuan (dvd)
    Running Time: 99 minutes
    Price: $29.95

Gin Soon Tai Chi Chuan Federation - Curriculum

I. **Tai Chi Chuan Fundamentals**
   a. Tai Chi Kung
   b. Center Harmony Qigong
   c. Three Circles Exercise
   d. San Feng Yi Jin Jing

II. **Tai Chi Chuan for Beginners**
   a. 8 Techniques Medium Frame Solo Form
   b. 11 Techniques AJ Tai Chi Chuan
   c. 12 Techniques Large Frame Solo Form
   d. 12 Techniques Returning Tai Chi Chuan
   e. 14 Techniques Middle Frame Solo Form
   f. 15 Techniques Small Frame Solo Form
   g. 22 Techniques Medium Frame Solo Form

III. **Comparative Tai Chi Chuan**
   a. 41 Techniques Returning Tai Chi Chuan
   b. 42 Techniques Application Solo Form
   c. 42 Techniques Medium Frame Solo Form
   d. 43 Techniques Large Frame Solo Form
   e. 43 Techniques Middle Frame Solo Form
   f. 45 Techniques A.J. Tai Chi Chuan/ Returning Tai Chi Chuan
   g. 48 Techniques Small Frame Solo Form

IV. **Traditional Tai Chi Chuan Solo Forms**
   a. Middle Frame Solo Form (Medium Circle Form)
   b. Large Frame Solo Form (Large Circle Form)
   c. Middle Frame Solo Form (Middle Circle Form)
   d. Small Frame Solo Form (Small Circle Form)
   e. Crane Form
   f. Tiger Form
   g. Snake Form
   h. Tai Chi Chung Chuan
   i. 108 Techniques Tai Chi Chuan
   j. Pre-arranged Sparring Set (San Sou)
   k. 13 Animals Forms (chicken, monkey, crane, tiger, bear, snake, phoenix, toad, lion, dragon, magpie, horse, and lynx)

V. **Push Hand Exercises**
   a. Stationary Step Single Join Hands
   b. Stationary Step Double Join Hands
   c. Dynamic Stepping (Stepping on the Flowers)
   d. Dynamic Step Single Join Hands
   e. Dynamic Step Double Join Hands
   f. Great Pulling (Da Lu)
   g. Opening and Closing
   h. Four Corners and Four Directions
   i. Dynamic Push Hands

VI. Weapons
   a.   Tai Chi Staff
   b.   Tai Chi Knife
   c.   Tai Chi Sword
   d.   Tai Chi 13 Spears Set

The Gin Soon Tai Chi Chuan Federation

The Gin Soon Tai Chi Club was founded in 1969 with permission from Grandmaster Yeung Sau Chung to propagate the Classical Yang Family Style Tai Chi Chuan in North America. It is the oldest school teaching Tai Chi Chuan in the Greater Boston Area today.

Although there are many schools of Tai Chi Chuan available in the United States, the Gin Soon Tai Chi Club is different from others because its founder, Grandmaster Gin Soon Chu, is a disciple who studied with and was authorized to teach by Grandmaster Yang Sau-Chung, firstborn and heir of the legendary Yang Cheng-Fu. Grandmaster Chu received a deep and well-rounded training, first from Master Lai Hok Soon and then from Grandmaster Yang Sau-Chung, a training that covered all aspects of Classical Yang Family Style Tai Chi Chuan.

The school has attracted many students from around the world with its traditional approach to training characterized by personal individualized attention, emphasis on correct forms, personal development, integration of body, *chi*, and intent, repetition, mutual respect, and hard work.

Over the years, many students have graduated from the school and become instructors themselves. In 1995, the Gin Soon Tai Chi Chuan Federation was established to better serve our members who come from different countries.

We are receptive to teaching workshops and seminars (private or group) at the headquarters or abroad. All of the instruction is given by Grandmaster Gin Soon Chu and his sons, Master Vincent Chu and Master Gordon Chu.

Gin Soon Tai Chi Chuan Federation
33 Harrison Avenue, 2nd floor
Boston, MA 02111
Tel: (617) 542-4442
Website: www.gstaichi.org

Classical Yang Style Tai Chi Chuan Video Series by Vincent Chu

1. Tai Chi Chuan For Beginners (vcd)
   Running Time: 55 Minutes
   Price: $29.95

2. Yang Family Tai Chi Chuan: Large Frame Short Form (vcd)
   Running Time: 52 Minutes
   Price: $39.9

3. Center Harmony Qigong (vhs or vcd)
   Running Time: 45 Minutes
   Price: $29.95

4. Three Circles Exercise (vhs or vcd)
   Running Time: 45 Minutes
   Price: $29.95

5. Yang Style Tai Chi Chuan (two dvd set)
   Running Time: 3 hours 10 minutes
   Price: $99.95

6. Tai Chi Chuan For Beginners: Fifteen Techniques Small Frame Solo Form (dvd)
   Running Time: 57:58 minutes
   Price: $24.95

7. Tai Chi Chuan For Beginners: Twelve Techniques Large Frame Solo Form (dvd)
   Running Time: 74 minutes
   Price: $24.95

8. Tai Chi Chuan For Beginners: Eight Techniques Medium Frame Solo Form (dvd)
   Running Time: 59 minutes
   Price: $19.95

9. Tai Chi Chuan For Beginners: Fourteen Techniques Middle Frame Solo Form (dvd)
   Running Time: 87 minutes
   Price: $24.95

10. Tai Chi Chuan For Beginners: Twelve Techniques Returning Tai Chi Chuan (dvd)
    Running Time: 99 minutes
    Price: $29.95